Epilepsy

Editor

STEVEN C. SCHACHTER

NEUROLOGIC CLINICS

www.neurologic.theclinics.com

Consulting Editor
RANDOLPH W. EVANS

November 2022 • Volume 40 • Number 4

ELSEVIER

1600 John F. Kennedy Boulevard • Suite 1800 • Philadelphia, Pennsylvania, 19103-2899

http://www.theclinics.com

NEUROLOGIC CLINICS Volume 40, Number 4
November 2022 ISSN 0733-8619, ISBN-13: 978-0-323-84916-6

Editor: Stacy Eastman
Developmental Editor: Hannah Almira Lopez

Neurologic Clinics (ISSN 0733-8619) is published quarterly by Elsevier Inc., 360 Park Avenue South, New York, NY 10010–1710. Months of issue are February, May, August, and November. Periodicals postage paid at New York, NY, and additional mailing offices. Subscription prices are $343.00 per year for US individuals, $916.00 per year for US institutions, $100.00 per year for US students, $420.00 per year for Canadian individuals, $953.00 per year for Canadian institutions, $475.00 per year for international individuals, $953.00 per year for international institutions, $210.00 for foreign students/residents, and $100.00 for Canadian students/residents. To receive student/resident rate, orders must be accompanied by name of affiliated institution, date of term, and the *signature* of program/residency coordinator on institution letterhead. Orders will be billed at individual rate until proof of status is received. Foreign air speed delivery is included in all *Clinics* subscription prices. All prices are subject to change without notice. **POSTMASTER:** Send address changes to *Neurologic Clinics*, Elsevier Health Sciences Division, Subscription Customer Service, 3251 Riverport Lane, Maryland Heights, MO 63043. **Customer Service: Telephone: 1-800-654-2452 (U.S. and Canada); 314-447-8871 (outside U.S. and Canada). Fax: 314-447-8029. E-mail: journalscustomerservice-usa@elsevier.com (for print support); journalsonlinesupport-usa@elsevier.com (for online support).**

Reprints. For copies of 100 or more of articles in this publication, please contact the Commercial Reprints Department, Elsevier Inc., 360 Park Avenue South, New York, New York, 10010-1710; Tel.: +1-212-633-3874; Fax: +1-212-633-3820, and E-mail: reprints@elsevier.com.

Neurologic Clinics is also published in Spanish by Nueva Editorial Interamericana S.A., Mexico City, Mexico.

Neurologic Clinics is covered in *Current Contents/Clinical Medicine, MEDLINE/PubMed (Index Medicus), EMBASE/Excerpta Medica, and PsycINFO, and ISI/BIOMED.*

Contributors

CONSULTING EDITOR

RANDOLPH W. EVANS, MD
Clinical Professor, Department of Neurology, Baylor College of Medicine, Houston, Texas, USA

EDITOR

STEVEN C. SCHACHTER, MD
Department of Neurology, Beth Israel Deaconess Medical Center, Massachusetts General Hospital, Harvard Medical School, Chief Academic Officer, Consortia for Improving Medicine with Innovation & Technology (CIMIT), Boston, Massachusetts, USA

AUTHORS

TYLER J. BALL, MD
Fellow, Department of Neurological Surgery, Vanderbilt University Medical Center, Nashville, Tennessee, USA

NICHOLAS J. BEIMER, MD
Clinical Assistant Professor, Departments of Neurology and Psychiatry, Michigan Medicine, University of Michigan, Ann Arbor, Michigan, USA

MARTIN BRODIE, MD
Epilepsy Unit, West Glasgow Ambulatory Care Hospital-Yorkhill, Glasgow, United Kingdom

MONICA B. DHAKAR, MD, MS
Assistant Professor, Department of Neurology, The Warren Alpert Medical School of Brown University, Providence, Rhode Island, USA

BARBARA A. DWORETZKY, MD
Professor of Neurology, Department of Neurology, Brigham and Women's Hospital, Boston, Massachusetts, USA

DARIO J. ENGLOT, MD, PhD
Assistant Professor, Department of Neurological Surgery, Vanderbilt University Medical Center, Nashville, Tennessee, USA

BEHNAZ ESMAEILI, MD
Assistant Professor, Department of Neurology, University of Washington, Seattle, Washington, USA

NANCY FOLDVARY-SCHAEFER, DO, MS
Professor, Department of Neurology, Cleveland Clinic Lerner College of Medicine, Director, Sleep Disorders Center, Cleveland Clinic Neurological Institute, Cleveland, Ohio, USA

BARRY E. GIDAL, PharmD
University of Wisconsin-Madison School of Pharmacy, Madison, Wisconsin, USA

CLOE L. GRAY, PhD
BioSerenity, Atlanta, Georgia, USA

MADELEINE M. GRIGG-DAMBERGER, MD
Professor, Department of Neurology, University of New Mexico, Albuquerque, New Mexico, USA

BABITHA HARIDAS, MBBS
Assistant Professor, Departments of Neurology and Pediatrics, Johns Hopkins University, Johns Hopkins Hospital, Baltimore, Maryland, USA

SMITHA K. HOLLA, MD
Assistant Professor, Department of Neurology, University of Wisconsin-Madison, Madison, Wisconsin, USA

NATHALIE JETTÉ, MD, MSc, FRCPC
Professor, Department of Neurology, Icahn school of Medicine at Mount Sinai, New York, New York, USA

MARIUS KLØVGAARD, MD, PhD
Department of Neurology, Herlev Hospital, Herlev, Copenhagen, Denmark; Department of Neurology, The Epilepsy Clinic, Copenhagen University Hospital/Rigshospitalet, Copenhagen, Denmark

ERIC H. KOSSOFF, MD
Professor, Departments of Neurology and Pediatrics, Johns Hopkins University, Johns Hopkins Hospital, Baltimore, Maryland, USA

ROBERT J. KOTLOSKI, MD, PhD
Department of Neurology, University of Wisconsin-Madison School of Medicine and Public Health, Department of Neurology, William S Middleton Memorial Veterans Hospital, Madison, Wisconsin, USA

PARIMALA VELPULA KRISHNAMURTHY, MD
Department of Neurology, University of Wisconsin-Madison, Madison, Wisconsin, USA

CHURL-SU KWON, MD, MPH, FRSPH
Assistant Professor, Department of Neurosurgery, Department of Neurology, Icahn School of Medicine at Mount Sinai, New York, New York, USA

WILLIAM CURT LAFRANCE Jr, MD, MPH
Professor of Psychiatry and Neurology, The Warren Alpert Medical School of Brown University, Director of Neuropsychiatry and Behavioral Neurology, Rhode Island Hospital, Providence, Rhode Island, USA

BRUCE LAVIN, MD, MPH
BioSerenity, Atlanta, Georgia, USA

KIMFORD J. MEADOR, MD, FAAN, FAES, FRCPE
Professor, Department of Neurology and Neurological Sciences, Stanford University, Stanford University School of Medicine, Palo Alto, California, USA

BRUCE D. NEARING, PhD
Department of Medicine, Beth Israel Deaconess Medical Center, Harvard Medical School, Boston, Massachusetts, USA

TRUDY D. PANG, MD, MMSc
Department of Neurology, Beth Israel Deaconess Medical Center, Harvard Medical School, Boston, Massachusetts, USA

DANIKA L. PAULO, MD
Resident Physician, Department of Neurological Surgery, Vanderbilt University Medical Center, Nashville, Tennessee, USA

KURUPATH RADHAKRISHNAN, MD, DM, FAMS, FAAN, FANA
Senior Consultant, Department of Neurosciences, Avitis Institute of Medical Sciences, Palakkad, Kerala, India

CHATURBHUJ RATHORE, MD, DM
Department of Neurology, Smt. B. K. Shah Medical Institute and Research Center, Sumandeep Vidyapeeth, Vadodara, Gujarat, India

CLAUS REINSBERGER, MD, PhD
Professor of Sport Medicine, Institute of Sports Medicine, Paderborn University, Paderborn, Germany; Department of Neurology, Brigham and Women's Hospital, Boston, Massachusetts, USA

MICHELE ROMOLI, MD, PhD, FEBN
Neurology and Stroke Unit, Department of Neuroscience, Bufalini Hospital, Cesena, Italy

PHILIPPE RYVLIN, MD, PhD
Professor, Department of Neurology, The Epilepsy Clinic, Copenhagen University Hospital/Rigshospitalet, Copenhagen, Denmark

ANNE SABERS, MD, DMSc
Department of Neurology, The Epilepsy Clinic, Copenhagen University Hospital/Rigshospitalet, Copenhagen, Denmark

STEVEN C. SCHACHTER, MD
Department of Neurology, Beth Israel Deaconess Medical Center, Massachusetts General Hospital, Harvard Medical School, Chief Academic Officer, Consortia for Improving Medicine with Innovation & Technology (CIMIT), Boston, Massachusetts, USA

ARJUNE SEN, MD, PhD, FRCPE
Associate Professor and Head, Oxford Epilepsy Research Group, NIHR Biomedical Research Centre, Nuffield Department of Clinical Neurosciences, University of Oxford, Oxford, United Kingdom

AARON F. STRUCK, MD
Assistant Professor, Department of Neurology, University of Wisconsin-Madison, William S Middleton Veterans Hospital, Madison, Wisconsin, USA

THANUJAA SUBRAMANIAM, MD
Clinical Fellow, Department of Neurology, Yale School of Medicine, New Haven, Connecticut, USA

MAGDALENA SZAFLARSKI, PhD
Associate Professor and Director of Graduate Studies, Department of Sociology, The University of Alabama at Birmingham, Birmingham, Alabama, USA

SOFIA TONIOLO, MD, FEBN
Cognitive Neurology Group, Nuffield Department of Clinical Neurosciences, University of Oxford, John Radcliffe Hospital, Oxford, United Kingdom

RICHARD L. VERRIER, PhD, FHRS
Department of Medicine, Beth Israel Deaconess Medical Center, Harvard Medical School, Boston, Massachusetts, USA

SOLVEIG VIELUF, PhD
Research Fellow, Division of Epilepsy and Clinical Neurophysiology, Boston Children's Hospital, Harvard Medical School, Boston, Massachusetts, USA; Institute of Sports Medicine, Paderborn University, Paderborn, Germany

ELAINE C. WIRRELL, MD, FRCPC
Professor, Divisions of Epilepsy and Child and Adolescent Neurology, Department of Neurology, Mayo Clinic, Rochester, Minnesota, USA

Contents

A dire complication associated with chronic epilepsy is abrupt premature death, currently referred to as sudden unexpected death in epilepsy (SUDEP). Although the traditional view has been that SUDEP is due primarily to peri-ictal respiratory failure leading to cardiac asystole, mounting evidence implicates accelerated heart disease, leading to an "epileptic heart" condition, especially after age 40, as another potential cause of abrupt premature death, although cardiac death is specifically excluded by the standard definition of SUDEP. Sudden cardiac death in epilepsy carries a 2.8-fold greater risk than in the general population and is 4.5 times more frequent than SUDEP. This review will discuss the rationale for routine use of electrocardiograms to assess cardiac risk in patients with epilepsy and the impact of epilepsy treatments, namely antiseizure medications and chronic vagus nerve stimulation.

Telemedicine is a method of health care delivery well suited for epilepsy care, where there is an insufficient supply of trained specialists. The telemedicine "Hub and Spoke" approach allows patients to visit their local health clinic ('Spokes') to establish appropriate care and monitoring for their seizure disorder or epilepsy, and remotely connect with epileptologists or neurologists at centralized centers of expertise ('Hubs'). The COVID-19 pandemic resulted in an expansion of telemedicine capabilities and use, with favorable patient and provider experience and outcomes, allowing for its wide scale adoption beyond COVID-19.

Wearable devices and mobile health software applications have a great potential for improving epilepsy-related health outcomes and contributing to personalized medical care for persons with epilepsy. With limitations and challenges, they can be used for tracking seizure occurrence and for seizure detection, prediction, and forecasting in hospital and ambulatory settings. They can also help promote self-monitoring and self-management and thereby contribute to patient empowerment. In this review, we provide an overview of current wearable devices and mobile health software applications for epilepsy. We focus on clinically validated devices, their clinical applications, the challenges faced when using these devices in real-world settings, and how these devices may be optimized in the future.

Marius Kløvgaard, Anne Sabers, and Philippe Ryvlin

Persons with epilepsy (PWE) have an up to 34-fold increased risk of dying suddenly and unexpectedly compared with the general population. Despite being potentially preventable by optimal care, sudden unexpected death in epilepsy (SUDEP) is one of the most frequent causes of death in PWE, especially in children and younger adults. The incidence of SUDEP in the general epilepsy population is rather consistent at 1.2 to 1.3 per 1000 person-year across series. Several risk factors for SUDEP have been identified, but with focal-to-bilateral or generalized tonic-clonic seizures and sleeping alone as the most significant. Thereby, optimal care and nocturnal surveillance might decrease the risk of SUDEP. Finally, PWE wants information about SUDEP, and providing this information might increase adherence to the treatment and thereby good seizure control. This narrative review provides an update on SUDEP.

Kimford J. Meador

Most children born to women with epilepsy (WWE) are normal, but have increased risks for malformations and poor neuropsychological outcomes. Antiseizure medications (ASMs) are among the most commonly prescribed teratogenic medications in women of childbearing age. However, WWE typically cannot avoid using ASMs during pregnancy. Teratogenic risks vary across ASMs. Valproate poses a special risk for anatomic and behavioral teratogenic risks compared with other ASMs. The risks for many ASMs remain uncertain. Women of childbearing potential taking ASMs should be taking folic acid. Breastfeeding while taking ASMs seems safe. WWE should receive informed consent outlining risks before conception.

Madeleine M. Grigg-Damberger and Nancy Foldvary-Schaefer

Sleep is a restorative balm for many, often less so for people with epilepsy. Complex bidirectional interactions between sleep and epilepsy can be detrimental to sleep, epilepsy and those affected. Sleep is a state of variable activation of the EEG and seizure occurrence in people with epilepsy. Sleep disorders are highly prevalent and portend worse seizure and epilepsy-related outcomes. Randomized clinical trials of sleep interventions in epilepsy populations are few, yet warranted, given the effects of sleep dysfunction on quality of life and the risk of SUDEP in people with epilepsy.

with epilepsy have a higher risk of ASD, as compared with the general population. Diagnosing epilepsy in those with ASD can be challenging. For example, stereotyped behaviors could be mistaken as ASD stereotypies, when in fact, they may be due to seizures. Fortunately, in recent years, we have gained a better understanding of the best antiseizure medications (ASMs) to use in this vulnerable population. However, more studies are needed to understand how best to screen for ASD in epilepsy, what the various ASD phenotypes are in people with epilepsy, especially those due to de novo genes/mutations, as well as factors influencing the fluctuating nature of ASD symptoms (eg, seizure type, frequency, syndromes, ASMs).

Patients with medically refractory epilepsy, as defined by failure to achieve seizure freedom after adequate trials of 2 antiseizure medications, should be considered for early surgical evaluation. Achieving seizure freedom or meaningful seizure reduction, the goals of surgical treatment, can significantly improve quality of life while decreasing disease-related morbidity and mortality. Preoperative work up and imaging modalities aid in localization of epileptogenic zones that can be targeted in surgery. Resection of a seizure focus yields highest chances of seizure freedom; however, many promising minimally invasive or noninvasive treatment options have been developed in recent years that are closely intertwined with technological advancements and serve as viable alternatives to resection, particularly neuromodulation and ablation procedures. There are also new treatment options being developed and new neuromodulation targets being studied. Surgical treatment options should be thoughtfully selected based on each patient's individual disease process and preferences.

Even though sexual dysfunction occurs in about half of people with epilepsy (PWE), it is mostly under-reported, under-recognized, and under-treated. Sexual dysfunctions are more common in patients with uncontrolled epilepsy, frequent seizures, and those receiving enzyme-inducing antiseizure medicines (ASMs). The presence of underlying anxiety or depression is associated with a higher frequency of sexual dysfunction in PWE. Even though the evidence is limited, the newer and non–enzyme-inducing ASMs do not largely cause sexual dysfunction. A multidisciplinary and multipronged approach is required for the comprehensive evaluation and management of sexual dysfunction in PWE.

Epilepsy is most common in older people and yet optimizing the management of seizures in this demographic has often been somewhat overlooked. With populations aging across the world and those with complex early-onset epilepsies thankfully living into later life, the prevalence of epilepsy in older people is escalating rapidly. Assessment and management in this age group can be challenging. Seizures may present in unusual ways and the complex comorbidities and polypharmacy that often characterize older age, might make establishing a diagnosis of epilepsy in older persons difficult. Drug choices and treatment options are often more limited and need to be specifically tailored to the older individual with careful consideration of relevant comorbidities. The complex inter-relationship between epilepsy, dementia, and vascular disease in older people would seem a research priority, as there might be interventions to help reduce adverse outcomes in a growing and potentially vulnerable group.

 Video content accompanies this article at http://www.neurologic. theclinics.com.

Identifying and treating critically ill patients with seizures can be challenging. In this article, the authors review the available data on patient populations at risk, seizure prognostication with tools such as 2HELPS2B, electrographic seizures and the various ictal-interictal continuum patterns with their latest definitions and associated risks, ancillary testing such as imaging studies, serum biomarkers, and invasive multimodal monitoring. They also illustrate 5 different patient scenarios, their treatment and outcomes, and propose recommendations for targeted treatment of electrographic seizures in critically ill patients.

Treatment of seizure clusters endeavors to prevent additional seizures and avoid progression to conditions such as prolonged seizures and status epilepticus. Rescue therapies are key components of seizure action plans (SAPs) for individuals with seizure clusters. Three rescue therapies are approved in the United States for the treatment of seizure clusters: diazepam rectal gel, midazolam nasal spray, and diazepam nasal spray. Diazepam rectal gel is an effective rescue therapy for seizure clusters, though adults and adolescents may have social reservations regarding its administration. Intranasal delivery of midazolam or diazepam is a promising alternative to rectal administration because these formulations offer easy, socially acceptable administration exhibit a rapid onset, and allow for the possibility of self-administration. Off-label benzodiazepines, such as orally disintegrating lorazepam and intranasal use of an intravenous (IV) formulation of midazolam via nasal atomizer, are less well characterized regarding bioavailability and tolerability compared with approved agents.

NEUROLOGIC CLINICS

THE CLINICS ARE AVAILABLE ONLINE!
Access your subscription at:
www.theclinics.com

Preface
Epilepsy

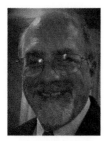

Steven C. Schachter, MD
Editor

The increasing variety of technologies under development and entering clinical practice offer new opportunities to enhance the diagnosis and treatment of patients with epilepsy. While recent experience with these tools by researchers, care providers, and patients has begun to inform treatment options and testing paradigms, there remain many unmet needs in epilepsy that could potentially be solved through the application of technologies.

The current issue of *Neurologic Clinics* addresses this situation through a series of articles written by renowned experts. Technologies are described that support diagnosis, characterize heart function, facilitate remote clinical visits, enhance epilepsy surgery, and provide urgent treatment. The other articles are state-of-the-art reviews of topics that remain challenging at this time, and which therefore are potential targets for novel technologies to accelerate progress.

Steven C. Schachter, MD
Departments of Neurology
Harvard Medical School
Beth Israel Deaconess Medical Center
Massachusetts General Hospital
Consortia for Improving Medicine with
Innovation & Technology
125 Nashua Street, Suite 3228, Boston
MA 02114, USA

E-mail address:
sschacht@bidmc.harvard.edu

Neurol Clin 40 (2022) xiii
https://doi.org/10.1016/j.ncl.2022.03.007
0733-8619/22/© 2022 Published by Elsevier Inc.

neurologic.theclinics.com

The Epileptic Heart and the Case for Routine Use of the Electrocardiogram in Patients with Chronic Epilepsy

Richard L. Verrier, PhD[a],*, Trudy D. Pang, MD, MMSc[b],
Bruce D. Nearing, PhD[a], Steven C. Schachter, MD[b,c,d]

KEYWORDS

- Sudden cardiac death • Vagus nerve stimulation • Electrocardiogram • Guidelines
- T-wave alternans • T-wave heterogeneity • Sudden unexpected death in epilepsy
- Antiseizure medications

KEY POINTS

- Cardiovascular comorbidities are common in people with chronic epilepsy.
- Drug-resistant epilepsy is associated with accelerated heart disease leading to vulnerability to sudden cardiac death (SCD), especially after age 40.
- SCD incidence is 2.8-fold greater among patients with epilepsy than in the general population and is 4.5 times more frequent than sudden unexpected death in epilepsy.
- The involvement of cardiac factors provides a strong rationale for routine use of electrocardiograms in establishing baseline cardiovascular risk and monitoring the ongoing impact of epileptic seizures and antiseizure medications.
- Crescendo in T-wave heterogeneity may serve as a novel ECG-based marker capable of forecasting GTCS.

PUBLIC HEALTH BURDEN OF CHRONIC EPILEPSY

Chronic epilepsy afflicts more than 50 million individuals worldwide, including 3 million adults and 470,000 children in the United States alone.[1] Sudden unexpected death in

Funding: No funds were received for preparation of this article.
[a] Department of Medicine, Beth Israel Deaconess Medical Center, Harvard Medical School, 99 Brookline Avenue, RN-301, Boston, MA 02215, USA; [b] Department of Neurology, Beth Israel Deaconess Medical Center, Harvard Medical School, 185 Pilgrim Road, Boston, MA 02215, USA; [c] Department of Neurology, Massachusetts General Hospital, Harvard Medical School, 55 Fruit Street, Boston, MA, 02114, USA; [d] Consortia for Improving Medicine with Innovation & Technology (CIMIT), 125 Nashua Street, Suite 324, Boston, MA 02114, USA
* Corresponding author. Department of Medicine, Division of Cardiovascular Medicine, Harvard Medical School, Beth Israel Deaconess Medical Center, 99 Brookline Avenue, RN-301, Boston, MA 02215.
E-mail address: rverrier@bidmc.harvard.edu

epilepsy (SUDEP) accounts for one death per 1000 adult epilepsy patients each year or 2750 to 3600 deaths in the United States annually.[1,2] The International League Against Epilepsy defines SUDEP as "a sudden, unexpected death in a person with epilepsy, with or without evidence of a seizure preceding the death, in which there is no evidence of other disease, injury, or drowning that caused the death."[1] Although multiple pathophysiologic mechanisms including congenital brain and heart channelopathies have been implicated in SUDEP,[3,4] pulmonary failure in the postictal period leading to cardiac asystole is best characterized and therefore most often invoked.[5,6] The determination of SUDEP is not made in deaths due to cardiac causes, by definition.[7] Sudden cardiac death (SCD), however, constitutes a 4.5-fold greater risk for premature demise in patients with epilepsy than SUDEP.

GOALS OF THIS REVIEW

The objectives of this review are 3-fold. The first is to review succinctly the evidence implicating cardiac factors in premature death among people with epilepsy. The second is to examine the clinical evidence supporting the use of the electrocardiogram (ECG) as standard of care in individuals with chronic epilepsy. The third is to discuss the potential utility of ECG markers in evaluating the impact of antiseizure medications (ASMs) as well as the therapeutic effect of chronic vagus nerve stimulation (VNS) on cardiac risk. Based on the evidence, we propose that ECG assessments should be standard of care in the evaluation of patients with newly diagnosed epilepsy to assess cardiac disease status and risk for SCD as well as for the longitudinal management of those with chronic epilepsy.

CARDIAC PATHOGENESIS IN CHRONIC EPILEPSY

Mounting evidence implicates cardiac involvement as a major factor in sudden premature death in epilepsy.[8,9] This reappraisal has been bolstered by reports of cardiovascular comorbidities in 62% to 82% of individuals with an epilepsy diagnosis.[10–12] The presumed catalysts are accelerated atherosclerosis, altered lipid profiles, and side effects of enzyme-inducing ASMs.[13–15] Recurrent seizures and the attendant hyperadrenergic activity can lead to structural damage to the heart, which in turn can increase cardiac electrical instability and susceptibility to serious arrhythmias. Proarrhythmic actions of some ASMs, particularly sodium channel blocking agents, have been invoked.[16] The incidence of myocardial infarction is 1.5 to 4.8 times greater in patients with epilepsy than in the general population.[17,18]

Exclusion of patients with cardiovascular comorbidities including structural heart disease or coronary artery disease from epilepsy investigations[19] may account in part for the underestimation of cardiac arrhythmia incidence and cardiovascular mortality in chronic drug-resistant epilepsy. The greater than 3000-subject Amsterdam Resuscitation Studies reported that the risk of cardiac arrest due to ventricular fibrillation was 2.8-fold greater in people with epilepsy (95% CI: 1.4–5.3) and 5.8-fold (95% CI: 2.1–15.6) greater in symptomatic epilepsy cases than in the general population.[16] In the Oregon Sudden Unexpected Death Study, Stecker and colleagues[20] found an SCD rate of 4.4% per year in patients with epilepsy, an incidence that is 4.5-fold that of SUDEP (Fig. 1). These investigators determined that patients with epilepsy experienced sudden cardiac arrest at a younger age, 55 ± 25 years, compared with those without epilepsy, who died suddenly at 63 ± 19 years ($P < .0001$). It is noteworthy that in the majority (66%) of sudden cardiac arrests among individuals with epilepsy, there was no evidence of an antecedent or concomitant seizure, as confirmed by witnesses who were familiar with the victim's seizure characteristics. Recent

Cardiac Mortality in Epilepsy: Beyond SUDEP

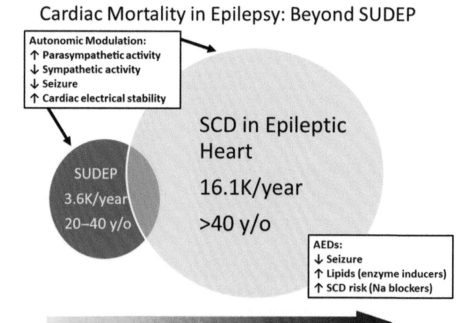

Fig. 1. Venn diagram of the interrelationship between sudden cardiac death (SCD) in patients with epilepsy and sudden unexpected death in epilepsy (SUDEP). SUDEP incidence data of 3600 adults/y are from Harden and colleagues[1] and Thurman and colleagues.[2] SCD incidence data of 16,100 adults/y are from Bardai and colleagues,[16] Stecker and colleagues,[20] Zack and Kobau,[56] and Benjamin and colleagues[57]. AEDs, antiepileptic drugs; Na, sodium (*From* Verrier RL, Pang TD, Nearing BD, et al. The Epileptic Heart: Concept and clinical evidence. Epilepsy Behav 2020;105:106946; with permission.)

analysis of 5 years of claims among ~82,000 Medicaid beneficiaries with epilepsy identified cardiac dysrhythmias in greater than 37% of cases.[21] An illustrative case of the SCD scenario is provided (**Fig. 2**).[22]

Collectively, this evidence has led to the concept of "The Epileptic Heart," which we defined as "a heart and coronary vasculature damaged by chronic epilepsy as a result of repeated surges in catecholamines and hypoxemia leading to electrical and mechanical dysfunction."[8] The Epileptic Heart condition with its attendant augmented risk for SCD gains greater importance after the age of 40 due to accelerated atherosclerosis in individuals with pharmacoresistant epilepsy (**Box 1, Fig. 3, Tables 1 and 2**). Accordingly, age is a critical factor and should be considered in evaluating apparent pathologic mechanisms.

CLINICAL EVIDENCE OF UTILITY OF CONVENTIONAL ELECTROCARDIOGRAM MARKERS

Recently, Chahal and colleagues[23] demonstrated that QT interval prolongation, a well-established marker associated with increased risk for all-cause mortality in the general population and in cohorts with established coronary artery disease, predicts all-cause mortality in patients evaluated for epilepsy (**Fig. 4**). This finding is consistent with prior observations that cardiac repolarization abnormalities are relatively common in patients with drug-resistant epilepsy. Significantly, one-third of patients with epilepsy

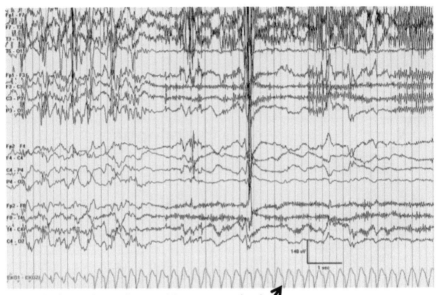

Ventricular tachycardia requiring countershock ↗

Fig. 2. Case report of 75-year-old woman with history of generalized tonic/clonic seizures, hypertension, coronary artery disease managed by right coronary artery stent, and no recurring ischemia. On the day of hospital admission, she had a seizure during breakfast and was admitted to hospital, where she experienced another seizure with self-terminating but rapid ventricular tachycardia. Subsequently, left ventricular ejection fraction was 30% with evidence of neurogenic stunning. (*From* Espinosa PS, Lee JW, Tedrow UB, et al. Sudden unexpected near death in epilepsy: malignant arrhythmia from a partial seizure. Neurology 2009;72:1702–3; with permission.)

have been found to exhibit cardiac repolarization abnormalities, specifically QT-interval prolongation and/or dispersion, interictally.[8,12,24–26]

Chahal and colleagues[23] performed a 16,250-patient retrospective study of QT intervals in 12-lead ECGs of all patients evaluated across 15 years at the Mayo Clinic (Rochester MN, USA) during their index presentation of possible seizure or epilepsy including atypical spells. It is surprising in this large cohort that only 57% of all patients and 44% of those with a likely epilepsy diagnosis underwent a resting 12-lead ECG recording at index hospital visit, highlighting the underutilization of a tool that is important not only in establishing baseline cardiac status but also in differential diagnosis of epilepsy. The limited use of ECG in the initial evaluation of patients with a new diagnosis of epilepsy is a probable consequence of the absence of guidelines in the United States.

Chahal and colleagues[23] raised several additional reasons for routine use of the 12-lead ECG for patients at evaluation for first seizure. Specifically, patients with channelopathies associated with prolonged QT interval such as the long QT and Brugada syndromes can exhibit a dual pattern of seizure-like episode with secondary arrhythmia and may be misdiagnosed. Failure to detect telltale QT prolongation may culminate in SCD.

APPLICATION OF NEWER ELECTROCARDIOGRAM TOOLS FOR CARDIAC RISK ASSESSMENT

Standard 12-lead and ambulatory ECG (AECG) recordings remain among the most valuable tools in monitoring of repolarization abnormalities and assessing SCD risk in the general population.[27–29] There is growing evidence that these tools have

---

Box 1
Criteria for Epileptic Heart*

- Chronic Epilepsy with or without Drug-Resistance
  - Use standard diagnostic criteria

- Myocardial Injury and Arrhythmia Risk on ECG
  - Clinical signs and symptoms such as effort intolerance, chest pain, irregular pulse and palpitations
  - Atrial and/or ventricular arrhythmias
  - P waves greater than 2.5 mm tall and/or greater than 110 ms wide may indicate atrial enlargement
  - Q waves with large downward deflection may indicate prior myocardial infarction
  - QRS complex width greater than 150 ms may indicate conduction abnormalities and electrical dyssynchrony
  - Severe QT interval prolongation (>450 ms in men, >470 ms in women) may indicate repolarization abnormalities or ASM use
  - ST-segment depression or elevation
  - T_{peak}-T_{end} abnormality
  - T-wave alternans $\geq$47 μV

- Altered Autonomic Tone as Assessed by HRV Measures
  - rMSSD less than 27 ± 12 ms
  - LF/HF ratio greater than 1.5 to 2.0

- Diastolic Dysfunction on Echocardiography
  - Increased left ventricle stiffness[55]
  - Elevated left ventricle filling pressure
  - Increased left atrial volume

- Hyperlipidemia and Accelerated Atherosclerosis
  - Triglycerides greater than 150 mg/dL; low HDL (women <50, men <40) (equivalent to metabolic syndrome)

*Requires the presence of chronic epilepsy and any 2 other criteria. The major requirements are the presence of chronic epilepsy and ECG changes indicative of ventricular abnormalities (ie, prior myocardial infarction, left ventricular hypertrophy, and markers of potentially life-threatening arrhythmia risk), or echocardiographically determined myocardial dysfunction, and constitute the minimum requirements for diagnosis. Minor indicators are altered lipids and HRV changes. TWA testing by the modified moving average method is cleared by the US Food and Drug Administration and EU Medical Device Regulation. It is approved in the United States for reimbursement by local contractors by the Center for Medicare and Medicaid Services (CAG #00293R2) "for the evaluation of patients at risk for SCD." *Abbreviations:* ASM, antiseizure medication; ECG, electrocardiogram; HDL, high-density lipoprotein; HRV, heart rate variability; LF/HF ratio, low- to high-frequency ratio; rMSSD, root mean square of successive differences of R-R intervals; TWA, T-wave alternans.

From Verrier RL, Pang TD, Nearing BD, et al. The Epileptic Heart: a clinical syndromic approach. Epilepsia 2021;62:1780-9; with permission.

---

potential merit for assessing arrhythmia risk in patients with chronic epilepsy. Among the most extensively studied markers is T-wave alternans (TWA), a microvolt-level beat-to-beat fluctuation in ST-segment or T-wave morphology (**Fig. 5**).[30] TWA's fundamental connection with arrhythmia risk is based on its reflection of heterogeneity of repolarization and establishing the substrate and propensity for unidirectional conduction block and reentry.[31,32] The capacity of TWA analysis to stratify risk for SCD and cardiovascular mortality with odds ratios of 4.8 to 22.6 has been confirmed by investigations in general populations as well as in ∼5500 patients with diverse cardiac conditions[30,33] including ischemic heart disease, heart failure, and the long QT

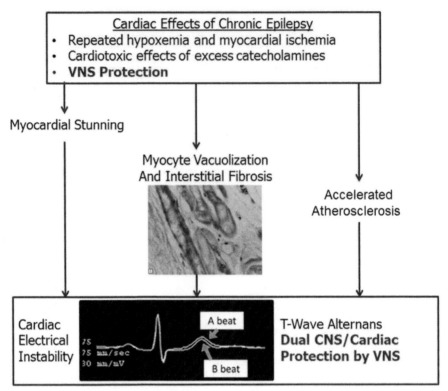

Fig. 3. Conceptual framework of the link between chronic epilepsy and development of the "Epileptic Heart." Cardiotoxic effects of catecholamines, repeated hypoxemia, with increased cardiac electrical instability manifest as T-wave alternans, a repeating ABAB beat-to-beat pattern in the ST-segment and T wave of the ECG. CNS, central nervous system; VNS, vagus nerve stimulation. (Richard L. Verrier, Steven C. Schachter, Is heart disease in chronic epilepsy a consequence of seizures or a fellow traveler?, Epilepsy & Behavior, 86, 2018, 211–213, https://doi.org/10.1016/j.yebeh.2018.06.027.)

Table 1
Comparison of Definitions of SUDEP and SCD

SUDEP	SCD
• Sudden unexpected death in a person with epilepsy with or without evidence of a preceding seizure and without evidence of injury, drowning, or other disease	• Witnessed natural death heralded by abrupt loss of consciousness, within 1 h of onset of acute symptoms, presumed due to cardiac arrest; • OR: Unwitnessed, unexpected death of someone seen in a stable medical condition <24 h previously with no evidence of a noncardiac cause
Walczak et al,[7] Nashef et al[53]	Huikuri et al[54]

Abbreviations: SCD, sudden cardiac death; SUDEP, sudden unexpected death in epilepsy.
From Verrier RL, Pang TD, Nearing BD, et al. The Epileptic Heart: a clinical syndromic approach. Epilepsia 2021;62:1780-9; with permission.

Table 2
Comparison of mode of death and risk factors: SUDEP versus SCD in patients with epilepsy

SUDEP	SCD in Patients with Epilepsy
• Peri-ictal event likely triggered by a convulsive seizure	• Patients usually die during daily activities
• Patients usually found dead in bed, often prone	○ Two-thirds of deaths are not associated with seizure
• Patient characteristics:	• Patient characteristics:
○ Chronic epilepsy	○ Coronary artery atherosclerosis, myocardial ischemia, myocardial infarction
○ Poor seizure control (especially GTCS)	
○ ASM polytherapy	
○ Youth	○ Sodium channel blocking ASMs
○ Early age at seizure onset	○ Diastolic dysfunction
○ Male	○ Myocardial fibrosis
○ Medication noncompliance	○ Left ventricular hypertrophy
○ Postictal pulmonary failure	○ Hyperadrenergic activity
○ Inherited and possibly acquired channelopathies	○ Conduction or repolarization abnormalities
	○ Inherited and possibly acquired channelopathies
Harden et al,[1] Thurman et al[2]	Verrier et al[9]

Abbreviations: ASM, antiseizure medication; GTCS, generalized tonic-clonic seizure; SCD, sudden cardiac death; SUDEP, sudden unexpected death in epilepsy.
From Verrier RL, Pang TD, Nearing BD, et al. The Epileptic Heart: a clinical syndromic approach. Epilepsia 2021;62:1780-9; with permission.

syndrome.[34] TWA was also found to be capable of tracking effects of antiarrhythmic and proarrhythmic effects of medications.[35]

A TWA ladder of risk revealed that drug-resistant epilepsy registers a surprisingly high level of SCD risk comparable to prevalent cardiac conditions with the highest risk of cardiac arrhythmia (**Fig. 6**).[33] TWA's relationship to acute complex partial seizures or secondary generalized tonic-clonic seizures (GTCS) was investigated by Strzelczyk and colleagues,[36] who found that TWA increased significantly during the immediate postictal phase following GTCS.

Pang and coworkers[37] carried out a side-by-side comparison of TWA and heart rate variability (HRV) measurements with both traditional AECG monitors and state-of-the-art lightweight, wearable, wireless ECG patches in patients with newly diagnosed and chronic drug-resistant epilepsy but without known heart disease to address key questions. TWA levels in drug-resistant epilepsy patients were significantly greater than in those with newly diagnosed epilepsy, which did not differ from healthy control adults (**Fig. 7**). In all subjects with established epilepsy, TWA exceeded the $\geq$47-μV cut point of abnormality for cardiac risk, likely due to cumulative effects of recurrent seizure-induced cardiac injury from catecholamine insults and the atherosclerotic effects of years of lipid-altering ASM therapy. One of the study patients without a prior history of cardiac disease or arrhythmia had an interictal crescendo in TWA level preceding a brief run of ventricular tachycardia (**Fig. 8**). Because this arrhythmia occurred on the 4th day of monitoring, it was captured on the ECG patch but would have been missed by standard AECG monitoring, which is typically limited to 1 or 2 days.

Autonomic dysfunction as indicated by depressed HRV analyzed by root mean square of successive differences (rMSSD) has long been recognized in patients with chronic epilepsy. Interestingly, Pang and colleagues[37] found HRV to be inversely

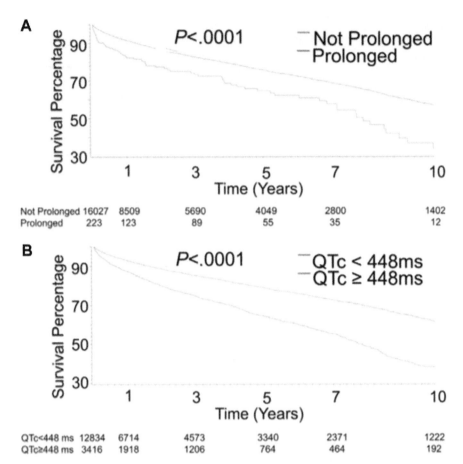

Fig. 4. Kaplan–Meier survival plots as predicted by a prolonged QT interval in patients with index evaluation for seizure or epilepsy based on the optimized cut point. (*From* Chahal CAA, Gottwald JA, St. Louis EK, et al. QT prolongation in patients with index evaluation for seizure or epilepsy is predictive of all-cause mortality. Heart Rhythm 2022;19:578–584. https://doi.org/10.1016/j.hrthm.2021.11.013; with permission.)

related to TWA levels in chronic epilepsy patients. Thus, decreases in HRV, which reflect reductions in vagal tone, are associated with simultaneous significant elevations in TWA.

EPILEPSY MONITORING UNIT EXPERIENCE WITH NOVEL ELECTROCARDIOGRAM MARKERS

Pang and coworkers conducted follow-up studies in the epilepsy monitoring unit (EMU), which provides an opportune venue to exploit the ECG to gain insights into the impact of acute seizure and ASMs on cardiac electrical stability, because ASMs are routinely and rapidly adjusted in this controlled setting. Patients with chronic epilepsy exhibited elevated TWA at EMU admission, presumably due to the behavioral stress of this novel environment.[38] Heightened sympathetic nerve activity is implicated by the fact that heart rate was markedly elevated on admission day and by the

Modified Moving Average Method

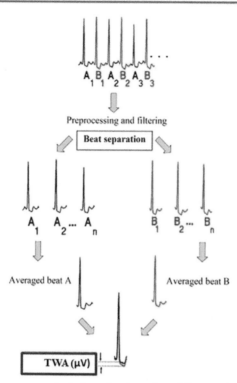

Fig. 5. Modified moving average technique for detection of T-wave alternans (TWA). Alternate beats are dichotomized into bins of "A" beats (*blue*) and "B" beats (*red*), and the T-wave morphologies in each bin are averaged. The averaged beats are then superimposed, and the difference in the magnitude of the T waves of the A and B averaged beats is quantified in microvolts. This difference is the TWA level, which indicates the degree of cardiac risk. (*Modified from* Verrier RL, Ikeda T. Ambulatory ECG-based T-wave alternans monitoring for risk assessment and guiding medical therapy: Mechanisms and clinical applications. Prog Cardiovasc Dis 2013;56:172–85; with permission.)

incidental observation that in the sole patient who was receiving a beta-adrenergic blocking agent, TWA was not elevated. These observations suggest that the stress of hospital admission with the presumed attendant elevations in catecholamines acts on a vulnerable cardiac substrate to provoke repolarization abnormalities that have been linked to increased risk for cardiovascular mortality.[29,39] The respective elevations in TWA are consistent with the well-known finding of greater mortality risk associated with GTCS.[26]

Recently, Pang and colleagues demonstrated that a crescendo in the TWH level occurs at 30-min prior to seizure (**Fig. 9**).[40] By comparison, heart rate was not elevated until 10 min prior to seizure onset, and patients with PNES did not exhibit the TWH crescendo pattern. Thus, TWH may constitute a new biomarker that could be used to forecast GTCS. Clearly, more work needs to be done to establish definitively the clinical utility of TWH in forecasting GTCS as well as its capacity to assess SCD risk in patients with chronic epilepsy.

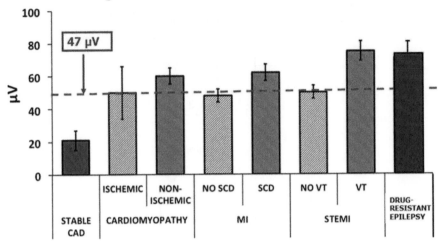

Fig. 6. T-wave alternans (TWA) ladder of sudden cardiac death (SCD) risk. Patients with chronic epilepsy exhibit TWA in the severely abnormal range, ≥ 60 μV, similar to patients who experience ventricular tachycardia following myocardial infarction. AECG, ambulatory electrocardiogram; CAD, coronary artery disease; MI, myocardial infarction; STEMI, ST-segment elevation myocardial infarction; VT, ventricular tachycardia (*Modified from* Verrier RL, Ikeda T. Ambulatory ECG-based T-wave alternans monitoring for risk assessment and guiding medical therapy: Mechanisms and clinical applications. Prog Cardiovasc Dis 2013;56:172–85; with permission.)

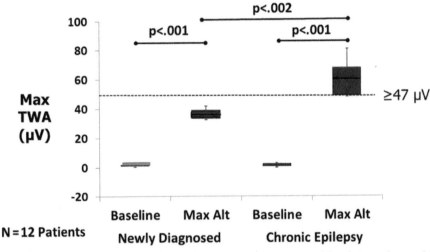

Fig. 7. Box plot displaying maximum (max) T-wave alternans (TWA) levels in patients with newly diagnosed or chronic epilepsy. Data are from day 1 recordings on ambulatory ECG monitors. The lower line of the box represents the 25th percentile, the middle line the 50th percentile, and the top line the 75th percentile. The whiskers represent the lowest and highest values. Although the baseline TWA levels did not differ, the maximum levels achieved during the day were significantly lower in patients with newly diagnosed than chronic epilepsy (35 ± 1.3 vs 62 ± 5.4 μV, $P < .002$). In all 6 patients with chronic epilepsy, the maximum TWA level exceeded the ≥ 47 μV cut point of abnormality (*dashed horizontal line*) during the monitoring period. Values are expressed as means ± SEM. (*From* Pang TD, Nearing BD, Krishnamurthy KB, et al. Cardiac electrical instability in newly diagnosed/chronic epilepsy tracked by Holter and ECG patch. Neurology 2019;93:450-8; with permission.)

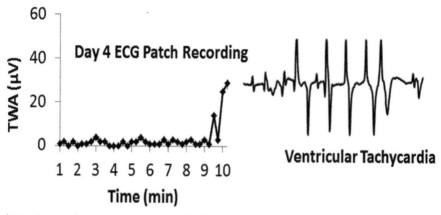

Fig. 8. Crescendo in T-wave alternans (TWA) level heralded onset of ventricular tachycardia in a patient with chronic epilepsy on the 4th day of the wireless ECG patch recording. (*From* Pang TD, Nearing BD, Krishnamurthy KB, et al. Cardiac electrical instability in newly diagnosed/chronic epilepsy tracked by Holter and ECG patch. Neurology 2019;93:450-8; with permission.)

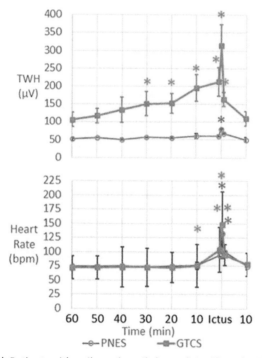

Fig. 9. Upper panel: Patients with epilepsy (n = 6) showed significantly elevated T-wave heterogeneity (TWH) levels starting at 30 min before generalized tonic-clonic seizure (GTCS) with an acute spike during GTCS and return to baseline at 10 min after GTCS. Patients with psychogenic nonepileptic seizure (PNES) (n = 3) showed no significant change in TWH prior to ictus, with mild TWH elevation during the event. Lower panel: Patients with epilepsy did not show significant heart rate changes (>2 beats/min) until 10 min before GTCS followed by significant ictal tachycardia and return nearly to baseline by 10 min after seizure. Patients with PNES showed no significant increase in heart rate prior to ictus. *significant (p<0.05) elevation above baseline.

USE OF THE 12-LEAD ELECTROCARDIOGRAM IN TRACKING EFFECTS OF ANTISEIZURE MEDICATIONS

Because ASMs can affect both cardiac autonomic function and myocardial ion channels, they have the potential to exhibit both antiarrhythmic and proarrhythmic influences. On the positive side, ASMs have the potential to exert antiarrhythmic actions through effects on the autonomic nervous system and cardiac ion channels. The proarrhythmic effects of certain ASMs, such as those with sodium channel-blocking effects, including carbamazepine, lamotrigine, and phenytoin, may exacerbate SCD risk.[16] Blockade of the cardiac sodium channels, particularly when cardiovascular disease is present, can cause conduction abnormalities and lead to malignant arrhythmias including wide-complex ventricular tachycardia. The link between sodium channel blockade and arrhythmia risk is supported by the milestone Cardiac Arrhythmia Suppression Trial (CAST).[41] This important trial revealed that the sodium channel blockers flecainide and encainide were significantly proarrhythmic and resulted in an increased incidence of death over placebo. Myocardial ischemia during seizures, particularly GTCS,[42] may compound the risk for malignant ventricular arrhythmias in individuals taking chronic ASMs with sodium channel-blocking properties. It is noteworthy that several ASMs, such as phenobarbital, phenytoin, carbamazepine, and lamotrigine, prolong the QT interval,[43] an action associated with proarrhythmic effects in the cardiology literature. However, there has been no systematic study of the potential proarrhythmic and antiarrhythmic actions of ASMs.

EFFECTS OF VAGUS NERVE STIMULATION ON SEIZURE, SUDDEN UNEXPECTED DEATH IN EPILEPSY, AND CARDIAC RISK

VNS therapy has been found generally to suppress seizures in a worldwide experience[44] and furthermore is associated with reduced SUDEP incidence.[45] Thus, the impact of VNS therapy on the pathogenesis of the Epileptic Heart is of interest given its cardioprotective effects.[46,47] Schomer and colleagues[48] demonstrated that VNS therapy increased HRV, indicating enhanced vagal tone, and substantially reduced TWA in patients with drug-resistant epilepsy. These findings were extended in subjects enrolled in the AspireSR E–36 trial, which demonstrated that VNS was associated with a highly significant decrease in interictal TWA levels in all patients studied (**Fig. 10**).[49] Nearly three-quarters (70%) of the patients with abnormal TWA levels converted from positive to negative TWA test results following 3 weeks after the VNS titration period. Because with each 20-μV increase in TWA, cardiac mortality and SCD risk in a general population increased by 55% and 58%, respectively,[50] a reduction in TWA levels in response to VNS in epilepsy patients is likely to be salutary. On a practical note, it should be appreciated that the QT-interval prolonging effects of VNS[49] do not adequately reflect its antiarrhythmic properties, as the main action of VNS is to reduce heterogeneity of repolarization, decreasing reentrant arrhythmias.[46,51]

PUTATIVE MECHANISMS OF VAGUS NERVE STIMULATION-MEDIATED CARDIOPROTECTION

VNS is likely to exert its cardioprotective action at 2 major sites. First, VNS acts at the level of the central nervous system to prevent or reduce seizure intensity. This action in turn reduces hyperadrenergic activity, thereby decreasing myocardial substrate injury and enhancing cardiac electrical stability. The second main locus of VNS action is at the neurocardiac level. In patients with severe heart failure, VNS resulted in parallel reductions in TWA, TWH, ventricular tachycardia incidence, and improvement in heart

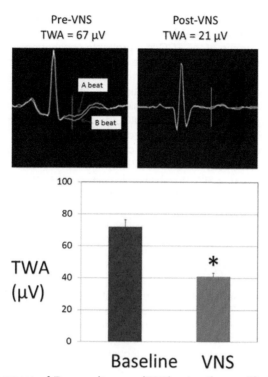

Fig. 10. Top: Assessment of T-wave alternans (TWA) using the modified moving average method in a representative patient with drug-resistant epilepsy performed before and after 4 weeks following vagus nerve stimulation (VNS) device implantation, when the device was operating at planned levels. Templates of QRS-complex-aligned superimposed beats reveal a separation in the morphology of the A and B beats, reflecting the ABABAB pattern of TWA between the J point and T wave. In this patient, tracings from before (*left*) and after VNS device implantation (*right*) indicate a reduction in maximum TWA from 67 μV, greater than the ≥47 μV cut point for abnormality, to 21 μV. Bottom: Summary data in 28 patients with interpretable ECGs in the E−36 study showing a significant reduction in maximum TWA from 72 ± 4.3 to 41 ± 2.3 μV (*P* < .0001) in response to magnet-mode VNS therapy. (*From* Verrier RL, Nearing BD, Olin B, et al. Baseline elevation and reduction in cardiac electrical instability assessed by quantitative T-wave alternans in patients with drug-resistant epilepsy treated with vagus nerve stimulation in the AspireSR E-36 trial. Epilepsy Behav 2016;62:85–9; with permission.)

failure status across 3 years.[46] Cardioprotection by chronic VNS is likely to be multi-factorial with a major effect of antagonizing cardiac-bound sympathetic nerve activity. This principle is illustrated in a study by Yuan and colleagues,[52] who assessed skin sympathetic activity using an innovative new technique to confirm salutary actions of VNS in drug-resistant epilepsy patients. Other cardioprotective effects of VNS are probably involved such as anti-inflammatory and antiapoptotic effects.[47]

SUMMARY AND RECOMMENDATIONS

The body of evidence reviewed supports the concept that chronic epilepsy exerts a significant adverse impact on the structural integrity of the heart and its vasculature, resulting in a condition termed "The Epileptic Heart."[8] The damaging influences of recurrent seizures lead to autonomic dysfunction, cardiac electrical instability, and vulnerability to life-threatening arrhythmias. Arrhythmia susceptibility can be worsened by ASMs that block sodium channels[16,43] or induce enzymes that increase lipid levels.[13,15] Underutilization of the ECG is a probable consequence of the absence of guidelines in the United States, at variance with the United Kingdom, where routine use of the 12-lead ECG is recommended "to help identify cardiac-related conditions that could mimic an epileptic seizure" [National Institute for Health and Care Excellence (NICE) Clinical Guidelines for Epilepsies: Diagnosis and Management, CG137] (www.nice.org.uk/guidance). The current NICE guideline draft (November 2021) indicates "a 12-lead ECG to help identify cardiac-related conditions that could mimic an epileptic seizure... or identify cardiac causes of seizure-like symptoms" (NICE share new drafted epilepsy guidelines | Epilepsy Research UK).

Currently, clinical care of patients with chronic epilepsy does not routinely include cardiac evaluations or longitudinal assessments using a standard ECG. The high incidence of cardiac disease in individuals with chronic epilepsy[14] underscores the need to incorporate cardiac care as part of the essential long-term management of patients with drug-resistant epilepsy. Recording 12-lead ECGs in all patients at EMU admission is now standard of care at our medical center. We further recommend a resting 12-lead ECG and/or an AECG patch recording to identify potential cardiac pathologic conditions. The 12-lead ECG can be a useful screening tool both at baseline and at regular intervals to monitor disease progression. In patients with drug-refractory epilepsy, particularly those with GTCS and/or concurrent cardiovascular risk factors, further evaluation with multiday AECG patch monitors could be highly informative. Clearly, the value of ECG monitoring merits intense investigation in patients with newly diagnosed or chronic epilepsy because it offers the potential for improved diagnosis and ultimately for guiding therapy and reducing cardiac-related morbidity and mortality.

CLINICAL CARE POINTS

- Clinical guidelines for electrocardiographic (ECG) monitoring of patients with epilepsy in the United States do not adequately reflect the need for information for differential diagnosis of epilepsy and insights on patients' cardiac status.

- The epilepsy monitoring unit provides an opportune venue for ECG monitoring of the impact of seizure or antiseizure medications (ASMs) on patients' cardiac status.

- T-wave alternans, an indicator of cardiovascular mortality and sudden cardiac death risk, can be accurately monitored from wired ambulatory ECG (AECG) monitors or state-of-the-art, lightweight, wearable, wireless AECG patch monitors.

- QT prolongation and T-wave heterogeneity can be readily identified from 12-lead resting ECGs to provide insights into cardiac risk, including potential proarrhythmic effects of ASMs.

- Standard 12-lead ECGs should be obtained at baseline in patients with newly diagnosed or suspected epilepsy, and at regular intervals to provide screening for cardiac pathologic conditions; full cardiac evaluations should be considered in patients with chronic drug-resistant epilepsy and concurrent cardiovascular risk factors.

CONFLICTS OF INTEREST

None of the authors has a conflict of interest relative to this review. Drs R.L. Verrier and T.D. Pang are members of the medical advisory board of StratusNeuro (Irving TX). Drs R.L. Verrier and B.D. Nearing receive research funding from LivaNova USA (Houston TX), Medtronic (Minneapolis MN), Preventice Solutions/Boston Scientific (Marlborough MA), and StratusNeuro (Irving TX). Dr T.D. Pang receives research funding from Beth Israel Deaconess Medical Center Department of Neurology. Dr S.C.

Schachter receives funding from Elsevier and National Institute of Biomedical Imaging and Bioengineering, National Institutes of Health (NIBIB, NIH).

REFERENCES

1. Harden C, Tomson T, Gloss D, et al. Practice guideline summary: sudden unexpected death in epilepsy incidence rates and risk factors: report of the Guideline Development, Dissemination, and Implementation Subcommittee of the American Academy of Neurology and the American Epilepsy Society. Epilepsy Curr 2017; 17:180–7.
2. Thurman DJ, Hesdorffer DC, French JA. Sudden unexpected death in epilepsy: assessing the public health burden. Epilepsia 2014;55:1479–85.
3. Myers KA, Sivathamboo S, Perucca P. Heart rate variability in epilepsy: a potential biomarker of sudden unexpected death in epilepsy risk. Epilepsia 2018;59: 1372–80.
4. Chahal CAA, Salloum MN, Alahdab F, et al. Systematic review of the genetics of sudden unexpected death in epilepsy: Potential overlap with sudden cardiac death and arrhythmia-related genes. J Am Heart Assoc 2020;9:e012264.
5. Ryvlin P, Nashef L, Lhatoo SD, et al. Incidence and mechanisms of cardiorespiratory arrests in epilepsy monitoring units (MORTEMUS): a retrospective study. Lancet Neurol 2013;12:966–77.
6. Ryvlin P. Update on SUDEP. Neurologic Clinics, current issue, in press.
7. Walczak TS, Leppik IE, D'Amelio M, et al. Incidence and risk factors in sudden unexpected death in epilepsy: a prospective cohort study. Neurology 2001;56: 519–25.
8. Verrier RL, Pang TD, Nearing BD, et al. The Epileptic Heart: Concept and clinical evidence. Epilepsy Behav 2020;105:106946.
9. Verrier RL, Pang TD, Nearing BD, et al. The Epileptic Heart: a clinical syndromic approach. Epilepsia 2021;62:1780–9.
10. Selassie AW, Wilson DA, GU Martz, et al. Epilepsy beyond seizure: a population-based study of comorbidities. Epilepsy Res 2014;108:305–15.
11. Lamberts RJ, Blom MT, Wassenaar M, et al. Sudden cardiac arrest in people with epilepsy in the community. Neurology 2015;85:212–8.
12. Lamberts RJ, Blom MT, Novy J, et al. Increased prevalence of ECG markers for sudden cardiac arrest in refractory epilepsy. J Neurol Neurosurg Psychiatr 2015; 86:309–13.
13. Mintzer S, Miller R, Shah K, et al. Long-term effect of antiepileptic drug switch on serum lipids and C-reactive protein. Epilepsy Behav 2016;58:127–32.
14. Zack M, Luncheon C. Adults with an epilepsy history, notably those 45–64 years old or at the lowest income levels, more often report heart disease than adults without an epilepsy history. Epilepsy Behav 2018;86:208–10.
15. Josephson CB, Wiebe S, Delgado-Garcia G, et al. Association of enzyme-inducing antiseizure drug use with long-term cardiovascular disease. JAMA Neurol 2021;78:1367–74.
16. Bardai A, Blom MT, van Noord C, et al. Sudden cardiac death is associated both with epilepsy and with use of antiepileptic medications. Heart 2015;101:17–22.
17. Janszky I, Hallqvist J, Tomson T, et al. Increased risk and worse prognosis of myocardial infarction in patients with prior hospitalization for epilepsy—The Stockholm Heart Epidemiology Program. Brain 2009;132:2798–804.

18. Wilson DA, Wannamaker BB, Malek AM, et al. Myocardial infarction after epilepsy onset: a population-based retrospective cohort study. Epilepsy Behav 2018;88: 181–8.

19. Serdyuk S, Davtyan K, Burd S, et al. Cardiac arrhythmias and sudden unexpected death in epilepsy: Results of long-term monitoring. Heart Rhythm 2021; 18:221–8.

20. Stecker EC, Reinier K, Uy-Evanado A, et al. Relationship between seizure episode and sudden cardiac arrest in patients with epilepsy. Circ Arrhythm Electrophysiol 2013;6:912–6.

21. Bensken WP, Fernandez-Baca Vaca G, Jobst BC, et al. Burden of chronic and acute conditions and symptoms in people with epilepsy. Neurology 2021;97: e2368–80.

22. Espinosa PS, Lee JW, Tedrow UB, et al. Sudden unexpected near death in epilepsy: malignant arrhythmia from a partial seizure. Neurology 2009;72:1702–3.

23. Chahal CAA, Gottwald JA, St. Louis EK, et al. QT prolongation in patients with index evaluation for seizure or epilepsy is predictive of all-cause mortality. Heart Rhythm 2022;19(4):578–84. https://doi.org/10.1016/j.hrthm.2021.11.013. S1547-5271(21)02346-8.

24. Feldman AE, Gidal BE. QTc prolongation by antiepileptic drugs and the risk of torsade de pointes in patients with epilepsy. Epilepsy Behav 2013;26:421–6.

25. Kishk NA, Sharaf Y, Ebraheim AM, et al. Interictal cardiac repolarization abnormalities in people with epilepsy. Epilepsy Behav 2018;79:106–11.

26. Thijs RD, Ryvlin P, Surges R. Autonomic manifestations of epilepsy: emerging pathways to sudden death? Nat Rev Neurol 2021;17:774–88.

27. Porthan K, Viitasalo M, Toivonen L, et al. Predictive value of electrocardiographic T-wave morphology parameters and T-wave peak to T-wave end interval for sudden cardiac death in the general population. Circ Arrhythm Electrophysiol 2013; 6:690–6.

28. Kenttä TV, Nearing BD, Porthan K, et al. Prediction of sudden cardiac death with automated high throughput analysis of heterogeneity in standard resting 12-lead electrocardiogram. Heart Rhythm 2016;13:713–20.

29. Verrier RL, Huikuri HV. Tracking interlead heterogeneity of R- and T-wave morphology to disclose latent risk for sudden cardiac death. Heart Rhythm 2017;14:1466–75.

30. Verrier RL, Klingenheben T, Malik M, et al. Microvolt T-wave alternans: Physiologic basis, methods of measurement, and clinical utility. Consensus guideline by the International Society for Holter and Noninvasive Electrocardiology. J Am Coll Cardiol 2011;44:1309–24.

31. Verrier RL, Kumar K, Nearing BD. Basis for sudden cardiac death prediction by T-wave alternans from an integrative physiology perspective. Heart Rhythm 2009; 6:416–22.

32. Verrier RL, Nearing BD, D'Avila A. Spectrum of clinical applications of interlead ECG heterogeneity assessment: From myocardial ischemia detection to sudden cardiac death risk stratification. Ann Noninvasive Electrocardiol 2021;26:e12894.

33. Verrier RL, Ikeda T. Ambulatory ECG-based T-wave alternans monitoring for risk assessment and guiding medical therapy: Mechanisms and clinical applications. Prog Cardiovasc Dis 2013;56:172–85.

34. Takasugi N, Goto H, Takasugi M, et al. Prevalence of microvolt T-wave alternans in patients with long QT syndrome and its association with torsade de pointes. Circ Arrhythm Electrophysiol 2016;9:e003206.

35. Verrier RL, Nieminen T. T-wave alternans as a therapeutic marker for antiarrhythmic agents. J Cardiovasc Pharmacol 2010;55:544–54.

36. Strzelczyk A, Adjei P, Scott CA, et al. Postictal increase in T-wave alternans after generalized tonic–clonic seizures. Epilepsia 2011;52:2112–7.

37. Pang TD, Nearing BD, Krishnamurthy KB, et al. Cardiac electrical instability in newly diagnosed/chronic epilepsy tracked by Holter and ECG patch. Neurology 2019;93:450–8.

38. Pang TD, Nearing BD, Olin B, et al. Uncovering ictal and interictal cardiac electrical instability in the EMU using high-resolution dynamic EKG recording [abstract]. Epilepsy Currents 2019;19(6).

39. Monteiro FR, Rabelo Evangelista AB, Nearing BD, et al. T-wave heterogeneity in standard resting 12-lead ECGs is associated with 90-day cardiac mortality in women following emergency department admission: A nested case-control study. Ann Noninvasive Electrocardiol 2021;26:e12826.

40. Pang TD, Nearing BD, Verrier RL, et al. T-wave heterogeneity crescendo in the surface EKG is superior to heart rate acceleration for seizure prediction. Epilepsy Behav 2022;130. 108670.

41. Echt DS, Liebson PR, Mitchell LB, et al. Mortality and morbidity in patients receiving encainide, flecainide, or placebo. The Cardiac Arrhythmia Suppression Trial. N Engl J Med 1991;324:781–8.

42. Tigaran S, Molgaard H, McClelland R, et al. Evidence of cardiac ischemia during seizures in drug-refractory epilepsy patients. Neurology 2003;60:491–5.

43. Zaccara G, Lattanzi S. Comorbidity between epilepsy and cardiac arrhythmias: Implication for treatment. Epilepsy Behav 2019;97:304–12.

44. Wasade VS, Schultz L, Mohanarangan K, et al. Long-term seizure and psychosocial outcomes of vagus nerve stimulation for intractable epilepsy. Epilepsy Behav 2015;53:31–6.

45. Ryvlin P, So EL, Gordon CM, et al. Long-term surveillance of SUDEP in drug-resistant epilepsy patients treated with VNS therapy. Epilepsia 2018;59:562–72.

46. Nearing BD, Anand IS, Libbus I, et al. Vagus nerve stimulation provides multiyear improvements in autonomic function and cardiac electrical stability in the ANTHEM-HF study. J Card Fail 2021;27:208–16.

47. De Ferrari GM, Schwartz PJ. Vagus nerve stimulation: from pre-clinical to clinical application: challenges and future directions. Heart Fail Rev 2011;16:195–203.

48. Schomer AC, Nearing BD, Schachter SC, et al. Vagus nerve stimulation reduces cardiac electrical instability assessed by quantitative T-wave alternans analysis in patients with drug-resistant focal epilepsy. Epilepsia 2014;55:1996–2002.

49. Verrier RL, Nearing BD, Olin B, et al. Baseline elevation and reduction in cardiac electrical instability assessed by quantitative T-wave alternans in patients with drug-resistant epilepsy treated with vagus nerve stimulation in the AspireSR E-36 trial. Epilepsy Behav 2016;62:85–9.

50. Leino J, Verrier RL, Minkkinen M, et al. Importance of regional specificity of T-wave alternans in assessing risk for cardiovascular mortality and sudden cardiac death during routine exercise testing. Heart Rhythm 2011;8:385–90.

51. Verrier RL, Fuller H, Justo FA, et al. Unmasking atrial repolarization to assess alternans, spatio-temporal heterogeneity, and susceptibility to atrial fibrillation. Heart Rhythm 2016;13:953–61.

52. Yuan Y, Hassel JL, Doytchinova A, et al. Left cervical vagal nerve stimulation reduces skin sympathetic nerve activity in patients with drug resistant epilepsy. Heart Rhythm 2017;14:1771–8.

53. Nashef L, So EL, Ryvlin P, et al. Unifying the definitions of sudden unexpected death in epilepsy. Epilepsia 2012;53:227–33.
54. Huikuri HV, Castellanos A, Myerburg RJ. Sudden death due to cardiac arrhythmias. N Engl J Med 2001;345:1473–82.
55. Fialho GL, Wolf P, Walz R, et al. Increased cardiac stiffness is associated with autonomic dysfunction in patients with temporal lobe epilepsy. Epilepsia 2018; 59:e85–90.
56. Zack MM, Kobau R. National and state estimates of the numbers of adults and children with active epilepsy — United States, 2015. MMWR Morb Mortal Wkly Rep 2017;11:821–5.
57. Benjamin EJ, Virani SS, Callaway CW, et al. American Heart Association Council on Epidemiology and Prevention Statistics Committee and Stroke Statistics Subcommittee. Heart disease and stroke statistics— 2018 update: a report from the American Heart Association. Circulation 2018;137:e67–492.

Telemedicine and Epilepsy Care

Bruce Lavin, MD, MPH[a], Cloe L. Gray, PhD[a],*, Martin Brodie, MD[b,1]

KEYWORDS

- Telemedicine • Teleconsultation • Epilepsy care • Remote EEG • COVID-19

KEY POINTS

- Epilepsy is on the rise, especially in health resource-limited areas, worsening a shortfall in the number of neurologists available to treat patients.
- Telemedicine bridges the gap in health care services, permitting access for neurologists to consult with people with epilepsy
- During the COVID-19 pandemic, teleconsultation use increased by people with epilepsy

INTRODUCTION

Telehealth, often used interchangeably with telemedicine, involves the use of telecommunication technology for the exchange of medical information from one location to another to provide health care services. Telemedicine, more narrowly defined, relates to the exchange of health information to provide remote clinical services and medical care by a provider for a patient. Both telehealth and telemedicine may offer a wide range of services that can be delivered by any or all the following modalities:

- Asynchronous/store and forward
- Synchronous/live
- Remote physiologic monitoring
- Data collected and sent in batches after information is gathered
- Data collected and sent real time as it is being collected
- Continuous physiologic monitoring with wearable devices

Epilepsy is a chronic neurologic disorder amenable to care and management via telemedicine services. Since the invention of the electroencephalograph and the use of electroencephalography (EEG) a century ago, the diagnosis of seizure disorders and epilepsy is possible through the assessment of EEGs. The usual assessment of a patient presenting with a seizure disorder can be accomplished by obtaining the

a BioSerenity, 3330 Cumberland Boulevard, Suite 800, Atlanta, GA 30339, USA; b Epilepsy Unit, West Glasgow Ambulatory Care Hospital-Yorkhill, Glasgow, United Kingdom
1 Present address: 11 Somerset Place, Glasgow G3 7JT, Scotland, United Kingdom.
* Corresponding author.
E-mail address: cloe.gray@bioserenity.com

Neurol Clin 40 (2022) 717–727
https://doi.org/10.1016/j.ncl.2022.03.004
neurologic.theclinics.com
0733-8619/22/

patient history and ambulatory EEG with video, often accompanied by electrocardiography as well as neuroimaging studies when appropriate. The earliest form of telemedicine for epilepsy involved asynchronous/store and forward of diagnostic information obtained by EEGs. The EEG recordings were transmitted in stored batches to trained specialists for the interpretation and diagnosis of possible seizure disorders. As technology progressed and the level of comfort grew with the use of telemedicine, EEG data were subsequently live streamed, allowing specialists to directly monitor and assess patient seizure disorders. The subsequent digitalization and real-time transmission of the EEG recordings and signals make sharing of the data more efficient and more effective for remote live continuous or intermittent patient monitoring of patients located over great distances from the specialist.

TELEMEDICINE-EPILEPSY CARE

Today, the majority (at least 80%) of the world's population of people with seizure disorders and epilepsy reside in areas with limited health care resources around the world, and three-quarters of these individuals have not received appropriate diagnosis or treatment.[1] Those living in poor, developing countries, low- or middle-income countries (LMIC), or rural areas, where medical resources may be limited, often must travel great distances or endure lengthy medical appointment delays in seeking trained specialists to receive their health care. Many LMIC areas of the world have no neurologists or less than one per 10,000 population, although the United States and many European Countries have from 5 to 10 specialists per 100,000.[2] In either case, the number of specialists is far outpaced by the growing number of people having or developing seizure disorders with approximately 1.2% of the US population having epilepsy[3] and 1 in 26 people developing epilepsy worldwide.

The World Health Organization and the Pan American Health Organizations realize that limited access to epilepsy care represents a significant public health concern. According to the World Health Assembly Resolution on the Global Fight against Epilepsy in the resulting Global Action report entitled "Epilepsy: A Public Health Imperative", people living with epilepsy need to be better connected with experienced health care providers and have better access to care despite limitations in resources.[4] To address the issue of delay in diagnosis and treatment of people with epilepsy, the Global Action Plan suggests that primary care physicians and allied health professionals be provided with the necessary tools to better recognize and manage seizure disorders and epilepsy in such remote areas. Telemedicine for Epilepsy Care has the potential to deliver on the global mandate and provide high-quality, convenient, and cost-effective epilepsy management for all.[5]

With almost 3.5 million people suffering from epilepsy in the United States and an estimated 230 specialized epilepsy centers in the United States (NAEC membership), a recent study revealed that between 58% and 72% of adults with epilepsy or uncontrolled seizures engaged with a neurologist or an epileptologist although approximately 23% saw a generalist or primary care physician. As many as 12% saw no physician at all over a 1-year period from the onset of their seizures.[3] There have been many studies illustrating the negative impact on health outcomes because of diagnostic and treatment delays for epilepsy care, particularly in children having focal epilepsy.[6,7]

Telemedicine's impact on epilepsy care is influenced by the patient journey in seeking or connecting with medical care for their seizure disorder and may in turn directly influence the outcome of their journey. The nature and complexity of the seizure disorders and the proximity and availability of appropriate medical services will contribute to the best use of telemedicine and virtual care versus in-person care (**Fig. 1**). Despite the latest antiseizure medicines available, the drug response rate for people with epilepsy remains at roughly 2/3 being seizure free when properly treated. A third of patients are treatment refractory or drug resistant, therefore requiring additional and continued intervention.[8] The identification of this population can be better achieved with the support of telemedicine and remote patient monitoring.[9,10] It is reasonable to expect that those patients presenting with complex medical issues, including drug resistance, will require interventions necessitating face-to-face consultations.

PATIENT JOURNEY INFLUENCES MODALITY OF PROVIDER ENGAGEMENT

True virtual care telemedicine, used for many acute illnesses and some chronic disorders, is where the patient may receive their medical care remotely without the need to visit the provider in person or travel to traditional "brick and mortar" health care facilities. This may be appropriate in the routine management of people with known or previously diagnosed epilepsy where medication adjustments and refills may be required. It may also be useful for follow-up visits requiring occasional episodic monitoring or medical surveillance of patients while also obtaining EEGs and other vital sign telemetry. The initial diagnosis of de novo seizure disorders or the further medical evaluation of more difficult epilepsy disorders resistant to medication may require a more hybrid approach with telemedicine.

Comprehensive epilepsy care with telemedicine may be best addressed by a hybrid "Hub and Spoke" model where there is a comprehensive Epilepsy Center with trained specialists, serving as the primary Epilepsy Center or "Hub". Local clinics and less specialized health care facilities, as the "Spokes" may serve as the in-person intermediaries between the patient, their provider, and the remote specialist at the "Hub". Veterans Affairs epilepsy care services successfully use the "Hub and Spoke" telemedicine model to manage the care of veterans with

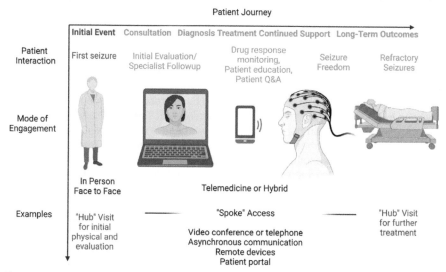

Fig. 1. Patient journey influences modality of provider engagement. (Created with BioRender.com.)

seizure disorders. There are 17 Epilepsy Centers of Excellence (ECoE) located in major urban medical centers across the United States providing comprehensive epilepsy care and consultation to the over 150 VA Medical Centers and approximately 1400 community-based outpatient clinics in the community.[11] The VA system uses telemedicine services, along with an eConsultation between patients, primary care providers, and epilepsy specialists, to help provide education, research, counseling, and clinical services, linking the many local clinics and medical centers to the ECoE. The advantage of eConsultations is the timely access to the specialist's expertise and medical opinion when the face-to-face patient examination is not required or possible due to distance.

IMPACT OF CORONAVIRUS DISEASE 2019 (COVID-19) ON EPILEPSY AND TELEMEDICINE

COVID-19 and the ensuing lockdown caused profound issues in people with epilepsy. The earliest experiences in China, Italy, Kuwait and Spain revealed an increase in the number of breakthrough seizures during the lockdown.[12–16] Other reports showed that patients experienced worse availability of medical services,[17] and delays in getting epilepsy-related tests or prescriptions filled during the pandemic lockdown.[18] In a survey of patients with Dravet syndrome, there were no increases in seizures, but behavior and sleep–wake patterns worsened, and clinic appointments were postponed.[19,20] Similarly, pediatric patients with epilepsy and neurocognitive disorders had worsened behavioral issues, such as deficits in attention and increased aggression.[21] These studies indicate a need for continued access using alternative methods to specialists and trained providers.

INSTRUMENTATION OF TELEMEDICINE IN EPILEPSY CARE

The COVID-19 pandemic has spurred innovation in mobile apps and Internet programs to help people manage their epilepsy.[22] In Colombia, an open-source epilepsy telehealth electronic health record was combined with an algorithm to automatically detect abnormal brain activity in EEG records.[23] Combined with the electronic health record, the algorithm has been proposed to be used by neurologists combined with trained technologists in rural areas to perform EEGs for patients. An ePortal called Providing Individualized Services and Care in Epilepsy was developed to allow the patient or caregiver the ability to collaborate with doctors on their care and treatment.[24]

In Italy, during the initial COVID-19 surge and health resource burden, telemedicine was used to assess and monitor patients with epilepsy.[25] Teleconsultation was able to determine that patients did not experience an increase in seizure frequency, but they did have higher levels of stress and poor sleep quality. Patients reported high levels of satisfaction with the telephone visit, and they supported the ability of teleconsultations to interact with a health care provider despite the pandemic. Patients with epilepsy were also able to receive their basic neurologic exams using videoconferencing if they did not require more complex studies.[24]

At the New York University Langone Health system, virtual visits were implemented to evolve from the traditional neurologic outpatient model.[26] Using cameras, the neurologist could ask the patient to perform physiologic, physical coordination, and memory tests. The assessment of the cognitive effects of epilepsy can also be performed with a virtual visit. People with epilepsy may often be impacted in their learning, memory, and verbal abilities, as well as reductions in processing speed, executive function, language, and anterograde memory with a higher risk for depression and generalized anxiety disorders.[27]

EFFECTIVENESS OF TELEMEDICINE FOR EPILEPSY

Telemedicine for childhood epilepsy allowed providers to identify issues requiring modification of antiepileptic drugs, and such changes did not cause medication errors or other issues in patients.[28] Studies have been done to determine the effectiveness of telemedicine epilepsy care using the ketogenic diet as a treatment.[29] Providers used WhatsApp to help families manage their epilepsy symptoms following the diet, and families felt that video calls helped them understand how to prepare a ketogenic diet.

Telemedicine was used in the United States to diagnose childhood focal epilepsy.[30,31] Through telemedicine, children were able to be diagnosed by remote video with EEG and hyperventilation studies to receive their treatment, resulting in a significant reduction in their seizures.

MEDICAL RECORD SURVEYS

In several retrospective studies, the impact of telehealth was affirmed by examining medical records. In one study, the outcome of telemedicine was compared with in-person visits in childhood epilepsy.[32] There were no determined differences in seizure frequency or changes of oral antiepileptic drugs between patients who met in person with practitioners and those who were assessed by telephone. It affirmed that telemedicine consultations could be successfully used to assess children with epilepsy.

In Ohio, the epilepsy center at the Cleveland Clinic began to use telemedicine through Cleveland Clinic Express Care Online, commercial videoconferencing tools such as FaceTime or GoogleDuo, or telephone communication.[33] The clinic experienced more no-shows to clinic appointments once the COVID-19 pandemic began, but outpatient care transitioned favorably to video or telephone communication with the specialists.

Telemedicine visits did not increase the number of hospital admissions by patients.[34] Telemedicine also allowed staff to accurately assess and document new epilepsy symptoms, indicating that telemedicine can fulfill the needs of patients and staff during COVID.[35]

CLINICIAN PERSPECTIVES ON TELEHEALTH

Clinicians found the switch to telehealth a positive experience.[36] One survey found that two-thirds of clinicians would continue to use telehealth in the future if it was an option.[37] In another survey, over 90% of clinicians expressed satisfaction using telemedicine.[38] Epilepsy, where medical history is often the key to diagnosis, was considered more suitable for telemedicine than disorders that required detailed physical examinations.[39] Some did express reservations about telemedicine for first-time patients, those with indeterminate seizure frequencies, and complex or drug-resistant patients who needed surgery.[40,41] Clinicians cited difficulties with connecting to patients (especially in rural areas) and patients being unfamiliar with the technology. However, many neurologists believed that they could spend more quality time with each patient while also allowing them to provide care to a greater number of patients. Additionally, telemedicine allows the provider to interact and assess the patient in a more familiar setting, such as at home (where the evaluation of sleep, emotional, or other precipitating causes of seizure disorders are more reliable).

CAREGIVER PERSPECTIVES ON TELEHEALTH

Caregivers of patients with epilepsy surveyed about using telehealth stated it was an overall positive experience; two-thirds of participants stated that telehealth was a valuable tool for routine visits but did not believe it was acceptable for the initial evaluation of neurologic disorders.[42] Many caregivers believed telehealth visits allowed them to save time and travel, but they still preferred in-person appointments for their consultations.[43] Those with prior experience with telehealth expressed a desire to continue using telehealth after the COVID-19 pandemic.[44] However, in countries with large rural populations with communication barriers, caregivers lacked awareness of telehealth, and as a result, epilepsy outcomes were found to worsen.[45]

PATIENTS' PERSPECTIVES ON TELEHEALTH

Most surveyed patients stated that telehealth fulfilled their needs for follow-up care and was satisfied with using telemedicine.[46–49] A majority felt telemedicine visits were more convenient,[40] and they were more willing to contact their provider via teleconsultation for their care.[50] Patients who had teleconsultation via phone or video conference indicated that it allowed them to avoid travel, it reduced waiting times and time away from work or school, they were more comfortable with the privacy of the encounters, and they were willing to continue using telemedicine if given the option.[18,37,51] However, some patients indicated that they were dissatisfied with telemedicine[52] as it felt less intimate or personal and those with treatment-resistant epilepsy expressed a preference for face-to-face visits.[18]

BENEFITS OF TELEMEDICINE

During the COVID-19 pandemic, the risk of infection transmission due to in-person visits is eliminated by telemedicine, and beyond the pandemic, those who are immunocompromised can use telemedicine as an alternative to an in-person visit. Additionally, people with epilepsy whose seizures are not well controlled cannot drive, making telemedicine vital for access to care without relying on someone to provide transportation.[53] One study reported that the societal impact of telemedicine was the potential reduction in carbon emissions calculated to be 35,000–40,000 kg of carbon dioxide.[54]

LIMITATIONS OF TELEMEDICINE

Telemedicine does have some limitations that can affect patients' experiences with the technology. Patients, especially in rural areas, may not have high-speed Internet access, making video consultation difficult.[55] Patients, caregivers, and even some health care providers may not be competent or comfortable with telemedicine technology, limiting the effectiveness of telehealth. Patient and data privacy, while well protected with the latest advancements in telehealth cybersecurity technology that has emerged since the COVID-19 pandemic started, can remain a concern, as health-related data can still be corrupted or inappropriately obtained by others. Finally, future equitable reimbursement to providers for telemedicine visits after the COVID-19 pandemic will be uncertain.

REIMBURSEMENT FOR TELEMEDICINE

Before the COVID-19 pandemic, telemedicine reimbursement was inconsistent between third-party payers and Medicare, often equated to a simple telephone call. Providers were also reluctant to embrace telemedicine as a routine means of patient

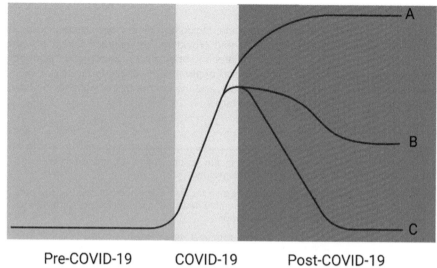

Pre-COVID-19   COVID-19   Post-COVID-19

Fig. 2. Future directions of telemedicine. (Created with BioRender.com.)

engagement. As a result, patients primarily visited their providers in person to receive their epilepsy care. In March 2020, Health and Human Services and the Center for Medicaid and Medicare Services relaxed regulations regarding telemedicine, allowing patients to schedule and conduct virtual visits.[56] Specifically, new patients could schedule visits for evaluation and management virtually, send prerecorded images or videos to their practitioners in advance and communicate by telephone or by e-visit (such as via video with an online portal). Parity was established in the payment for a visit, meaning that telehealth visits were reimbursed at in-person rates.[57] As a result of the public health emergency of COVID-19, and the success of telemedicine in addressing the health care crisis, these improvements in care by telehealth services are projected to remain permanent as the pandemic continues and likely beyond.[58]

FUTURE DIRECTIONS OF TELEMEDICINE

The possible course of telemedicine in the future could take several paths (**Fig. 2**). (A) The use of telemedicine for epilepsy could increase if patients, providers, and caretakers see the benefits of telemedicine and expand the adoption of remote health care. This could be due to the demonstration of health care cost reduction, innovation in the quality of the health care service and its outcomes, and/or the reduction in the risk of infection. Internet infrastructure and connectivity platforms will also improve, especially in rural areas that might not be able to take advantage of telemedicine due to the lack of high-speed Internet access. Reimbursement would also need to continue for the adoption of telemedicine to increase. (B) The use of telemedicine could decrease slightly if reimbursement policies remain in place, but patients prefer to return to in-person visits to a greater degree. Some surveys, in fact, suggest this to be the case.[59] (C) Telemedicine use could decrease to pre-COVID pandemic levels if office visit parity reimbursements for telemedicine are reduced or eliminated, there are disincentives for physicians to offer telemedicine visits, or it becomes more difficult or costly for patients to use telemedicine.

SUMMARY

The development of tools for telemedicine, including online portals and the use of smartphone technology to link patients and providers, has enabled continued care for patients separated from their physicians and specialists. Outcomes of telemedicine include reduced time to diagnosis and treatment, the ability to titrate or change medicines quickly (vs frequent office visits), and the connection of patients in underserved communities with physician shortages.

CLINICS CARE POINTS

- Telemedicine may be most appropriate in the routine follow-up and management of previously identified seizure disorders and epilepsy.
- Asynchronous data uploading is most effective for specialist preconsultation assessments, although live videoconferencing and live remote patient monitoring are most effective for real-time patient engagement and evaluation.
- Telemedicine visits should be conducted as though it were a face to face in a clinic visit, with patient privacy, lack of distractions, and proper patient and provider preparation.
- Health care policies impacting reimbursement, physician–patient engagement, and remote Internet/mobile technologies will either enable or inhibit further telemedicine adoption
- There has been a significant growth in telehealth technology and use with the onset of the COVID-19 pandemic due to health safety concerns, overburdening of in-facility health care services, and the continued lack of health care provider resources. It has since leveled off but remains high compared with pre-COVID levels.

DISCLOSURE

The authors declare that they have no relevant or material financial interests that relate to the research described in this article.

REFERENCES

1. Espinosa-Jovel C, Toledano R, Aledo-Serrano Á, et al. Epidemiological profile of epilepsy in low income populations. Seizure 2018;56:67–72.
2. Dall TM, Storm MV, Donofrio PD, et al. Supply and demand analysis of the current and future US neurology workforce. Neurology 2013;81(5):470–8.
3. Zack MM, Kobau R. National and State Estimates of the Numbers of Adults and Children with Active Epilepsy - United States, 2015. MMWR Morb Mortal Wkly Rep 2017;66(31):821–5.
4. Guekht A, Brodie M, Secco M, et al. The road to a World Health Organization global action plan on epilepsy and other neurological disorders. Epilepsia 2021;62(5):1057–63.
5. Lavin B, Dormond C, Scantlebury MH, et al. Bridging the healthcare gap: Building the case for epilepsy virtual clinics in the current healthcare environment. Epilepsy Behav 2020;111:107262.
6. Parviainen L, Kälviäinen R, Jutila L. Impact of diagnostic delay on seizure outcome in newly diagnosed focal epilepsy. Epilepsia Open 2020;5(4):605–10.
7. Berg AT, Loddenkemper T, Baca CB. Diagnostic delays in children with early onset epilepsy: impact, reasons, and opportunities to improve care. Epilepsia 2014;55(1):123–32.

8. Chen Z, Brodie MJ, Liew D, et al. Treatment Outcomes in Patients With Newly Diagnosed Epilepsy Treated With Established and New Antiepileptic Drugs: A 30-Year Longitudinal Cohort Study. JAMA Neurol 2018;75(3):279–86.
9. Brunnhuber F, Slater J, Goyal S, et al. Past, present and future of home video-electroencephalographic telemetry: a review of the development of in-home video-electroencephalographic recordings. Epilepsia 2020;61(Suppl 1):S3–10.
10. Mumford V, Rapport F, Shih P, et al. Promoting faster pathways to surgery: a clinical audit of patients with refractory epilepsy. BMC Neurol 2019;19(1):29.
11. Epilepsy Centers of Excellence. https://www.epilepsy.va.gov/. Accessed January 2, 2022.
12. Si Y, Sun L, Sun H, et al. Epilepsy management during epidemic: A preliminary observation from western China. Epilepsy Behav 2020;113:107528.
13. Assenza G, Lanzone J, Brigo F, et al. Epilepsy Care in the Time of COVID-19 Pandemic in Italy: Risk Factors for Seizure Worsening. Front Neurol 2020; 11:1–11.
14. Abokalawa F, Ahmad SF, Al-Hashel J, et al. The effects of coronavirus disease 2019 (COVID-19) pandemic on people with epilepsy (PwE): an online survey-based study. Acta Neurol Belg 2022;122(1):59–66.
15. Conde-Blanco E, Centeno M, Tio E, et al. Emergency implementation of telemedicine for epilepsy in Spain : Results of a survey during SARS-CoV-2 pandemic. Epilepsy Behav 2020;107211.
16. Puteikis K, Mameniškienė R. Epilepsy care and COVID-19: A cross-sectional online survey from Lithuania. Acta Neurol Scand 2021;143(6):666–72.
17. Puteikis K, Jasionis A, Mameniškienė R. Recalling the COVID-19 lockdown: Insights from patients with epilepsy. Epilepsy Behav 2020;115:107573.
18. Fonseca E, Quintana M, Lallana S, et al. Epilepsy in time of COVID-19: A survey-based study. Acta Neurol Scand 2020;142(6):545–54.
19. Brambilla I, Aibar JÁ, Hallet AS, et al. Impact of the COVID-19 lockdown on patients and families with Dravet syndrome. Epilepsia Open 2021;6(1):216–24.
20. Cardenal-Muñoz E, Nabbout R, Boronat S, et al. Impact of COVID-19 on Spanish patients with Dravet syndrome and their caregivers: consequences of lockdown. Revista de neurologia 2021;73(2):57–65.
21. Pasca L, Paola M, Grumi S, et al. Impact of COVID-19 pandemic in pediatric patients with epilepsy with neuropsychiatric comorbidities : A telemedicine evaluation. Epilepsy Behav 2021;115:107519.
22. Choi SA, Lim K, Baek H, et al. Impact of mobile health application on data collection and self-management of epilepsy. Epilepsy Behav 2021;119:107982.
23. Molina E, Torres CES, Salazar-Cabrera R, et al. Intelligent telehealth system to support epilepsy diagnosis. J Multidisciplinary Healthc 2020;13:433–45.
24. Power K, McCrea Z, White M, et al. The development of an epilepsy electronic patient portal: Facilitating both patient empowerment and remote clinician-patient interaction in a post-COVID-19 world. Epilepsia 2020;61(9):1894–905.
25. Olivo S, Cheli M, Dinoto A, et al. Telemedicine during the SARS-Cov-2 pandemic lockdown: Monitoring stress and quality of sleep in patients with epilepsy. Epilepsy Behav 2021;118:107864.
26. Grossman SN, Han SC, Balcer LJ, et al. Rapid implementation of virtual neurology in response to the COVID-19 pandemic. Neurology 2020;94(24): 1077–87.
27. Tailby C, Collins AJ, Vaughan DN, et al. Teleneuropsychology in the time of COVID-19: The experience of The Australian Epilepsy Project. Seizure 2020;83: 89–97.

28. Kumar P, Dawman L, Panda P, et al. Feasibility and effectiveness of teleconsultation in children with epilepsy amidst the ongoing COVID-19 pandemic in a resource-limited country. Seizure 2020;81:29–35.

29. Semprino M, Fasulo L, Fortini S, et al. Telemedicine, drug-resistant epilepsy, and ketogenic dietary therapies: a patient survey of a pediatric remote-care program during the COVID- 19 pandemic. Epilepsy Behav 2020;112:7–12.

30. Stafstrom CE, Sun LR, Kossoff EH, et al. Diagnosing and managing childhood absence epilepsy by telemedicine. Epilepsy Behav 2021;115:107404.

31. Kessler SK, McGinnis E. A practical guide to treatment of childhood absence epilepsy. Paediatr Drugs 2019;21(1):15–24.

32. Kikuchi Kenjiro, Hamano Shin-Ichiro, Horiguchi Ayumi, et al. Telemedicine in epilepsy management during the coronavirus disease 2019 pandemic. Pediatr Int official J Jpn Pediatr Soc 2021. In press.

33. Punia V, Nasr G, Zagorski V, et al. Evidence of a rapid shift in outpatient practice during the COVID-19 pandemic using telemedicine. Telemed J E Health 2020; 26(10):1301–3.

34. Joshi C, Jacobson M, Silveira L, et al. Risk of Admission to the emergency room/inpatient service after a neurology telemedicine visit during COVID-19 Pandemic. Pediatr Neurol 2021;122:15–9.

35. Moura LMVR, Donahue MA, Smith JR, et al. Telemedicine Can Support Measurable and High-Quality Epilepsy Care During the COVID-19 Pandemic. Am J Med Qual 2021;36(1):5–16.

36. Kuchenbuch M, Onofrio GD, Wirrell E, et al. An accelerated shift in the use of remote systems in epilepsy due to the COVID-19 pandemic. Epilepsy Behav 2020;112:107376.

37. Casares M, Wombles C, Skinner HJ, et al. Telehealth perceptions in patients with epilepsy and providers during the COVID-19 pandemic. Epilepsy Behav 2020; 112:107394.

38. Rametta SC, Fridinger SE, Gonzalez AK, et al. Analyzing 2,589 child neurology telehealth encounters necessitated by the COVID-19 pandemic. Neurology 2020;95(9):e1257–66.

39. Cross JH, Kwon S, Akbar A, et al. Epilepsy care during the COVID-19 pandemic. Epilepsia 2021;62(10):2322–32.

40. Banks J, Corrigan D, Grogan R, et al. LoVE in a time of CoVID : Clinician and patient experience using telemedicine for chronic epilepsy management. Epilepsy Behav 2021;115:107675.

41. Teng T, Sareidaki DE, Chemaly N, et al. Physician and patient satisfaction with the switch to remote outpatient encounters in epilepsy clinics during the Covid-19 pandemic. Seizure 2021;91:60–5.

42. Trivisano M, Specchio N, Pietrafusa N, et al. Impact of COVID-19 pandemic on pediatric patients with epilepsy – The caregiver perspective. Epilepsy Behav 2020;113:107527.

43. Dozières-Puyravel B, Auvin S. Usefulness, limitations, and parental opinion about teleconsultation for rare pediatric epilepsies. Epilepsy Behav 2021;115:107656.

44. Klotz KA, Borlot F, Scantlebury MH, et al. Telehealth for children with epilepsy is effective and reduces anxiety independent of healthcare setting. Front Pediatr 2021;9:1–8.

45. Saleem T, Sheikh N, Hassan M, et al. COVID-19 containment and its unrestrained impact on epilepsy management in resource-limited areas of Pakistan. Epilepsy Behav 2020;(January):107476.

46. Millevert C, van Hees S, Siewe Fodjo JN, et al. Impact of COVID-19 on the lives and psychosocial well-being of persons with epilepsy during the third trimester of the pandemic: Results from an international, online survey. Epilepsy Behav 2021; 116:107800.
47. Mostacci B, Licchetta L, Cacciavillani C, et al. The Impact of the COVID-19 Pandemic on People With Epilepsy. An Italian Survey and a Global Perspective. Front Neurol 2020;11:1–9.
48. Nair PP, Aghoram R, Thomas B, et al. Video teleconsultation services for persons with epilepsy during COVID-19 pandemic: An exploratory study from public tertiary care hospital in Southern India on feasibility, satisfaction, and effectiveness. Epilepsy Behav 2021;117:107863.
49. Willems LM, Balcik Y, Noda AH, et al. SARS-CoV-2-related rapid reorganization of an epilepsy outpatient clinic from personal appointments to telemedicine services : A German single-center experience. Epilepsy Behav 2020;112:107483.
50. Rathore C, Baheti N, Ram A, et al. Impact of COVID-19 pandemic on epilepsy practice in India: A tripartite survey. Seizure 2020;86:60–7.
51. Von Wrede R, Moskau-Hartmann S, Baumgartner T, et al. Counseling of people with epilepsy via telemedicine : Experiences at a German tertiary epilepsy center during the COVID-19 pandemic. Epilepsy Behav 2020;112:107298.
52. Lallana S, Fonseca E, Restrepo JL, et al. Medium-term effects of COVID-19 pandemic on epilepsy: a follow-up study. Acta Neurol Scand 2021;144:99–108.
53. Burton A. How do we fix the shortage of neurologists? Lancet Neurol 2018;17(6): 502–3.
54. Blenkinsop S, Foley A, Schneider N, et al. Carbon emission savings and short-term health care impacts from telemedicine: An evaluation in epilepsy. Epilepsia 2021;62(11):2732–40.
55. Gursky JM, Boro A, Escalante S, et al. Disparities in access to neurologic telemedicine during the COVID-19 Pandemic: a bronx tale. Neurol Clin Pract 2021; 11(2):e97–101.
56. Cohen BH, Busis NA, Ciccarelli L. Coding in the World of COVID-19: Non-Face-to-Face Evaluation and Management Care. Continuum (Minneap Minn) 2020; 26(3):785–98.
57. Bajowala SS, Milosch J, Bansal C. Telemedicine Pays: Billing and Coding Update. Curr Allergy Asthma Rep 2020;20(10):60.
58. Trump administration finalizes permanent expansion of medicare telehealth services and improved payment for time doctors spend with patients. 2020. Available at: https://www.cms.gov/newsroom/press-releases/trump-administration-finalizes-permanent-expansion-medicare-telehealth-services-and-improved-payment. Accessed September 7, 2021.
59. Brigo F, Bonavita S, Leocani L, et al. Telemedicine and the challenge of epilepsy management at the time of COVID-19 pandemic. Epilepsy Behav 2020;110: 107164.

The Potential of Wearable Devices and Mobile Health Applications in the Evaluation and Treatment of Epilepsy

Behnaz Esmaeili, MD[a],*, Solveig Vieluf, PhD[b,c,1],
Barbara A. Dworetzky, MD[d], Claus Reinsberger, MD, PhD[c,d]

KEYWORDS

- Wearables • Biosensors • Mobile health • Mobile applications • Seizure detection
- Seizure prediction • Epilepsy

KEY POINTS

- Wearable devices can detect generalized onset and focal to bilateral generalized tonic-clonic seizures (GTCS) accurately.
- There are currently 2 Food and Drug Administration (FDA)-approved wearable devices for detecting GTCS during the resting state.
- There are yet no FDA-approved wearable devices for reliable detection of other seizure types besides GTCS.
- It remains to be elucidated whether using wearable devices can significantly improve epilepsy-related health outcomes.

INTRODUCTION

Wearable devices and mobile health (mHealth) software applications (apps) have the potential to optimize personalized medical care for persons with epilepsy (PWE).[1] There has been a rapid growth of wearable devices and mHealth apps during the past decade that aim to address seizure detection, seizure prediction, seizure forecasting, and epilepsy self-management.[1–5] With regard to epilepsy clinical care, both technologies have worked toward facilitating seizure reporting.[1,6] Accurate

[a] Department of Neurology, University of Washington, 325 9th Avenue, Box 359745, Seattle, WA 98104, USA; [b] Division of Epilepsy and Clinical Neurophysiology, Boston Children's Hospital, Harvard Medical School, Boston, MA, USA; [c] Institute of Sports Medicine, Paderborn University, Paderborn, Germany; [d] Department of Neurology, Brigham and Women's Hospital, 60 Fenwood Rd, Boston, MA 02115, USA
[1] Present address: Department of Neurology, Boston Children's Hospital, 1 Autumn St, Boston, MA 02215, USA.
* Corresponding author.
E-mail address: Behnaz.esmaeili@gmail.com

Neurol Clin 40 (2022) 729–739
https://doi.org/10.1016/j.ncl.2022.03.005
0733-8619/22/© 2022 Elsevier Inc. All rights reserved.

neurologic.theclinics.com

seizure reporting is needed to use seizure frequency as a clinical outcome measure. The standard reporting tools are paper-based seizure diaries. As the digitization of medical applications continues, an increasing number of apps offer diary functions,[6] which provide several advantages: transmission errors are eliminated and transmission time is reduced because the data is stored directly in digital form[7]; the data format is comparable between patients, easing the development of effective analysis tools; online visualizations and near real-time evaluations of the diary entries are possible; and patients can receive automatic reminders to fill out the diary, which can improve adherence. Despite these advantages, there currently remains a need for active data entry, which can be especially challenging for the pediatric population. Wearable devices nevertheless have the potential to overcome the difficulties with manual data entry and provide objective physiologic data.

Wearable technologies or biosensors, often referred to as wearables, are small electronic devices that are typically worn on the body and record personal data. Compared with traditional monitoring devices, wearables are easy-to-use, noninvasive or minimally invasive, fashionable, affordable, and the recorded data volume is lower. They have potential to close a long-existing gap in continuous telemonitoring, particularly to detect and predict seizures.[8–11] In addition, wearables have the potential to identify patients at a high risk of seizure-related morbidity and mortality, including sudden unexpected death in epilepsy (SUDEP), and to trigger responses from caregivers to potentially prevent death.[12] Despite the advancement of technology and interest from patients and caregivers, wearables and apps have yet to be integrated into epilepsy care where more clinical data will contribute in the future.

Here, we review the commonly used wearables and apps, focusing on devices approved by the United States Food and Drug Administration (FDA) and potential clinical applications. We consider their limitations, challenges, and future direction.

BIOSIGNALS AND SENSORS

Wearable biosensors can record long-term physiologic signals, making them potentially suitable for applications in epilepsy care. Autonomic alterations are common findings in both peri-ictal and interictal states.[13–16] Wearables can measure changes in autonomic function, allowing for seizure detection and prediction.[16] Many commercially available biosensors measure electroencephalogram (EEG) and non-EEG signals including accelerometry (ACC), electromyogram (EMG), electrocardiogram (ECG), photoplethysmography, electrodermal activity (EDA), and skin temperature (TEMP).[4,17–19] Generalized tonic-clonic seizures (GTCS) are associated with more intense ictal movements and peri-ictal autonomic findings including changes in ECG, EDA, TEMP, and other autonomic measures, making it easier to detect using biosensors.[20] There are currently 2 FDA-approved wearable devices with applications for the detection of GTCS using non-EEG biosensors: Embrace 2 (E2, Empatica Embrace, Boston MA) and SPEAC (Brain Sentinel SPEAC, San Antonio TX). Empatica E2 is a wristwatch with biosensors to measure and log long-term EDA, TEMP, and ACC, which provide data to assess the sympathetic autonomic drive and movements. Machine learning (ML) models embedded in Embrace analyze these data in real-time to detect GTCS.[10] The SPEAC sensor is worn on one arm with a surface EMG monitor patch attached to the biceps muscle. It uses surface EMG signals to measure even subtle movements and analyzes the data in real-time to detect tonic-clonic activity that indicates GTCS.[21] Both devices can send an alert to the patient's caregiver and save data on cloud servers.

There is an ongoing search for wearables to reliably detect other seizure types, including focal impaired awareness seizures,[18] but no such devices currently have FDA approval. One area of active research on these devices focuses on the types of biosignals to use, which may include both EEG and non-EEG data. There are currently many devices under development to detect other seizure types, but validation has not yet been achieved to justify regular clinical use. To improve the quality of studies focusing on seizure detection devices, researchers have proposed standards for clinical validation to clarify the level of evidence provided for each device.[22] This is extremely important considering the rapid growth of wearables claiming seizure detection. Clinical validation trials are classified into 5 phases ranging from phase 0, intended for initial studies of a new seizure detection technique, to phase 4, which includes follow-up studies on the feasibility and utility of the new devices in patients' home environments.[22] There are many phase 0 to 1 validation studies of seizure detection devices compared with fewer phase 2 to 4 studies.[19] The latter devices are summarized in recent review articles.[17,19] The 2 above-mentioned devices currently have FDA approval for very specific applications. Here, we will review studies on clinical validation of the FDA-approved devices.

CLINICAL VALIDATION OF FDA-APPROVED WEARABLE DEVICES
E2 Wristwatch

The E2 wristwatch (Empatica) uses multimodal biosensors to detect GTCS. The device was cleared by the FDA in 2018 for detecting GTCS during the resting state for adults and in 2019 for children aged 6 years and older.[10] The ML models used for seizure detection in E2 are detailed in previous studies.[20] Gold-standard video-EEG data, obtained from PWE admitted to epilepsy monitoring units (EMUs) and annotated by epileptologists, were used to train the seizure detection models. An inpatient study of 69 patients including 22 patients with seizures showed 94.55% sensitivity and a false alarm rate (FAR) of 0.2, but no false alarms during sleep.[20] The same group reported a prospective EMU study of 135 patients including 22 with seizures showing a sensitivity of 100% with FAR of 0.42[10]. In outpatient settings where annotations are made by patients/caregivers, FARs are higher. Studies using ambulatory data on 27 patients including 14 with seizures reported 93% sensitivity with FAR of 0.58.[23] Long-term ambulatory data over 1 year with only 3 patients showed an improvement of sensitivity to greater than 97% with FAR less than 0.4.[24] Overall, wearables using EDA and ACC sensors have high sensitivity to detect GTCS. The high FAR during wakefulness in real life remains challenging and requires future studies.

SPEAC

The SPEAC device (Brain Sentinel) uses surface EMG to detect GTCS. It was cleared by the FDA in 2017 for detecting GTCS during the resting state in adults. Surface EMG from unilateral biceps/triceps was recorded in 33 patients with epilepsy admitted for video-EEG monitoring including 11 patients with seizures.[25] The ML model applied to offline data detected 95% of GTCS identified by video-EEG with FAR of 0.017 but no false alarms during sleep. In a prospective multicenter study with 199 patients with a history of GTCS admitted to EMUs, including 61 patients with seizures, the detection algorithm showed 76% sensitivity and a mean FAR of 2.52.[26] Other studies using surface EMG biosensors in EMUs also showed high sensitivity for the detection of GTCS. Using surface EMG-based seizure detection for fully automated real-time data analysis of 73 patients in EMUs showed 93.8% sensitivity with FAR of 0.67 for the detection of GTCS.[27]

APPLICATIONS OF WEARABLES IN EPILEPSY CLINICAL CARE
Seizure Detection and Prediction

Clinicians and PWE aim to achieve the goal of zero seizures by optimizing medical management of epilepsy guided by reported seizure frequency. Seizure diaries are not always reliable.[28] Patients may underreport their seizures for multiple reasons including the nature of their seizure or recall bias.[29,30] Witness reports are also inaccurate.[31] Therefore, self-reported seizure diaries tend to underestimate seizure burden, limiting optimal care. Previous studies have already raised questions about the reliability of seizure diaries in research studies.[32] Wearables, however, could identify the occurrence of seizures in long-term ambulatory monitoring, providing objective data to track seizure frequency more accurately.[11,20,33–35] These data can be used to optimize medical management as well as neuromodulation parameters in patients with implanted intracranial devices.

Among the different effects of seizures/epilepsy on quality of life, the unpredictability of seizures is quite distressing for PWE and their caregivers.[36] They usually try to identify triggering factors for seizures in order to avoid them; however, these connections are often not reliable. Circadian and multidien patterns of seizure risk have been shown to inform about phases of high seizure likelihood for individual patients.[37] Long-term recording of biosignals using wearables may facilitate seizure prediction and seizure forecasting,[8,38,39] which can improve patients' quality of life. For patients with cyclic variations in seizure occurrence, reliable seizure forecasting may also allow for targeted medical management at the time the patient is at the highest risk for seizure.

DIAGNOSIS OF EPILEPSY: EPILEPTIC VERSUS NONEPILEPTIC SEIZURES

Functional seizures or psychogenic nonepileptic seizures and convulsive syncope are the top differential for epileptic seizures. Despite attempting to capture habitual episodes using video-EEG monitoring, indeterminate results occur regularly adding to diagnostic delay.[40] Difficulty bringing patients into the EMU include insurance-related, family-related, or work-related issues, or availability. The development of wearables using ultralong-term monitoring could meet an important clinical need if it were comparable in accuracy to gold standard video-EEG monitoring. Previous studies have shown surface EMG and ACC data recorded by wearables in the EMUs can distinguish GTCS from nonepileptic convulsive seizures with an accuracy exceeding 80% to 90%[41,42] and 70%,[43,44] respectively. For patients with both epileptic and nonepileptic seizures, wearables may identify the frequency of episodes to guide treatment.

Full-montage ambulatory scalp EEG monitoring is integral to epilepsy care, typically providing EEG data over days. It is commonly used for assessing ictal/interictal burden. Full-montage ambulatory EEG, even short term, is potentially stigmatizing and uncomfortable. Wearables have tried to overcome these disadvantages by using limited electrodes, subcutaneous electrodes, and/or using biosignals other than EEG.[35,45,46]

EPILEPSY-RELATED MORTALITY

Frequent GTCS increase risk of SUDEP and other epilepsy-related mortality.[47] Despite advancement in understanding risk factors (RFs) and mechanisms, there are still no reliable biomarkers for SUDEP. Postictal EEG suppression, postictal cardiorespiratory changes including postictal central apnea and asystole, prolonged QT interval, and reduced heart rate variability are potential RFs associated with

SUDEP.[48–53] Although EMU-based studies offer valuable RF information, wearables may provide superior long-term ambulatory monitoring data because some RFs are not consistently present after every GTCS in a single individual.[12] Chronic monitoring by wearables may even provide further information about the pathophysiology of fatal seizures as with SUDEP. Embrace data from one SUDEP showed an unusually large EDA surge after the fatal GTCS compared with nonfatal seizures.[54] Such data may help establish a risk profile for each patient to inform prevention.

Lower incidence of SUDEP has been shown in residential care centers that have a higher level of nocturnal supervision,[55] suggesting an alarm notification system may decrease SUDEP by allowing the caregiver to turn the patient away from prone position (which may result in fatal airway obstruction), provide cardiorespiratory resuscitation, or apply home oxygen. Despite these potential benefits, there is uncertainty whether using wearables can result in an effective intervention to prevent SUDEP.[19,54] Wearables may be used to optimize medical management in response to more accurate seizure burden, which may also help prevent SUDEP or other seizure-related mortality.

The International League Against Epilepsy and The International Federation of Clinical Neurophysiology Working Group recently published clinical practice guidelines on the use of wearables for seizure detection for PWE in ambulatory settings.[19] These guidelines recommend clinically validated wearables for the detection of GTCS in the presence of significant safety concerns, especially in unsupervised patients where alarms can trigger a rapid intervention (within 5 minutes). Currently, there is limited evidence supporting the clinical applications of wearables and decreasing seizure-related mortality and injury in PWE. Therefore, these recommendations currently remain weak and conditional.

MOBILE HEALTH APPLICATIONS IN EPILEPSY

Although a variety of approaches have been used to promote epilepsy self-management for decades,[56,57] recent advancements in the field of mHealth have made it possible to improve these approaches by providing a single means for collecting health care data, delivering medical information, and making health care available to more patients.[5,6,58,59] The patient education and epilepsy self-management enabled by mHealth may improve epilepsy-related health outcomes. Examples of this are apps that track symptoms, maintain seizure history, educate patients, and help change behaviors, including using reminders to take medications, exercise sleep hygiene, and self-manage stress, all of which can help improve seizure control and quality of life.[6] Compared with earlier techniques, the advantage of using mHealth for epilepsy self-management and patient education is improved accessibility, decreased burden on health care providers, and lower cost.[5] The health data collected by apps bears the potential to personalize epilepsy care based on observed patterns in seizures and potential triggers. Some of these apps have been used in clinical trials for the collection of self-reported data.[60]

There are many epilepsy-related apps available on different mobile platforms; however, recent systematic reviews[6,61,62] each reported on a subset of these (20–22 apps), focusing on patient education and self-management. Although not all studies have the same inclusion criteria for which apps to include, there is at least a 50% overlap between the lists of apps reported on by each study. The studies assessed whether apps covered any of the self-management domains: health-care communication, treatment management, social support, medication adherence, seizure response, wellness, stress management, safety, coping, seizure tracking, proactivity, and the transition of care from childhood and adolescence to adulthood. Some studies also rated apps on the Mobile App Rating Scale (MARS) and reported whether they offer behavioral change techniques.[6,62] Most apps focus on patient education, treatment management, and how to track seizures, whereas few apps focus on pro-activity, meaningful communication with health-care providers, wellness, transition of care, or stress management, and no apps provide comprehensive coverage of all self-management domains. The most common features offered by apps to change behaviors include prompts for to self-monitor behavior, plans for social support, education on using prompts or cues, information about the behavior-health link and its consequences, and time management assistance.[6] Overall, the studied apps scored highest on MARS for functionality and esthetics, with lower scores on the engagement of users and information provision.[6,62]

Despite a proliferation of apps, there are limited data validating clinical application, their effectiveness on outcomes and quality of life, and user acceptability and engagement.[6] There is a need for apps with comprehensive coverage of different self-management domains. Mobile apps are overall underutilized by PWE with the number of installations ranging ~10 to ~10,000 per app.[61] Among epilepsy apps focused on self-management, the ones with the most installations on both the App Store and Google Play include Epilepsy Tool Kit, Young Epilepsy, Seizure Log, and My Seizure Diary.[61] Most epilepsy centers do not use or support epilepsy-related apps. The main barriers include the lack of cultural acceptability, lack of infrastructure to prescribe apps, concerns regarding patient data privacy and liability, and a lack of strong evidence supporting the role of these apps in clinical practice.[5]

LIMITATIONS AND CHALLENGES

The rapidly evolving field of wearables and mHealth poses several challenges for the development of clinical applications. One limitation regarding mHealth apps is the large number of competing apps, each with its own set of user data. This is relevant because a large data set is crucial for the development of reliable ML models, and it is more difficult to aggregate and analyze data from a disparate set of apps. Many apps are new and require further evaluation. The question of whether digital or paper-based diaries are more suitable depends on patient preferences. Regardless of the type of diary, the information entered must be of high quality, making patient adherence a key point. Lack of awareness likely contributes to a high number of missed seizures.[7] Wearables linked with apps provide a possible solution for overcoming these limitations.

Wearables also have limitations compared with existing monitoring devices. They are very sensitive to motion artifacts, especially those obtaining extracerebral biosignals at the body periphery. Battery life, data storage, and processing capacities are also limited. These limitations force compromises for which signals are recorded and to what fidelity. Recording and storing personal data also comes with liability challenges. For any technology that stores data digitally and, if necessary, analyzes it together with data from other users, data security and protection remain an important and difficult challenge.

Besides technological difficulties, studies evaluating the usefulness of wearables and mHealth apps are insufficient. Among these studies, a common set of challenges can be observed.[8,11,20,35,38,63,64] First, the selection of patients is biased. Often the accessible patient groups are themselves very selective, with participation mainly from tech-savvy patients and caregivers. Currently, it is challenging to enroll patients who can easily operate the wearable and are willing to use it over a long period of time; however, such use is necessary to generate data sets large enough for ML applications. Annotations are also a major challenge. Because diaries can be inaccurate, and only a highly selective set of patients carry an implanted EEG, the gold standard for ambulatory data collection is not yet settled.

Although devices using ACC and surface EMG data have a high sensitivity for detecting GTCS, achieving an acceptable balance between sensitivity and FAR in ambulatory settings remains challenging. In addition to high FAR, the uncomfortable fit or undesirable appearance of devices (which may include wires and electrodes), and difficulty using the technology can prevent PWE from consistent use.[65]

FUTURE DIRECTIONS

Designing a seizure monitoring system based on mobile seizure tracking apps and wearables is a collaborative, interdisciplinary effort. Many position articles propose pathways for achieving this goal.[66–69] The interest and acceptance of patients and caregivers as well as the interest of the data science community is a prerequisite for a successful development. On a research level, seizure-related mechanisms are not fully understood, especially considering the interindividual variance of clinical seizures, seizure provoking factors, and underlying epilepsy syndromes. One area of ongoing research models the brain as a physical system that can transition from one stable state to another. In this interpretation, a seizure is considered such a brain state, and the preictal phase of the seizure can be considered either as a transitional phase or another brain state in itself. In both cases, the preictal phase would be characterized by measurable changes in brain activity that also affects autonomic function.

Based on these considerations, the question is how to detect these changes– what are the relevant biomarkers to reliably detect preictal phase? A seizure prediction system may also need to consider other factors, such as personal characteristics, vigilance states, and seizure types. Due to rapid, ongoing advances in ML, the development of complex models that include these factors is now in the realm of possibility. Another area of research and development is focused on devices that can continuously and reliably record physiologic signals in outpatient settings, requiring a step from offline to real-time data analysis. These areas of ongoing development are interdependent and inform each other. They differ in their need for medical and technical input, again illustrating the interdisciplinary nature of this study.

Successful long-term monitoring with wearables will not only contribute to our ability to detect, count, predict, and forecast seizures, but will also lead to more personalized epilepsy care. To achieve that goal, we need to know which devices are suitable for which patients and which signals are most informative for which seizure types. We likely need to select individual algorithms that adapt to a patient over time. With more accurate seizure tracking and forecasting, the patient's response to medications can be monitored, which can assist in the adjustment of medications and dosages. Furthermore, this information can facilitate chronotherapy, allowing targeted therapies during periods of high seizure risk.[70] Continuous EEG data could also detect and quantify interictal epileptiform abnormalities, thereby supporting seizure diagnosis and management.

SUMMARY

The use of wearables for real-time seizure monitoring will gain more importance because of the interdisciplinary advancement of theory-based biomarkers, ML algorithms, and sensor technologies. There is already high-quality evidence showing that wearables reliably detect GTCS; however, there are only a few studies focused on feasibility and false alarms in home environments. We await evidence confirming that wearables will improve epilepsy outcomes and quality of life in PWE.

DISCLOSURE

B. Esmaeili and B.A. Dworetzky report no disclosures relevant to the article. S. Vieluf is part of a patent application covering technology for seizure forecasting. C. Reinsberger receives research funds from the German Institute of Sports Sciences for projects using wearables.

REFERENCES

1. Beniczky S, Karoly P, Nurse E, et al. Machine learning and wearable devices of the future. Epilepsia 2021;62(S2):S116–24.
2. Brinkmann BH, Karoly PJ, Nurse ES, et al. Seizure diaries and forecasting with wearables: epilepsy monitoring outside the clinic. Front Neurol 2021; 12:1128.
3. Baud M, Schindler K. Forecasting seizures: not unthinkable anymore. Epileptologie 2018;35:156–61.
4. Bruno E, Viana PF, Sperling MR, et al. Seizure detection at home: do devices on the market match the needs of people living with epilepsy and their caregivers? Epilepsia 2020;61(S1):S11–24.
5. Hixson JD, Braverman L. Digital tools for epilepsy: opportunities and barriers. Epilepsy Res 2020;162:106233.
6. Escoffery C, McGee R, Bidwell J, et al. A review of mobile apps for epilepsy self-management. Epilepsy Behav 2018;81:62–9.
7. Fisher RS, Blum DE, DiVentura B, et al. Seizure diaries for clinical research and practice: limitations and future prospects. Epilepsy Behav 2012;24(3):304–10.
8. Meisel C, El Atrache R, Jackson M, et al. Machine learning from wristband sensor data for wearable, noninvasive seizure forecasting. Epilepsia 2020;61(12): 2653–66.
9. Ulate-Campos A, Coughlin F, Gaínza-Lein M, et al. Automated seizure detection systems and their effectiveness for each type of seizure. Seizure 2016;40:88–101.
10. Regalia G, Onorati F, Lai M, et al. Multimodal wrist-worn devices for seizure detection and advancing research: Focus on the Empatica wristbands. Epilepsy Res 2019;153:79–82.
11. Tang J, El Atrache R, Yu S, et al. Seizure detection using wearable sensors and machine learning: setting a benchmark. Epilepsia 2021;62(8):1807–19.
12. Ryvlin P, Ciumas C, Wisniewski I, et al. Wearable devices for sudden unexpected death in epilepsy prevention. Epilepsia 2018;59:61–6.
13. Nagaraddi V, Lüders HO. Autonomic seizures: localizing and lateralizing value. In: Lüders HO, editor. Textbook of epilepsy surgery. London (UK): Informa Healthcare; 2008. p. 443–9.
14. Ansakorpi H, Korpelainen JT, Suominen K, et al. Interictal cardiovascular autonomic responses in patients with temporal lobe epilepsy. Epilepsia 2000; 41(1):42–7.
15. Esmaeili B, Kaffashi F, Theeranaew W, et al. Post-ictal modulation of baroreflex sensitivity in patients with intractable epilepsy. Front Neurol 2018;9:793.
16. Vieluf S, El Atrache R, Hammond S, et al. Peripheral multimodal monitoring of ANS changes related to epilepsy. Epilepsy Behav 2019;96:69–79.

17. Hubbard I, Beniczky S, Ryvlin P. The challenging path to developing a mobile health device for epilepsy: the current landscape and where we go from here. Front Neurol 2021;12:1737.
18. Ryvlin P, Cammoun L, Hubbard I, et al. Noninvasive detection of focal seizures in ambulatory patients. Epilepsia 2020;61(S1):S47–54.
19. Beniczky S, Wiebe S, Jeppesen J, et al. Automated seizure detection using wearable devices: a clinical practice guideline of the International League Against Epilepsy and the International Federation of Clinical Neurophysiology. Clin Neurophysiol 2021;132(5):1173–84.
20. Onorati F, Regalia G, Caborni C, et al. Multicenter clinical assessment of improved wearable multimodal convulsive seizure detectors. Epilepsia 2017; 58(11):1870–9.
21. Whitmire L, Voyles S, Cardenas D, et al. Diagnostic Utility of Continuous sEMG Monitoring in a Home Setting - Real-world use of the SPEAC® System (P4.5-012). Neurology 2019;92(15 Supplement). P4.5-012.
22. Beniczky S, Ryvlin P. Standards for testing and clinical validation of seizure detection devices. Epilepsia 2018;59(S1):9–13.
23. Caborni C, Migliorini M, Onorati F, et al. Tuning decision thresholds for active/rest periods significantly improves seizure detection algorithm performance: an evaluation using embrace smartwatch on outpatient settings. Epilepsia 2017; 58(Supplement 5):S98–9.
24. Onorati F, Caborni C, Guzman MF, et al. Performance of a wrist worn multimodal seizure detection system for more than a year in real life settings. Epilepsia 2018; 59(S3):S81.
25. Szabó CÁ, Morgan LC, Karkar KM, et al. Electromyography-based seizure detector: Preliminary results comparing a generalized tonic–clonic seizure detection algorithm to video-EEG recordings. Epilepsia 2015;56(9):1432–7.
26. Halford JJ, Sperling MR, Nair DR, et al. Detection of generalized tonic–clonic seizures using surface electromyographic monitoring. Epilepsia 2017;58(11): 1861–9.
27. Beniczky S, Conradsen I, Henning O, et al. Automated real-time detection of tonic-clonic seizures using a wearable EMG device. Neurology 2018;90(5): e428–34.
28. Fisher RS. Bad information in epilepsy care. Epilepsy Behav 2017;67:133–4.
29. Hoppe C, Poepel A, Elger CE. Epilepsy: accuracy of patient seizure counts. Arch Neurol 2007;64(11):1595–9.
30. Blum DE, Eskola J, Bortz JJ, et al. Patient awareness of seizures. Neurology 1996; 47(1):260–4.
31. Thijs RD, Wagenaar WA, Middelkoop HAM, et al. Transient loss of consciousness through the eyes of a witness. Neurology 2008;71(21):1713–8.
32. Blachut B, Hoppe C, Surges R, et al. Subjective seizure counts by epilepsy clinical drug trial participants are not reliable. Epilepsy Behav 2017;67:122–7.
33. Poh Y-Z, Loddenkemper Z, Reinsberger X, et al. Convulsive seizure detection using a wrist-worn electrodermal activity and accelerometry biosensor BRIEF COMMUNICATION e93. Int Leag Against Epilepsy Epilepsia 2012;53(5):93–7.
34. Böttcher S, Bruno E, Manyakov NV, et al. Detecting tonic-clonic seizures in multimodal biosignal data from wearables: methodology design and validation. JMIR mHealth Uhealth 2021;9(11). https://doi.org/10.2196/27674.
35. Cogan D, Birjandtalab J, Nourani M, et al. Multi-biosignal analysis for epileptic seizure monitoring. Int J Neural Syst 2017;27(1). https://doi.org/10.1142/S0129065716500313.

36. Berg AT, Kaiser K, Dixon-Salazar T, et al. Seizure burden in severe early-life epilepsy: perspectives from parents. Epilepsia Open 2019;4(2):293.
37. Baud MO, Kleen JK, Mirro EA, et al. Multi-day rhythms modulate seizure risk in epilepsy. Nat Commun 2018;9(1):88.
38. Yamakawa T, Miyajima M, Fujiwara K, et al. Wearable epileptic seizure prediction system with machine-learning-based anomaly detection of heart rate variability. Sensors (Basel) 2020;20(14):1–16.
39. Stirling RE, Grayden DB, D'Souza W, et al. Forecasting seizure likelihood with wearable technology. Front Neurol 2021;12:1170.
40. Reuber M, Fernandez G, Bauer J, et al. Diagnostic delay in psychogenic nonepileptic seizures. Neurology 2002;58(3):493–5.
41. Beniczky S, Conradsen I, Moldovan M, et al. Automated differentiation between epileptic and nonepileptic convulsive seizures. Ann Neurol 2015;77(2):348–51.
42. Husain AM, Towne AR, Chen DK, et al. Differentiation of epileptic and psychogenic nonepileptic seizures using single-channel surface electromyography. J Clin Neurophysiol 2021;38(5):432–8.
43. Kusmakar S, Karmakar CK, Yan B, et al. Improved detection and classification of convulsive epileptic and psychogenic non-epileptic seizures using FLDA and Bayesian Inference. Annu Int Conf IEEE Eng Med Biol Soc EMBS 2018;2018: 3402–5.
44. Naganur VD, Kusmakar S, Chen Z, et al. The utility of an automated and ambulatory device for detecting and differentiating epileptic and psychogenic nonepileptic seizures. Epilepsia Open 2019;4(2):309.
45. Gu Y, Cleeren E, Dan J, et al. Comparison between Scalp EEG and Behind-the-Ear EEG for development of a wearable seizure detection system for patients with focal epilepsy. Sensors (Basel) 2017;18(1). https://doi.org/10.3390/S18010029.
46. Viana PF, Duun-Henriksen J, Glasstëter M, et al. 230 days of ultra long-term subcutaneous EEG: seizure cycle analysis and comparison to patient diary. Ann Clin Transl Neurol 2021;8(1):288–93.
47. Harden C, Tomson T, Gloss D, et al. Practice guideline summary: Sudden unexpected death in epilepsy incidence rates and risk factors. Neurology 2017; 88(17):1674–80.
48. Lhatoo SD, Faulkner HJ, Dembny K, et al. An electroclinical case-control study of sudden unexpected death in epilepsy. Ann Neurol 2010;68(6):787–96.
49. Ryvlin P, Nashef L, Lhatoo SD, et al. Incidence and mechanisms of cardiorespiratory arrests in epilepsy monitoring units (MORTEMUS): a retrospective study. Lancet Neurol 2013;12(10):966–77.
50. Myers KA, Bello-Espinosa LE, Symonds JD, et al. Heart rate variability in epilepsy: a potential biomarker of sudden unexpected death in epilepsy risk. Epilepsia 2018;59(7):1372–80.
51. Bleakley LE, Soh MS, Bagnall RD, et al. Are variants causing cardiac arrhythmia risk factors in sudden unexpected death in epilepsy? Front Neurol 2020;11:925.
52. Vilella L, Lacuey N, Hampson JP, et al. Association of peri-ictal brainstem posturing with seizure severity and breathing compromise in patients with generalized convulsive seizures. Neurology 2021;96(3):e352–65.
53. Park KJ, Sharma G, Kennedy JD, et al. Potentially high-risk cardiac arrhythmias with focal to bilateral tonic-clonic seizures and generalized tonic-clonic seizures are associated with the duration of periictal hypoxemia full-length original research. Epilepsia 2017;58(12):2164–71.

54. Picard RW, Migliorini M, Caborni C, et al. Wrist sensor reveals sympathetic hyperactivity and hypoventilation before probable SUDEP. Neurology 2017;89(6): 633–5.
55. Van Der Lende M, Hesdorffer DC, Sander JW, et al. Nocturnal supervision and SUDEP risk at different epilepsy care settings. Neurology 2018;91(16):e1508–18.
56. Bradley PM, Lindsay B. Care delivery and self-management strategies for adults with epilepsy. Cochrane Database Syst Rev 2008;1:CD006244.
57. Wagner JL, Modi AC, Johnson EK, et al. Self-management interventions in pediatric epilepsy: what is the level of evidence? Epilepsia 2017;58(5):743–54.
58. Silva BMC, Rodrigues JJPC, de la Torre Díez I, et al. Mobile-health: a review of current state in 2015. J Biomed Inform 2015;56:265–72.
59. Choi SA, Lim K, Baek H, et al. Impact of mobile health application on data collection and self-management of epilepsy. Epilepsy Behav 2021;119:107982.
60. Ernst L de L, Harden CL, Pennell PB, et al. Medication adherence in women with epilepsy who are planning pregnancy. Epilepsia 2016;57(12):2039.
61. Alzamanan MZ, Lim KS, Ismail MA, et al. Self-management apps for people with epilepsy: systematic analysis. JMIR mHealth uHealth 2021;9(5). https://doi.org/ 10.2196/22489.
62. Mohammadzadeh N, Khenarinezhad S, Gha-Zanfarisavadkoohi E, et al. Evaluation of M-Health applications use in epilepsy: a systematic review. Iran J Public Health 2021;50(3):459.
63. Nasseri M, Nurse E, Glasstetter M, et al. Signal quality and patient experience with wearable devices for epilepsy management. Epilepsia 2020;61(S1):S25–35.
64. Vieluf S, Hasija T, Schreier PJ, et al. Generalized tonic-clonic seizures are accompanied by changes of interrelations within the autonomic nervous system. Epilepsy Behav 2021;124:108321.
65. Simblett SK, Biondi A, Bruno E, et al. Patients' experience of wearing multimodal sensor devices intended to detect epileptic seizures: a qualitative analysis. Epilepsy Behav 2020;102. https://doi.org/10.1016/J.YEBEH.2019.106717.
66. Kuhlmann L, Lehnertz K, Richardson MP, et al. Seizure prediction — ready for a new era. Nat Rev Neurol 2018;14(10):618–30.
67. Teijeiro AE, Shokrekhodaei M, Nazeran H. The conceptual design of a novel workstation for seizure prediction using machine learning with potential ehealth applications. IEEE J Transl Eng Heal Med 2019;7. https://doi.org/10.1109/JTEHM. 2019.2910063.
68. Meisel C, Loddenkemper T. Seizure prediction and intervention. Neuropharmacology 2020;172:107898.
69. Freestone DR, Karoly PJ, Cook MJ. A forward-looking review of seizure prediction. Curr Opin Neurol 2017;30(2):167–73.
70. Khan S, Nobili L, Khatami R, et al. Circadian rhythm and epilepsy. Lancet Neurol 2018;17(12):1098–108.

Update on Sudden Unexpected Death in Epilepsy

Marius Kløvgaard, MD, PhD[a,b,*], Anne Sabers, MD, DMSc[b], Philippe Ryvlin, MD, PhD[c]

KEYWORDS

- Epilepsy • Mortality • Seizure • Sudden unexpected death in epilepsy • SUDEP

KEY POINTS

- Sudden unexpected death in epilepsy (SUDEP) is one of the most frequent causes of death in persons with epilepsy (PWE).
- The incidence of SUDEP is rather consistent at 1.2 to 1.3 per 1000 person-year in the general epilepsy population but increases with the severity of epilepsy.
- Focal-to-bilateral or generalized tonic-clonic seizures are together with sleeping alone the most significant risk factors for SUDEP.
- Preventive strategies for SUDEP are needed, but optimal care might decrease the risk.

INTRODUCTION

Persons with epilepsy (PWE) have a high risk of premature death with a two to fourfold increased standardized mortality ratios (SMR) compared with the background population.[1] SMR are highest in children with epilepsy, whose mortality rate is increased up to 36-fold,[2–4] and in adults younger than 50 years, whereby SMR are reported to be up to 10-fold higher compared with the general population.[4,5] This increased mortality in PWE seems stable over time,[1] and was even found to progress in the United States during 1999 to 2017 period.[6] Part of this trend might reflect an increased incidence of epilepsy due to dementia, brain tumors, and stroke.[6]

Indeed, many different causes of death contribute to the increased mortality in PWE, including lethal accidents, status epilepticus, suicide, pneumonia, cardiovascular diseases, neoplasms, and sudden unexpected death in epilepsy (SUDEP).[1,4–9] Overall, more than 60% of all deaths can be classified as epilepsy-related when including those triggered by seizures, such as seizure-related accidents, SUDEP and aspiration pneumonia, and those related to the underlying cause of epilepsy, such as brain tumors.[3,7,10,11]

[a] Department of Neurology, Herlev Hospital, Borgmester Ib Juuls Vej 1, Herlev 2730, Copenhagen, Denmark; [b] Department of Neurology, The Epilepsy Clinic, Copenhagen University Hospital / Rigshospitalet, Blegdamsvej 9, Copenhagen 2100, Denmark; [c] Service de Neurologie, Département des Neurosciences Cliniques, Centre Hospitalier Universitaire Vaudois (CHUV), Rue du Bugnon 46, Lausanne CH-1011, Switzerland
* Corresponding author. Department of Neurology, The Epilepsy Clinic, Copenhagen University Hospital / Rigshospitalet, Blegdamsvej 9, Copenhagen 2100.
E-mail address: marius.kloevgaard.soerensen@regionh.dk

Neurol Clin 40 (2022) 741–754
https://doi.org/10.1016/j.ncl.2022.06.001
neurologic.theclinics.com
0733-8619/22/© 2022 Elsevier Inc. All rights reserved.

In PWE younger than 50 years, SUDEP is the second most frequent cause of death next to cancer, comprising nearly one out of five deaths.[4] SUDEP also accounts for 80% of all seizure-related deaths, thus potentially preventable by optimal seizure control.[10,12] The aim of this narrative review is to provide an update on SUDEP.

DEFINITION AND CLASSIFICATION OF SUDDEN UNEXPECTED DEATH IN EPILEPSY

SUDEP, which has been described for more than hundred years,[13] includes all cases of death whereby no known cause can be identified by postmortem examination.[14] Cases of SUDEP has been classified according to the Annegers definition or the unified definition by Nashef and colleagues.[14] The Annegers definition includes the following criteria: The person with epilepsy should die suddenly and unexpectedly while in a reasonable state of health and during normal activities and under benign circumstances, and no obvious cause of death should be found.[14] SUDEP can be further classified as *definite*, when all criteria, including a postmortem examination, are met, *probable* when all criteria, except a postmortem examination, are fulfilled, and *possible* when SUDEP cannot be ruled out, but there is insufficient evidence regarding the circumstances of the death.[14] The possible SUDEP category includes both cases with competing causes of death and cases with insufficient information regarding the circumstances of death. Studies of SUDEP have tried to distinguish these cases by subdividing possible SUDEP cases into cases with the lack of information and cases with competing causes of death.[15]

According to the unified definition of SUDEP by Nashef and colleagues, the following criteria should be fulfilled: The death should be sudden, unexpected, witnessed or unwitnessed, nontraumatic, and nondrowning, and with or without a seizure. Status epilepticus should be excluded, and a postmortem examination should not reveal any cause of death.[14] SUDEP can be further categorized as *definite*, when all criteria are fulfilled, *definite SUDEP plus*, if a concomitant condition other than epilepsy is identified and if the death may have been due to the combined effect of both conditions, *probable*, when the criteria for SUDEP, except for the postmortem examination, are met, *possible*, when a competing cause of death is present, *near-SUDEP/ near-SUDEP plus*, when a patient with epilepsy survives resuscitation for more than 1 hour after a cardiorespiratory arrest that has no structural cause identified after investigation, and *unclassified*, in cases with incomplete information.[14] The rationale for introducing the near-SUDEP category was that these cases might share some of the same features as SUDEP cases and could thus be included in studies evaluating SUDEP. However, when studying the incidence of SUDEP, this category must be modified to include only fatal near-SUDEP cases, defined as cases that are resuscitated but suffered brain death and died afterward in intensive care.[4]

Despite unifying the SUDEP criteria, the identification and classification of SUDEP cases can still be difficult.

A further update by Devinsky and colleagues[16] was proposed in 2018, especially to help distinguishing definite SUDEP plus cases from possible SUDEP cases and near-SUDEP cases from SUDEP. The definition of definite SUDEP is in accordance with the unified SUDEP criteria. However, for clarification cases with concomitant conditions are called either *definite SUDEP plus comorbidity* or *probable SUDEP plus comorbidity* stressing that the concomitant condition should be a potentially synergistic cause of death, but not a competing or independent cause of death. Furthermore, the near-SUDEP category was renamed *resuscitated SUDEP* to distinguish these from fatal cases, and the near-SUDEP plus category was omitted.

SUDEP has been added as a cause of death in the 11th edition of the International Classification of Diseases (ICD) for mortality and morbidity statistics (ICD-11/MH15).

In this ICD-version, SUDEP is defined as sudden death in a person with epilepsy that occurs under benign circumstances and in the absence of a known structural cause of death, thereby ruling out drowning, fatal injuries, intoxication, or other internal or external factors.[17] Furthermore, the death could be preceded by a seizure but do not have to. Cases of SUDEP are further subcategorized as *definite* if a postmortem examination does not reveal an alternative cause of death, *probable*, if postmortem examinations are lacking but potentially lethal alternative causes are excluded and all other criteria are met, *possible* in cases with competing causes of death or when data are insufficient to reasonably allow their classification. The term *SUDEP plus* is used for cases whereby another comorbidity might have contributed to the death, but not truly caused it. Finally, *near-SUDEP* is used for cases whereby cardiopulmonary resuscitation prevented a SUDEP. This definition mixes the Annegers and the unified definition of SUDEP[14] by using *possible SUDEP* for cases with competing causes and insufficient data together with the categories *SUDEP plus* and *near-SUDEP*. Finally, the unclassified category has been omitted.

INCIDENCE OF SUDDEN UNEXPECTED DEATH IN EPILEPSY

Until the recent introduction of SUDEP in the ICD-11 classification, no specific ICD-codes were available to classify this type of sudden death.[1,17] Its identification of SUDEP is thus difficult in register-based studies and requires access to additional information, including death certificates, medical files, and autopsy reports including toxicology examinations. Furthermore, the identification of SUDEP depends on the autopsy rate, the quality of the information regarding the circumstances at death, and the way the SUDEP criteria are applied. For instance, distinguishing cases of definite SUDEP plus from possible SUDEP can be difficult, and therefore, interindividual differences in SUDEP adjudication are observed.[16,18,19] Likewise, the incidence of SUDEP is likely underestimated in national registers.[16]

Consequently, the incidence of SUDEP varies between study populations and study settings. The incidence of SUDEP has been reported to be higher in institutional or hospital-based studies than in register-based population-based studies whereby it usually accounts for a minority of deaths due to the lack of ICD-codes for SUDEP.[1]

Only a limited number of nationwide population-based studies of SUDEP is available (**Table 1**). In a review from 2011 including 2 population-based studies, the incidence of SUDEP was reported as 0.9 to 2.3 per 1000 person-years in the general epilepsy population, 1.1 to 5.9 per 1000 person-years in patients with chronic refractory epilepsy, and 6.3 to 9.3 per 1000 person-years in candidates for epileptic surgery.[20,21] In a later review of 3 studies from 2014, the incidence of SUDEP was estimated at 1.2 per 1000 person-years when a prevalence of epilepsy of 0.7% was used, making SUDEP the second leading neurologic cause of potential years of life lost after stroke.[22,23] In the 2017 American Academy of Neurology SUDEP guidelines, based on 12 studies, the incidence of SUDEP was estimated at 0.22 per 1000 person-years in children and at 1.2 per 1000 person-years in adults.[24] Thereby, the 1-year risk of SUDEP was estimated to 1 out of 4500 children and 1 out of 1000 adults.

Recent nationwide studies of SUDEP from Sweden and Iceland have reported the incidence of SUDEP at 1.2 to 1.3 per 1000 person-years in the general epilepsy population when including all ages.[25,26] The Swedish study reported a nonsignificantly lower incidence of SUDEP at 1.1 per 1000 persons-years in persons aged 16 to 50 years,[25] while the study from Iceland reported a nonsignificantly higher incidence of SUDEP at 1.7 per 1000 persons-years in persons aged 15 to 34 years and at 2.2 per 1000 persons-years in persons aged 35 to 54 years.[26] A recent nationwide study

Table 1
Population-based and nationwide studies of the incidence of SUDEP

Study (Country)	Study Setting	Year	Included Age Groups	Number of Definite, Definite Plus, and Probable SUDEP Cases	Person-Years	Crude SUDEP Incidence (95% CI) per 1000 Person-Years
Ficker et al.[21] (USA)	Population-based	1998	All ages	9	25,940	0.35
Langan et al.[23] (Ireland)	Population-based	1998	All ages	15	10,200	1.47
Holst et al.[15] (Denmark)	Nationwide	2013	1–35 y	50	120,096	0.42
Sveinsson et al.[25] (Sweden)	Nationwide	2017	All ages	68	56,799	1.20
Keller et al.[28] (Canada)	Population-based	2018	0–17 y	16	14,545	1.11
Einarsdottir et al.[26] (Iceland)	Nationwide	2019	All ages	37	27,205	1.36
Kløvgaard et al.[4] (Denmark)	Nationwide	2021	1–49 y	81	81,648	0.99

Abbreviations: CI, confidence interval; SUDEP, sudden unexpected death in epilepsy.

of SUDEP in Denmark reported the incidence of SUDEP in persons aged 18 to 49 years at 1.2 per 1000 person-years in the general epilepsy population.[4]

Overall, the incidence of SUDEP in adults with epilepsy does not seem to differ significantly between studies from different countries. In contrast, that in children has been less consistent as detailed later in discussion. Older studies reported a lower incidence of SUDEP in children than in adults,[15,24] a finding confirmed by recent studies from Iceland, the United States, and Denmark.[4,26,27] In Iceland the incidence of SUDEP in children aged 0 to 14 years was reported at 0.2 per 1000 person-years,[26] while it was reported at 0.3 per 1000 person-years in children aged 1 to 17 years in Denmark.[4] These estimates were in accordance with the American Academy of Neurology 2017 guidelines, whereby the incidence of SUDEP in children younger than 18 years was estimated at 0.2 per 1000 person-years.[24] However, the nationwide study of SUDEP from Sweden, using the Annegers SUDEP definition, reported a general incidence of definite and probable SUDEP of 1.1 per 1000 person-years in both children younger than 16 years and in adults aged 16 to 50 years.[25] Another study from Canada also reported a higher than expected incidence of SUDEP of 1.2 per 1000 person-years in children less than 18 years, when using the unified SUDEP definition, and a prevalence of epilepsy of 0.3%.[28]

The higher than expected incidences of SUDEP in children reported in both Sweden and Canada raised concern and have been explained by the shift from older to newer SUDEP definitions.[29] However, the recent studies from Iceland, the United States, and Denmark used that unified SUDEP definition,[4,26,27] while the study from Sweden used the Annegers SUDEP definition.[25] Furthermore, the study of SUDEP in Denmark reported identical incidences when using the Annegers or the unified SUDEP definition.[4] Thus, the reason for the observed variation in the SUDEP incidence in children remains unclear. Differences in the autopsy rates in children might explain some of the differing SUDEP incidences in children between different countries.[4] Another explanation could be a difference in the criteria used to ascertain epilepsy.[4] In register-based studies, prevalent epilepsy can be defined in different ways, including contacts to the health care sector due to epilepsy as well as the prescription of antiseizure medication (ASM).[30] Therefore, reporting both subgroups of SUDEP and the total number of SUDEP together with the autopsy rate, the prevalence of epilepsy, the included PWE, and other causes of death might be important for the interpretation of the estimates.

When considering all autopsy-verified sudden and unexplained deaths in the general Danish population aged 1 to 49 years, it was found that 23% of these deaths have occurred in PWEs, even though PWEs only account for 0.8% of the Danish population.[4] Adjusted for age and sex, PWE had a 34-fold increased risk of sudden and unexplained death compared with persons without epilepsy,[4] a figure higher than previous estimates.[20,21]

Of interest, recent studies have suggested that the incidence of SUDEP decreased with the duration of follow-up, a finding which remains to be explained.[31,32]

UNDERLYING MECHANISMS

A number of studies have investigated the impact of seizures on cardiac and respiratory functions with the hope to understand the mechanisms leading to SUDEP, and suggested the role of hypoventilation, central or obstructive apnea, cardiac dysrhythmia, and so-called cerebral electrical shutdown.[20,33–46] Yet, observed cases of SUDEP are sparse. In the largest multicenter study of patients who died of a SUDEP while being recorded in an epilepsy monitoring unit (EMU), 9 patients were collated with video, electrocardiogram (ECG), and electroencephalogram (EEG) recordings. All patients suffered a focal-to-bilateral tonic-clonic seizure with immediate postictal tachypnea, tachycardia, and generalized EEG suppression, followed within 3 minutes by apnea, then bradycardia and terminal asystole.[47] In all 9 cases, terminal apnea was observed before terminal asystole, while 8 of the 9 patients were in the prone position, head in pillow, which is likely to have contributed to respiratory failure. The ECGs showed sinus arrest with no escape rhythm, and the parallel worsening of cardiac and respiratory function suggested a central dysfunction of brainstem centers controlling respiration and heart rhythm.[47] Epilepsy-triggered chronic cardiac dysfunction might also contribute to the mechanisms of SUDEP.[48] Accordingly, a case-control study showed that SUDEP cases had an abnormal cardiac response to sympathetic stimulation.[49] Furthermore, SUDEP autopsy findings have reported some level of pulmonary edema and subendocardial fibrosis.[48] Yet, a recent study of SUDEP in the United States failed to show differences in these pathologic findings between SUDEP and non-SUDEP deaths in PWE.[50]

Previously, ictal asystole was seen as a possible explanation for SUDEP. However, several studies have indicated that ictal asystole is not associated with these sudden and unexpected deaths. Ictal asystole is usually self-limiting due to the associated cerebral hypoperfusion, resulting in shorter seizure duration without focal-to-bilateral tonic-clonic seizure.[51–54] Furthermore, a few SUDEP cases have been reported in persons with cardiac pacemakers implanted to prevent ictal asystole, suggesting that such prevention does not necessarily protect against SUDEP.[55,56]

Other links between seizures and cardiac arrhythmias have been proposed, including so-called cardio-cerebral channelopathies. Studies have found that genetic variants associated with cardiac arrhythmia are also expressed in the brain and thereby might cause both epileptic seizures and cardiac arrhythmias resulting in a dual cerebral and cardiac phenotype.[48,57–59] Accordingly, SUDEP cases might share genetic variants associated with sudden cardiac death and dysfunction of respiratory control.[60–63] This was reported for long QT syndrome (LQTS), a disorder characterized by ventricular arrhythmias that might lead to syncope or sudden cardiac death,[64] whereby genetic variants causing LQTS might also cause epilepsy.[57] Yet, no case of torsade de pointes was observed in monitored SUDEP cases.[47,48]

Other genetic variants might be responsible for SUDEP, in particular those responsible for epileptic encephalopathies such as Dravet syndrome,[65–68] whereby SUDEP incidence has been reported as high as 9.3 per 1000 person-years.[20,67] Furthermore, patients with Dravet syndrome have a more frequent pattern of peri-ictal respiratory abnormalities such as airway obstruction and paradoxic breathing compared with persons with focal epilepsy.[69] Yet, as the mutations in the voltage-gated sodium channel gene SCN1A responsible for Dravet syndrome also leads to severe seizure burden, it remains difficult to disentangle the direct role of the mutation from that of refractory seizures in promoting SUDEP.[70–72] Mice models with mutations in the SCN1A gene might help to clarify this issue.[70,73]

Prolonged postictal generalized EEG suppression (PGES) was found to be associated with an increased risk of SUDEP,[74] respiratory dysfunction, arousal impairment, and autonomic dysregulation.[75–78] Yet, its association with SUDEP has been debated.[79] PGES and SUDEP are also observed in mice models with mutations in potassium or sodium channels.[80,81] In these models, PGES was associated with a wave of depolarization, spreading from the cortex to the brainstem whereby it suppressed networks controlling cardiac rhythm and respiration.[81–84] Apnea during the tonic phase of the seizure was also associated with the occurrence of SUDEP.[85]

Although SUDEP most typically occurs postictally, cases with no preceding seizures have been reported in 3 patients undergoing video-EEG monitoring at the time of death.[86] Interestingly, in 2 of the cases, the pattern of cardiorespiratory failure was similar to that observed in monitored SUDEP cases preceded by a seizure.[47,86]

RISK FACTORS AND PREDICTORS OF SUDDEN UNEXPECTED DEATH IN EPILEPSY

The main risk factor for SUDEP is the presence and frequency of focal-to-bilateral or generalized tonic-clonic seizures (GTCS),[87–91] regardless of whether or not the SUDEP was known to be preceded by a seizure.[47,86] The occurrence of GTCS in the last year was associated with an increased risk of SUDEP of up to 27-fold.[87–90] Nocturnal seizures have also been associated with an increased risk of SUDEP,[92,93] though a recent Swedish case-control study showed that this only applied to GTCS.[87] Another major risk factor for SUDEP is the fact of sleeping or living alone, which increases the risk of SUDEP by up to fivefold.[87,90,92,93] Combining the presence of GTCS within the last year and sleeping alone was associated with an odds ratio (OR) for SUDEP of 67.[87]

In general, the risk of SUDEP increases with the severity of epilepsy, being higher in persons with refractory epilepsies compared with those with well-controlled seizures.[33] Yet, SUDEP might occur after a few seizures and in types of epilepsy otherwise considered benign.[94–96]

Young age at onset of epilepsy (<16 years), longer duration of epilepsy (>15 years), and male gender have been reported as potential SUDEP risk factors, though with small odds ratio.[22,48,88,97] Higher SUDEP rate has also been reported in persons aged 20 to 40 years, as compared with other age groups,[22] suggesting age as a risk factor for SUDEP. Sleeping in the prone position might also increase the risk of SUDEP.[98]

Polytherapy with ASM as well as lamotrigine use were reported as risk factors for SUDEP,[88,99] but these findings could not be reproduced, in particular when controlling for the presence and number of GTCS.[89] Furthermore, a recent case-control study from Sweden found that polytherapy with ASM was associated with a significantly decreased risk of SUDEP when compared with no treatment (OR of 0.3), and a numerically lower SUDEP rate when compared with monotherapy after adjustment on GTCS frequency. This study also failed to show an association between specific ASM, including lamotrigine, and the risk of SUDEP.[100]

Based on the above risk factors, predictive models of the risk of SUDEP have been recently developed, showing a more accurate risk prediction when including 22 clinical predictor variables (area under the receiver operating curve [AUC] of 0.71) compared with a model based solely on the frequency of GTCS (AUC of 0.63).[97]

CLINICAL PRACTICE AND PREVENTION OF SUDDEN UNEXPECTED DEATH IN EPILEPSY

Preventive strategies for SUDEP are badly needed.

First of all, optimal seizure control with antiseizure treatment is paramount. Importantly, no ASM has been consistently associated with an increased risk of SUDEP,[100] despite previous reports suggesting the potential aggravating role of sodium channel blockers, and in particular lamotrigine in women. Furthermore, studies have reported that adjunctive treatment with ASMs in persons with uncontrolled epilepsy may in fact decrease the risk of SUDEP.[100,101] A recent study found that treatment with fenfluramine was associated with a lower SUDEP incidence in persons with Dravet syndrome, though further studies are needed to elucidate this finding.[102] Some data suggest that vagus nerve stimulation might reduce the risk of SUDEP,[32,87] while evidence are lacking regarding the preventive impact of other neuromodulation therapies and epilepsy surgery.[87,103,104]

A considerable risk for worsened seizure control is lack of treatment adherence which emphasizes the importance of informing routinely about the risk of SUDEP. PWE, relatives, and caregivers actually seek information about premature death[105,106] but surveys demonstrate that most of the clinicians do not discuss this issue on a regular basis.[107–109] Yet, information on SUDEP should not result in increased anxiety in PWE and their caregivers, but rather be presented in a way that emphasizes the importance of treatment adherence to prevent SUDEP.[110–112] It has been proposed to primarily discuss SUDEP with persons at high risk, such as those with uncontrolled GTCS,[113,114] though persons at low risk of SUDEP also wish to be informed.

Sleeping under observation might also reduce the risk of SUDEP, though this conclusion remained based on low-level evidence.[90,93,115,116] The development of wearable seizure detection devices might improve the feasibility of nocturnal surveillance, but also requires gathering high-level evidence before concluding on their usefulness to prevent SUDEP.[117] Such devices might be especially useful in PWE with intellectual disabilities with nocturnal GTCS who are sleeping unsupervised at nursery homes.[118]

SUMMARY

Recent population-based studies provide consistent figures of SUDEP incidence in the general epilepsy population at 1.2 to 1.3 per 1000 person-year, while SUDEP rate in children varies between series. Focal-to-bilateral or generalized tonic-clonic seizures, together with sleeping alone, represent the most significant risk factors for SUDEP. Optimal care and nocturnal surveillance are important modifiable risk factors to reduce the risk of SUDEP, though further preventive strategies are needed. Regular communication of seizure risk and SUDEP might increase adherence to the treatment and thereby good seizure control.

CLINICS CARE POINTS

- Persons with epilepsy (PWE) and their caregivers want information about sudden unexpected death in epilepsy (SUDEP).
- The risk of SUDEP increases with the severity of epilepsy but might occur after a few seizures and in all types of epilepsy.
- In children and younger adults, SUDEP is the second most frequent cause of death.

DISCLOSURES

The authors have nothing to disclose.

REFERENCES

1. Watila MM, Balarabe SA, Ojo O, et al. Overall and cause-specific premature mortality in epilepsy: a systematic review. Epilepsy Behav 2018;87:213–25.
2. Christensen J, Pedersen CB, Sidenius P, et al. Long-term mortality in children and young adults with epilepsy–A population-based cohort study. Epilepsy Res 2015;114:81–8.
3. Mbizvo GK, Bennett K, Simpson CR, et al. Epilepsy-related and other causes of mortality in people with epilepsy: A systematic review of systematic reviews. Epilepsy Res 2019;157:106192.
4. Kløvgaard M, Lynge TH, Tsiropoulos I, et al. Sudden unexpected death in epilepsy in persons younger than 50 years: A retrospective nationwide cohort study in Denmark. Epilepsia 2021;62(10):2405–15.
5. Thurman DJ, Logroscino G, Beghi E, et al. The burden of premature mortality of epilepsy in high-income countries: A systematic review from the Mortality Task Force of the International League Against Epilepsy. Epilepsia 2017;58(1):17–26.
6. DeGiorgio CM, Curtis A, Carapetian A, et al. Why are epilepsy mortality rates rising in the United States? A population-based multiple cause-of-death study. BMJ Open 2020;10(8):e035767.
7. Devinsky O, Spruill T, Thurman D, et al. Recognizing and preventing epilepsy-related mortality: a call for action. Neurology 2016;86(8):779–86.
8. Neligan A, Bell GS, Johnson AL, et al. The long-term risk of premature mortality in people with epilepsy. Brain 2011;134(Pt 2):388–95.
9. Fazel S, Wolf A, Långström N, et al. Premature mortality in epilepsy and the role of psychiatric comorbidity: a total population study. Lancet 2013;382(9905):1646–54.
10. Kløvgaard M, Lynge TH, Tsiropoulos I, et al. Epilepsy-related mortality in children and young adults in denmark: a nationwide cohort study. Neurology 2022;98(3):e213–24.
11. Karlovich E, Devinsky O, Brandsoy M, et al. SUDEP among young adults in the San Diego County Medical Examiner Office. Epilepsia 2020;61(3):e17–22.
12. Kløvgaard M, Lynge TH, Tsiropoulos I, et al. Comparing Seizure-Related Death and Suicide in Younger Adults with Epilepsy. Ann Neurol 2021;90(6):983–7.
13. Munson JF. Deaths in epilepsy. Med Rec 2010;77:58–62.
14. Nashef L, So EL, Ryvlin P, et al. Unifying the definitions of sudden unexpected death in epilepsy. Epilepsia 2012;53(2):227–33.

15. Holst AG, Winkel BG, Risgaard B, et al. Epilepsy and risk of death and sudden unexpected death in the young: a nationwide study. Epilepsia 2013;54(9): 1613–20.
16. Devinsky O, Bundock E, Hesdorffer D, et al. Resolving ambiguities in SUDEP classification. Epilepsia 2018;59(6):1220–33.
17. Organization WH. ICD-11 for Mortality and Morbidity Statistics 2022. 2022. Available at: https://icd.who.int/browse11/l-m/en#/http%3a%2f%2fid.who.int%2ficd%2fentity%2f1370023741. Accessed June 22, 2022.
18. Verducci C, Friedman D, Donner EJ, et al. SUDEP classification: discordances between forensic investigators and epileptologists. Epilepsia 2020;61(11): e173–8.
19. Keller AE, Ho J, Whitney R, et al. Autopsy-reported cause of death in a population-based cohort of sudden unexpected death in epilepsy. Epilepsia 2021;62(2):472–80.
20. Shorvon S, Tomson T. Sudden unexpected death in epilepsy. Lancet 2011; 378(9808):2028–38.
21. Ficker DM, So EL, Shen WK, et al. Population-based study of the incidence of sudden unexplained death in epilepsy. Neurology 1998;51(5):1270–4.
22. Thurman DJ, Hesdorffer DC, French JA. Sudden unexpected death in epilepsy: assessing the public health burden. Epilepsia 2014;55(10):1479–85.
23. Langan Y, Nolan N, Hutchinson M. The incidence of sudden unexpected death in epilepsy (SUDEP) in South Dublin and Wicklow. Seizure 1998;7(5):355–8.
24. Harden C, Tomson T, Gloss D, et al. Practice guideline summary: sudden unexpected death in epilepsy incidence rates and risk factors: report of the guideline development, dissemination, and implementation subcommittee of the american academy of neurology and the american epilepsy society. Neurology 2017;88(17):1674–80.
25. Sveinsson O, Andersson T, Carlsson S, et al. The incidence of SUDEP: a nationwide population-based cohort study. Neurology 2017;89(2):170–7.
26. Einarsdottir AB, Sveinsson O, Olafsson E. Sudden unexpected death in epilepsy. A nationwide population-based study. Epilepsia 2019;60(11):2174–81.
27. Cihan E, Devinsky O, Hesdorffer DC, et al. Temporal trends and autopsy findings of SUDEP based on medico-legal investigations in the United States. Neurology 2020;95(7):e867–77.
28. Keller AE, Whitney R, Li SA, et al. Incidence of sudden unexpected death in epilepsy in children is similar to adults. Neurology 2018;91(2):e107–11.
29. Harowitz J, Crandall L, McGuone D, et al. Seizure-related deaths in children: The expanding spectrum. Epilepsia 2021;62(3):570–82.
30. Thurman DJ, Beghi E, Begley CE, et al. Standards for epidemiologic studies and surveillance of epilepsy. Epilepsia 2011;52(Suppl 7):2–26.
31. Tomson T, Sveinsson O, Carlsson S, et al. Evolution over time of SUDEP incidence: A nationwide population-based cohort study. Epilepsia 2018;59(8): e120–4.
32. Ryvlin P, So EL, Gordon CM, et al. Long-term surveillance of SUDEP in drug-resistant epilepsy patients treated with VNS therapy. Epilepsia 2018;59(3): 562–72.
33. Tomson T, Nashef L, Ryvlin P. Sudden unexpected death in epilepsy: current knowledge and future directions. Lancet Neurol 2008;7(11):1021–31.
34. Serdyuk S, Davtyan K, Burd S, et al. Cardiac arrhythmias and sudden unexpected death in epilepsy: Results of long-term monitoring. Heart Rhythm 2021;18(2):221–8.

35. Liu J, Peedicail JS, Gaxiola-Valdez I, et al. Postictal brainstem hypoperfusion and risk factors for sudden unexpected death in epilepsy. Neurology 2020; 95(12):e1694–705.
36. Christiansen SN, Jacobsen SB, Andersen JD, et al. Differential Methylation in the GSTT1 Regulatory Region in Sudden Unexplained Death and Sudden Unexpected Death in Epilepsy. Int J Mol Sci 2021;22(6):2790.
37. Patodia S, Tachrount M, Somani A, et al. MRI and pathology correlations in the medulla in sudden unexpected death in epilepsy (SUDEP): a postmortem study. Neuropathol Appl Neurobiol 2021;47(1):157–70.
38. La A, Rm H, Guye M, Kumar R, et al. Altered brain connectivity in sudden unexpected death in epilepsy (SUDEP) revealed using resting-state fMRI. Neuroimage Clin 2019;24:102060.
39. Allen LA, Vos SB, Kumar R, et al. Cerebellar, limbic, and midbrain volume alterations in sudden unexpected death in epilepsy. Epilepsia 2019;60(4):718–29.
40. Vilella L, Lacuey N, Hampson JP, et al. Postconvulsive central apnea as a biomarker for sudden unexpected death in epilepsy (SUDEP). Neurology 2019;92(3):e171–82.
41. Mueller SG, Nei M, Bateman LM, et al. Brainstem network disruption: a pathway to sudden unexplained death in epilepsy? Hum Brain Mapp 2018;39(12): 4820–30.
42. Myers KA, Bello-Espinosa LE, Symonds JD, et al. Heart rate variability in epilepsy: a potential biomarker of sudden unexpected death in epilepsy risk. Epilepsia 2018;59(7):1372–80.
43. Sivathamboo S, Friedman D, Laze J, et al. Association of short-term heart rate variability and sudden unexpected death in epilepsy. Neurology 2021;97(24): e2357–67.
44. Somani A, El-Hachami H, Patodia S, et al. Regional microglial populations in central autonomic brain regions in SUDEP. Epilepsia 2021;62(6):1318–28.
45. Somani A, Perry C, Patodia S, et al. Neuropeptide depletion in the amygdala in sudden unexpected death in epilepsy: a postmortem study. Epilepsia 2020; 61(2):310–8.
46. Patodia S, Somani A, O'Hare M, et al. The ventrolateral medulla and medullary raphe in sudden unexpected death in epilepsy. Brain 2018;141(6):1719–33.
47. Ryvlin P, Nashef L, Lhatoo SD, et al. Incidence and mechanisms of cardiorespiratory arrests in epilepsy monitoring units (MORTEMUS): a retrospective study. Lancet Neurol 2013;12(10):966–77.
48. Devinsky O, Hesdorffer DC, Thurman DJ, et al. Sudden unexpected death in epilepsy: epidemiology, mechanisms, and prevention. Lancet Neurol 2016;15(10): 1075–88.
49. Szurhaj W, Leclancher A, Nica A, et al. Cardiac Autonomic Dysfunction and Risk of Sudden Unexpected Death in Epilepsy. Neurology 2021;96(21):e2619–26.
50. Devinsky O, Kim A, Friedman D, et al. Incidence of cardiac fibrosis in SUDEP and control cases. Neurology 2018;91(1):e55–61.
51. van der Lende M, Surges R, Sander JW, et al. Cardiac arrhythmias during or after epileptic seizures. J Neurol Neurosurg Psychiatry 2016;87(1):69–74.
52. Schuele SU, Bermeo AC, Locatelli E, et al. Ictal asystole: a benign condition? Epilepsia 2008;49(1):168–71.
53. Moseley BD, Ghearing GR, Benarroch EE, et al. Early seizure termination in ictal asystole. Epilepsy Res 2011;97(1–2):220–4.
54. Schuele SU, Bermeo AC, Alexopoulos AV, et al. Anoxia-ischemia: a mechanism of seizure termination in ictal asystole. Epilepsia 2010;51(1):170–3.

55. Bank AM, Dworetzky BA, Lee JW. Sudden unexpected death in epilepsy in a patient with a cardiac pacemaker. Seizure 2018;61:38–40.
56. Surges R, Adjei P, Kallis C, et al. Pathologic cardiac repolarization in pharmacoresistant epilepsy and its potential role in sudden unexpected death in epilepsy: a case-control study. Epilepsia 2010;51(2):233–42.
57. Li MCH, O'Brien TJ, Todaro M, et al. Acquired cardiac channelopathies in epilepsy: Evidence, mechanisms, and clinical significance. Epilepsia 2019;60(9): 1753–67.
58. Chahal CAA, Salloum MN, Alahdab F, et al. Systematic review of the genetics of sudden unexpected death in epilepsy: potential overlap with sudden cardiac death and arrhythmia-related genes. J Am Heart Assoc 2020;9(1):e012264.
59. Hamdy RM, Elaziz OHA, El Attar RS, et al. Evaluation of QT dispersion in epileptic patients and its association with SUDEP risk. Epilepsy Res 2022;180: 106860.
60. Bagnall RD, Crompton DE, Semsarian C. Genetic Basis of Sudden Unexpected Death in Epilepsy. Front Neurol 2017;8:348.
61. Goldman AM, Behr ER, Semsarian C, et al. Sudden unexpected death in epilepsy genetics: Molecular diagnostics and prevention. Epilepsia 2016; 57(Suppl 1):17–25.
62. Bagnall RD, Crompton DE, Petrovski S, et al. Exome-based analysis of cardiac arrhythmia, respiratory control, and epilepsy genes in sudden unexpected death in epilepsy. Ann Neurol 2016;79(4):522–34.
63. Bagnall RD, Crompton DE, Cutmore C, et al. Genetic analysis of PHOX2B in sudden unexpected death in epilepsy cases. Neurology 2014;83(11):1018–21.
64. Goldman AM, Glasscock E, Yoo J, et al. Arrhythmia in heart and brain: KCNQ1 mutations link epilepsy and sudden unexplained death. Sci Translational Med 2009;1(2):2ra6.
65. Young C, Shankar R, Palmer J, et al. Does intellectual disability increase sudden unexpected death in epilepsy (SUDEP) risk? Seizure 2015;25:112–6.
66. Kuchenbuch M, Barcia G, Chemaly N, et al. KCNT1 epilepsy with migrating focal seizures shows a temporal sequence with poor outcome, high mortality and SUDEP. Brain 2019;142(10):2996–3008.
67. Cooper MS, McIntosh A, Crompton DE, et al. Mortality in Dravet syndrome. Epilepsy Res 2016;128:43–7.
68. Bayat A, Kløvgaard M, Johannesen KM, et al. Deciphering the premature mortality in PIGA-CDG – An untold story. Epilepsy Res 2021;170:106530.
69. Kim Y, Bravo E, Thirnbeck CK, et al. Severe peri-ictal respiratory dysfunction is common in Dravet syndrome. J Clin Invest 2018;128(3):1141–53.
70. Griffin A, Hamling KR, Hong S, et al. Preclinical Animal Models for Dravet Syndrome: Seizure Phenotypes, Comorbidities and Drug Screening. Front Pharmacol 2018;9:573.
71. Auerbach DS, Jones J, Clawson BC, et al. Altered cardiac electrophysiology and SUDEP in a model of Dravet syndrome. PLoS One 2013;8(10):e77843.
72. Catterall WA. Dravet syndrome: a sodium channel interneuronopathy. Curr Opin Physiol 2018;2:42–50.
73. Han Z, Chen C, Christiansen A, et al. Antisense oligonucleotides increase Scn1a expression and reduce seizures and SUDEP incidence in a mouse model of Dravet syndrome. Sci Transl Med 2020;12(558):eaaz6100.
74. Lhatoo SD, Faulkner HJ, Dembny K, et al. An electroclinical case-control study of sudden unexpected death in epilepsy. Ann Neurol 2010;68(6):787–96.

75. Alexandre V, Mercedes B, Valton L, et al. Risk factors of postictal generalized EEG suppression in generalized convulsive seizures. Neurology 2015;85(18): 1598–603.
76. Kuo J, Zhao W, Li CS, et al. Postictal immobility and generalized EEG suppression are associated with the severity of respiratory dysfunction. Epilepsia 2016; 57(3):412–7.
77. Tao JX, Yung I, Lee A, et al. Tonic phase of a generalized convulsive seizure is an independent predictor of postictal generalized EEG suppression. Epilepsia 2013;54(5):858–65.
78. Sarkis RA, Thome-Souza S, Poh MZ, et al. Autonomic changes following generalized tonic clonic seizures: an analysis of adult and pediatric patients with epilepsy. Epilepsy Res 2015;115:113–8.
79. Bruno E, Richardson MP. Postictal generalized EEG suppression and postictal immobility: what do we know? Epileptic Disord 2020;22(3):245–51.
80. Wagnon JL, Korn MJ, Parent R, et al. Convulsive seizures and SUDEP in a mouse model of SCN8A epileptic encephalopathy. Hum Mol Genet 2015; 24(2):506–15.
81. Aiba I, Noebels JL. Spreading depolarization in the brainstem mediates sudden cardiorespiratory arrest in mouse SUDEP models. Sci Transl Med 2015;7(282): 282ra46.
82. Aiba I, Wehrens XH, Noebels JL. Leaky RyR2 channels unleash a brainstem spreading depolarization mechanism of sudden cardiac death. Proc Natl Acad Sci U S A 2016;113(33):E4895–903.
83. Jansen NA, Schenke M, Voskuyl RA, et al. Apnea Associated with Brainstem Seizures in Cacna1a (S218L) Mice Is Caused by Medullary Spreading Depolarization. J Neurosci 2019;39(48):9633–44.
84. Loonen ICM, Jansen NA, Cain SM, et al. Brainstem spreading depolarization and cortical dynamics during fatal seizures in Cacna1a S218L mice. Brain 2019;142(2):412–25.
85. Wenker IC, Teran FA, Wengert ER, et al. Postictal death is associated with tonic phase apnea in a mouse model of sudden unexpected death in epilepsy. Ann Neurol 2021;89(5):1023–35.
86. Lhatoo SD, Nei M, Raghavan M, et al. Nonseizure SUDEP: Sudden unexpected death in epilepsy without preceding epileptic seizures. Epilepsia 2016;57(7): 1161–8.
87. Sveinsson O, Andersson T, Mattsson P, et al. Clinical risk factors in SUDEP: a nationwide population-based case-control study. Neurology 2020;94(4): e419–29.
88. Hesdorffer DC, Tomson T, Benn E, et al. Combined analysis of risk factors for SUDEP. Epilepsia 2011;52(6):1150–9.
89. Hesdorffer DC, Tomson T, Benn E, et al. Do antiepileptic drugs or generalized tonic-clonic seizure frequency increase SUDEP risk? A combined analysis. Epilepsia 2012;53(2):249–52.
90. Langan Y, Nashef L, Sander JW. Case-control study of SUDEP. Neurology 2005; 64(7):1131–3.
91. Verducci C, Friedman D, Donner E, et al. Genetic generalized and focal epilepsy prevalence in the North American SUDEP Registry. Neurology 2020; 94(16):e1757–63.
92. Lamberts RJ, Thijs RD, Laffan A, et al. Sudden unexpected death in epilepsy: people with nocturnal seizures may be at highest risk. Epilepsia 2012;53(2): 253–7.

93. van der Lende M, Hesdorffer DC, Sander JW, et al. Nocturnal supervision and SUDEP risk at different epilepsy care settings. Neurology 2018;91(16): e1508–18.
94. Verducci C, Hussain F, Donner E, et al. SUDEP in the North American SUDEP Registry: The full spectrum of epilepsies. Neurology 2019;93(3):e227–36.
95. Hebel JM, Surges R, Stodieck SRG, et al. SUDEP following the second seizure in new-onset epilepsy due to limbic encephalitis. Seizure 2018;62:124–6.
96. Doumlele K, Friedman D, Buchhalter J, et al. Sudden unexpected death in epilepsy among patients with benign childhood epilepsy with centrotemporal spikes. JAMA Neurol 2017;74(6):645–9.
97. Jha A, Oh C, Hesdorffer D, et al. Sudden unexpected death in epilepsy: a personalized prediction tool. Neurology 2021;96(21):e2627–38.
98. Esmaeili B, Dworetzky BA, Glynn RJ, et al. The probability of sudden unexpected death in epilepsy given postictal prone position. Epilepsy Behav 2021; 116:107775.
99. Aurlien D, Gjerstad L, Taubøll E. The role of antiepileptic drugs in sudden unexpected death in epilepsy. Seizure 2016;43:56–60.
100. Sveinsson O, Andersson T, Mattsson P, et al. Pharmacologic treatment and SUDEP risk: A nationwide, population-based, case-control study. Neurology 2020; 95(18):e2509–18.
101. Ryvlin P, Cucherat M, Rheims S. Risk of sudden unexpected death in epilepsy in patients given adjunctive antiepileptic treatment for refractory seizures: a meta-analysis of placebo-controlled randomised trials. Lancet Neurol 2011;10(11): 961–8.
102. Cross JH, Galer BS, Gil-Nagel A, et al. Impact of fenfluramine on the expected SUDEP mortality rates in patients with Dravet syndrome. Seizure 2021;93:154–9.
103. Ryvlin P, Rheims S, Hirsch LJ, et al. Neuromodulation in epilepsy: state-of-the-art approved therapies. Lancet Neurol 2021;20(12):1038–47.
104. Ryvlin P, Cross JH, Rheims S. Epilepsy surgery in children and adults. Lancet Neurol 2014;13(11):1114–26.
105. Henning O, Nakken KO, Lossius MI. People with epilepsy and their relatives want more information about risks of injuries and premature death. Epilepsy Behav 2018;82:6–10.
106. Long L, Cotterman-Hart S, Shelby J. To reveal or conceal? Adult patient perspectives on SUDEP disclosure. Epilepsy Behav 2018;86:79–84.
107. Morton B, Richardson A, Duncan S. Sudden unexpected death in epilepsy (SUDEP): don't ask, don't tell? J Neurol Neurosurg Psychiatry 2006;77(2):199–202.
108. Asadi-Pooya AA, Trinka E, Brigo F, et al. Counseling about sudden unexpected death in epilepsy (SUDEP): A global survey of neurologists' opinions. Epilepsy Behav 2022;128:108570.
109. Barra SN, Providência R, Paiva L, et al. A review on advanced atrioventricular block in young or middle-aged adults. Pacing Clin Electrophysiol 2012;35(11): 1395–405.
110. Radhakrishnan DM, Ramanujam B, Srivastava P, et al. Effect of providing sudden unexpected death in epilepsy (SUDEP) information to persons with epilepsy (PWE) and their caregivers-Experience from a tertiary care hospital. Acta Neurol Scand 2018;138(5):417–24.
111. Shankar R, Henley W, Boland C, et al. Decreasing the risk of sudden unexpected death in epilepsy: structured communication of risk factors for premature mortality in people with epilepsy. Eur J Neurol 2018;25(9):1121–7.

112. Surges R, von Wrede R, Porschen T, et al. Knowledge of sudden unexpected death in epilepsy (SUDEP) among 372 patients attending a German tertiary epilepsy center. Epilepsy Behav 2018;80:360–4.

113. Brodie MJ, Holmes GL. Should all patients be told about sudden unexpected death in epilepsy (SUDEP)? Pros and Cons. Epilepsia 2008;49(Suppl 9):99–101.

114. Barbour K, Hesdorffer DC, Tian N, et al. Automated detection of sudden unexpected death in epilepsy risk factors in electronic medical records using natural language processing. Epilepsia 2019;60(6):1209–20.

115. Maguire MJ, Jackson CF, Marson AG, et al. Treatments for the prevention of Sudden Unexpected Death in Epilepsy (SUDEP). Cochrane Database Syst Rev 2020;4(4):Cd011792.

116. Schulz R, Bien CG, May TW. Decreasing SUDEP incidence in a tertiary epilepsy center between 1981 and 2016: Effects of better patient supervision. Epilepsy Behav 2019;92:1–4.

117. Ryvlin P, Ciumas C, Wisniewski I, et al. Wearable devices for sudden unexpected death in epilepsy prevention. Epilepsia 2018;59(Suppl 1):61–6.

118. Sun JJ, Perera B, Henley W, et al. Seizure and Sudden Unexpected Death in Epilepsy (SUDEP) characteristics in an urban UK intellectual disability service. Seizure 2020;80:18–23.

Effects of Maternal Use of Antiseizure Medications on Child Development

Kimford J. Meador, MD, FRCPE

KEYWORDS

- Epilepsy • Anticonvulsants • Pregnancy • Malformations
- Neurodevelopmental outcomes

KEY POINTS

- Women with epilepsy are at increased risks for poor anatomic and behavioral outcomes in their children, but most children born to these women are normal.
- Teratogenic risks vary across antiseizure medications (ASMs).
- Valproate poses a special risk for anatomic and behavioral teratogenic risks compared with other ASMs.
- The risks for many ASMs remain uncertain.
- Women of childbearing potential taking ASMs should be taking folic acid.

INTRODUCTION

Epilepsy is a common disorder with more than a half million women of childbearing age having epilepsy in the United States alone.[1] Antiseizure medications (ASMs) are the main therapeutic option for epilepsy and are among the most commonly prescribed teratogenic medications prescribed to women of childbearing age. The clinical dilemma is that drugs are generally contraindicated in pregnancy, but most women with epilepsy are unable to stop using ASMs because of risks of seizures with resultant consequences of injury, death, and loss of job or driving. Furthermore, seizures during pregnancy can result in fetal injury, miscarriage, or subsequent developmental delay. As a group, somatic and functional neurodevelopment outcomes are reduced in children of women with epilepsy, but it is important to remember that most children born to women with epilepsy are normal. The challenge to clinicians is to reduce these risks based on current knowledge. The challenge to basic and clinical researchers is to improve that inadequate evidence base.

Department of Neurology & Neurological Sciences, Stanford University, Stanford University School of Medicine, 213 Quarry Road, MC 5979, Palo Alto, CA 94304-5979, USA
E-mail address: kmeador@stanford.edu

Neurol Clin 40 (2022) 755–768
https://doi.org/10.1016/j.ncl.2022.03.006
0733-8619/22/© 2022 Elsevier Inc. All rights reserved.

BACKGROUND HISTORY

People with epilepsy have frequently suffered from stigma, which includes basic reproductive rights. In 1956, in the United States 17 states prohibited marriage in people with epilepsy; the last such state law in the United States was finally overturned in 1980.[2] Similar laws existed in other countries in the mid-twentieth century. For example, a similar law existed in the United Kingdom until 1970. In addition, 18 states in the United States in 1956 provided for the sterilization of people with epilepsy.[2] The justification of these sterilizations was poorly conceived, based on eugenics, and violated basic human rights; they had nothing to do with teratogenic risks of ASMs, which were not discovered until the 1960s.

Although the first modern ASM bromide was discovered in 1850s,[3] it would be more than 100 years before the teratogenic potential of ASMs were recognized. This recognition was shortly after the thalidomide tragedy, which highlighted the potential teratogenicity of pharmaceuticals. Thalidomide was introduced in the 1950s leading to approximately 10,000 children born with phocomelia (ie, missing or underdeveloped limbs) in just a few years, and thalidomide was banned in most countries by 1961.[4] In 1968, Meadow[5] published a letter-to-the-editor describing six children with congenital malformations who had been exposed in utero to ASMs; however, he was cautious noting "before creating anxiety about useful drugs, it would be helpful to know if other people have encountered the association." By 1974, multiple surveys were published, and Speidel and Meadow[6] noted that most authors estimated the risk of malformations from fetal ASM exposure to be two to three times the general population. Ironically, the letter by Meadow was a year after the discovery of the antiseizure effects of valproic acid, which is now known to be the most teratogenic ASM.[7] Spina bifida was linked to fetal valproate exposure in 1982,[8] but it would not be until early in the twenty-first century that full scope of valproate's risk would be recognized after the establishment of ASM pregnancy registries and other prospective studies. The risk could and should have been recognized earlier because a retrospective meta-analysis assessing the cumulative risk ratios for congenital malformations for each year beginning in 1983 showed risk as depicted by confidence intervals (CIs) separated for valproate from other ASMs in 1990 never to overlap again.[9] Unfortunately, this theme of many years passing as numerous fetal ASM exposures occur before the specific risks for specific ASMs are recognized continues today because the risks for most ASMs used today are unknown.[10]

ANATOMIC RISKS

Children of women with epilepsy, who are exposed to ASMs during pregnancy, are at increased risk for congenital malformations. Children of women with epilepsy who did not take ASM during pregnancy and the children of fathers with epilepsy are not at increased risk.[11] Thus, the risk seems to be caused by fetal ASM exposure because ASMs as a class are known to be teratogenic and produce birth defects in animals if given in high enough dosages. Given that major organs are formed during the first trimester, exposure during the first part of pregnancy poses risk for major congenital malformations (MCMs). Typical ASM-induced malformations include heart defects, orofacial clefts, skeletal deformities, urologic abnormalities, and neural tube defects.[12] However, these risks vary across ASMs. Risks for polytherapy seem higher than monotherapy, but the risks for specific combinations are unclear.

Multiple studies have consistently shown the increased risk of MCMs from fetal valproate exposure, and demonstrated that the risk for valproate is higher than any other ASMs, which have adequate data. Examples from the literature are offered. The North

American Antiepileptic Drug Pregnancy Registry has found that the risk for MCMs is 9.3% for valproate compared with phenobarbital 5.5%, topiramate 4.2%, phenytoin 2.9%, carbamazepine 3.0%, levetiracetam 2.4%, oxcarbazepine 2.2%, and lamotrigine 2.0%.[13] Similarly, the EURAP noted the risk of MCMs was valproate is 10.3% compared with phenobarbital 6.5%, phenytoin 6.4%, topiramate 3.9%, carbamazepine 5.5%, oxcarbazepine 3.0%, lamotrigine 2.9%, and levetiracetam 2.8%.[14] The same pattern has been seen in the UK-Ireland registry with MCMs occurring in 6.7% for valproate, 4.8% for topiramate, 2.6% for carbamazepine, 2.3% for lamotrigine, and 0.7% for levetiracetam.[15–17] A case-control study across 19 registries in 14 countries from 1995 to 2005 disclosed specific malformation risks for valproate (spina bifida, atrial septal defect, cleft palate, hypospadias, polydactyly, and craniosynostosis) and for carbamazepine (spina bifida).[18,19] A French national database study disclosed valproate was associated with eight specific MCMs (spina bifida, ventricular, atrial septal defects, pulmonary valve atresia, hypoplastic left heart syndrome, cleft palate, anorectal atresia, and hypospadias); specific defects were also seen for clonazepam (microcephaly), phenobarbital (ventricular septal defect), pregabalin (coarctation of aorta), and topiramate (cleft lip with or without cleft palate) but the findings for these other ASMs were based on a small number of MCMs.[20] A recent Danish population-based cohort study of individual-linked data of births 1997 to 2014 reported the valproate risk of MCMs was adjusted odds ratio of 2.44, 95% CI of 1.80 to 3.30, and separated from lamotrigine as early as 1997[21]; additionally, no significant differences were seen for lamotrigine, carbamazepine, oxcarbazepine, or levetiracetam versus unexposed.

Analyses of the US Medicaid Analytical eXtract dataset revealed no increased risk for gabapentin overall (relative risk, 1.07; 95% CI, 0.94–1.21), but an increased risk for cardiac defects was seen when more than two dispensed gabapentin prescriptions (relative risk, 1.40; 95% CI, 1.03–1.90), and an increased risk for pregabalin (1.80; 95% CI, 1.26–2.58) was seen for any use but not monotherapy (1.31; 95% CI, 0.80–2.14).[22]

Valproate poses an especially high risk for MCMs, and next highest for phenobarbital. The risks are intermediate for carbamazepine, gabapentin, phenytoin, pregabalin, and topiramate. The lowest risks of MCMs exists for levetiracetam, lamotrigine, and oxcarbazepine (**Fig. 1**). Data for other ASMs remain inadequate to accurately determination risks for MCMs (**Table 1**).

NEUROPSYCHOLOGICAL OUTCOMES
Valproate

Multiple studies have consistently shown the increased risk of neuropsychological impairments from fetal valproate exposure, and demonstrated that the risk for valproate is higher than any other ASMs that have adequate data.[23–40] Examples from the literature are offered. The Neurodevelopmental Effects of Antiepileptic Drugs (NEAD) study prospectively enrolled women with epilepsy and evaluated their children who had fetal ASM exposure to carbamazepine, lamotrigine, phenytoin, or valproate monotherapy. At age 3 years old, children exposed to valproate had mean IQ six to nine points lower than those exposed to the other ASMs.[26] At 6 years old, children exposed to valproate had mean IQ 8 to 11 points lower than those exposed to the other ASMs, and the valproate children demonstrated a dose-dependent decremental effect across multiple cognitive domains.[30] Other studies in the United Kingdom,[23–25,27,34,36] Australia,[28,29,38] and India[40] have confirmed the adverse effects of fetal valproate exposure on cognitive abilities. Population-based studies from Denmark, France, and Norway are discussed later. A Cochrane review in 2014 of 22

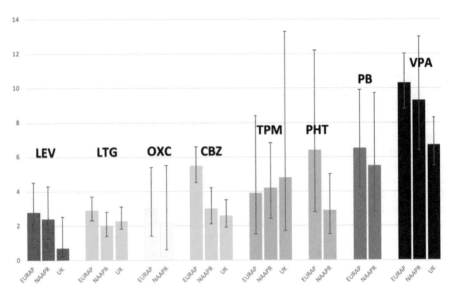

Fig. 1. Malformation rates (mean %, 95% CI) as function of ASM. CBZ, carbamazepine; LEV, levetiracetam; LTG, lamotrigine; OXC, oxcarbazepine; PB, phenobarbital; PHT, phenytoin; TPM, topiramate; VPA, valproate. (*Adapted from* Refs.[13–17])

prospective cohort studies and six registry-based studies confirmed the findings of adverse effects of valproate compared with unexposed children and with children exposed in utero to carbamazepine, lamotrigine, and phenytoin, but those three ASMs did not differ.[35] The review also noted valproate dose-dependent adverse effects in six studies. Given the dose-dependent effect, the question as to whether there is a safe dose has been raised, but valproate at less than 800 mg/d is associated with impaired verbal abilities (−5.6; 95% CI, -11.1 to −0.1; $P = .04$) and a six-fold increase in educational intervention (95% CI, 1.4–18.0; $P = .01$).[36]

Table 1
Risks of fetal ASM-induced major congenital malformations in humans based on current data

Data on Risks	Unknown Risks	
Highest Risks	Acetazolamide	Lacosamide
Phenobarbital	Brivaracetam	Lorazepam
Valproate	Cannabidiol	Midazolam
Intermediate Risks	Cenobamate	Perampanel
Carbamazepine	Clobazam	Primidone
Gabapentin	Clonazepam	Rufinamide
Phenytoin	Diazepam	Stiripentol
Pregabalin	Eslicarbazepine	Sultiame
Topiramate	Ethosuximide	Tiagabine
Lowest Risks	Everolimus	Vigabatrin
Lamotrigine	Felbamate	Zonisamide
Levetiracetam	Fenfluramine	
Oxcarbazepine		

Population-Based Studies

Danish population studies have demonstrated an increased risk of fetal valproate exposure for autism spectrum disorder (adjusted hazard ratio [aHR], 2.9; 95% CI, 1.7–4.9) and for childhood autism (aHR, 5.2; 95% CI, 2.7–10.0),[41] an increased risk for attentional-deficit/hyperactivity disorder (aHR, 1.48; 95% CI, 1.09–2.00),[42] and an increased risk for of intellectual disability (aHR, 4.48; 95% CI, 2.97–6.76) and intellectual disability with delayed childhood milestones (aHR, 6.07; 95% CI, 4.67–7.89), but also found increased risk of intellectual disability with prenatal exposure to maternal monotherapy use of carbamazepine (aHR, 3.84; 95% CI, 2.32–6.38), clonazepam (aHR, 2.41; 95% CI, 1.09–5.35), and oxcarbazepine (aHR, 3.70; 95% CI, 2.11–6.51) but not lamotrigine (aHR, 1.33; 95% CI, 0.71–2.48).[43] Another Danish study found that valproate-exposed children scored worse on the sixth-grade language tests (adjusted difference, 0.0.27; 95% CI, 0.0.42–0.0.12) and sixth-grade mathematics tests (adjusted difference, 0.0.33; 95% CI, 0.0.47–0.0.19); they also found clonazepam-exposed children scored worse in the sixth-grade language tests (adjusted difference, 0.0.07; 95% CI, 0.0.12–0.0.02).[39] Carbamazepine, lamotrigine, phenobarbital, and oxcarbazepine were not linked to poor school performance compared with unexposed children.

A French nationwide population-based cohort study found that fetal exposure to valproate was associated with increased risks of neurodevelopmental disorders (HR, 2.7; 95% CI, 1.8–4.0), pervasive developmental disorders (HR, 4.4; 95% CI, 2.1–9.3), mental retardation (HR, 3.1; 95% CI, 1.5–6.2), and visits to speech therapists (HR, 1.5; 95% CI, 1.1–1.9), with a dose-response relationship.[44] Among the other ASMs, pregabalin was associated with an increased risk of neurodevelopmental disorders (aHR, 1.5; 95% CI, 1.0–2.1), and phenobarbital was associated with higher risk of behavioral and emotional disorders (aHR, 7.6; 95% CI, 1.1–53.6).[45]

Other Antiseizure Medications

Although two studies have raised concerns,[33,46] most studies have not found neuropsychological impairments after fetal lamotrigine exosure.[26,28,30,32,34,36,37,39–44] Similarly, several studies have failed to find deficits from fetal levetiracetam exposure.[47–49] The Maternal Outcomes and Neurodevelopmental Effects of Antiepileptic Drugs (MONEAD) study, which is a continuation of the NEAD study with a new prospective cohort, recently reported age 2 years old cognitive outcomes for children who were mainly exposed to lamotrigine or levetiracetam or both.[50] The cohort of children exposed to ASMs did not differ from children of healthy women. In addition, no blood level or dose effects were seen for the primary outcome of language abilities. A secondary analysis did disclose a level-dependent effect of levetiracetam on the motor domain, but additional studies are needed to confirm this observation.

Some studies have reported adverse effects for carbamazepine[33,51] and phenytoin,[52,53] but others have not found an adverse signal for fetal exposures.[25,26,28,30,32,34,37,39,40,43,44] Similarly, there are mixed signals for oxcarbazepine.[33,39,43]

Several studies have demonstrated adverse effects of fetal phenobarbital exposure including two Danish studies with lower IQ scores in two adult men exposed in utero using different IQ measures,[54] two studies from India with reduced IQ and language abilities,[40,55] and a French population-based study with increased risk of intellectual disability.[45]

A Danish population-based study reported increased risk for intellectual disability in children with fetal clonazepam exposure,[43] and another Danish study found reduced language and math performance on sixth grade assessments.[39] In two small studies, fetal topiramate exposure has been reported with mixed results on neurodevelopmental effects.[49,56] A French nationwide population-based study noted increased risk for neurodevelopmental disorders from pregabalin exposure (aHR, 1.5; 95% CI, 1.0–2.1).[45] Gabapentin showed a marginal adverse effect on psychomotor development (odds ratio, 9.03; 95% CI, 1.00–62.78) in a systematic review and network meta-analysis.[57] It is obvious that data for some of the ASMs previously mentioned are inadequate. Furthermore, data for other ASMs are inadequate or completely lacking.

Periconceptional Folate

The NEAD study found that periconceptional folic acid supplementation was associated with higher IQ at age 6 in children exposed to ASM in utero; adjusted means were 108 (95% CI, 106–111) in those with folic acid exposure versus 102 (95% CI, 98–104) in those not exposed to folic acid.[30] The Norwegian Mother and Child Cohort Study found that periconceptional folic acid was associated with reduced risks for language delay and autism in children exposed to ASMs comprised primarily of lamotrigine, carbamazepine, and valproate.[58–60] Folate effects were related to exposure in the first 12 weeks of pregnancy. These researchers have also shown that higher ASM concentrations are correlated with higher concentrations of unmetabolized folic acid and inactive folate metabolites.[61] Additional research is needed to define the optimum dose of folic acid because concerns have been raised for risks of high-dose periconceptional folic acid.

Breastfeeding on Antiseizure Medications

Despite clear positive effects of breastfeeding for mother and child in the general population,[62] some have raised concerns for breastfeeding when taking ASMs. However, several studies in children who were previously exposed in utero have shown that breastfeeding while a woman is taking AMS is safe. The NEAD study and a Norwegian study found no adverse effects on cognition at 3 years old,[63,64] and the NEAD study actually showed that children exposed in utero who then breastfed actually had a mean IQ four points higher than those who did not breastfeed.[65] One reason why ASM exposure from breastmilk does not have adverse effects may be that ASM levels in breastfeeding children are much lower than their mothers in most cases.[66]

Conclusions for Neuropsychological Risks

Valproate poses an especially high risk, and there is also clear evidence of risk from phenobarbital. Risks for carbamazepine and phenytoin are less than valproate. The greatest safety in regards to behavioral teratogenesis seems to exist for lamotrigine and levetiracetam. There are some concerning but uncertain signals for clonazepam, oxcarbazepine, and pregabalin. Data for other ASMs are inadequate to accurately determination risks for cognitive and behavioral deficits from fetal exposure (**Table 2**). Periconceptional folate improves neuropsychological outcomes in children, and breastfeeding is safe while taking ASMs.

MECHANISMS OF ANTISEIZURE MEDICATION TERATOGENICITY

Several posited mechanisms for ASM teratogenic effects on fetal development have included suppression neuronal activity, folate-related mechanisms, ischemia/hypoxia, reactive intermediates, free radicals, arene oxides, neuronal apoptosis and synaptic dysfunction, and antagonism of neutropins and signal proteins. Teratogens are known to act in a dose-dependent manner on a susceptible genotype. In regards to ASMs,

Table 2 Risks of fetal ASM-induced neuropsychological developmental impairments in humans based on current data		
Data on Risks	**Unknown Risks**	
Highest Risks	Acetazolamide	Lacosamide
Phenobarbital	Brivaracetam	Lorazepam
Valproate	Cannabidiol	Midazolam
Intermediate Risks	Cenobamate	Perampanel
Carbamazepine	Clobazam	Primidone
Phenytoin	Diazepam	Rufinamide
Possible Risks	Eslicarbazepine	Stiripentol
Clonazepam	Ethosuximide	Sultiame
Oxcarbazepine	Everolimus	Tiagabine
Pregabalin	Felbamate	Topiramate
Lowest Risks	Fenfluramine	Vigabatrin
Lamotrigine	Gabapentin	Zonisamide
Levetiracetam		

the EURAP registry demonstrated dose-dependent effects for MCMs across all four of their most commonly used ASMs (ie, carbamazepine, lamotrigine, phenobarbital, valproate) (**Fig. 2**).[14] Furthermore, clear dose-dependent effects of valproate have been demonstrated across multiple cognitive domains for valproate.[30] Although the genetic substrate for ASM-induced teratogenesis is unknown, there is evidence for genetic influences on ASM-induced risks in humans. If a woman taking ASM during a pregnancy

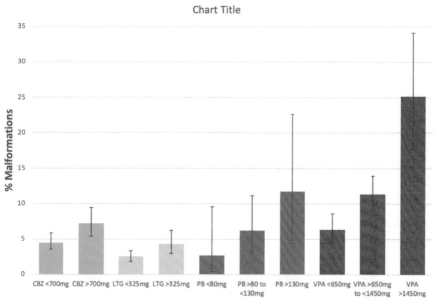

Fig. 2. Malformation rates (mean %, 95% CI) as function of ASM dose. Dosages given as mg/d. (*Adapted from* Ref.[14])

has a child with a malformation, her risk of having another child with a malformation when taking the same ASM (16.8%) is higher than a woman whose first child did not have a malformation in a prior pregnancy.[67,68]

There likely to be multiple teratogenic mechanisms. The mechanisms for anatomic and behavioral teratogenesis may differ because MCMs are the result of first-trimester exposures, whereas behavioral teratogenesis may be primarily caused by third-trimester exposures. The underlying mechanism for behavioral teratogenesis of ASMs may be similar to fetal alcohol effects on the immature brain, which produces neuronal apoptosis and synaptic dysfunction in the surviving neurons.[69] In fact, widespread neural apoptosis in the immature brains of animals has been demonstrated for clonazepam, diazepam, phenobarbital, phenytoin, valproate, and vigabatrin, but apoptosis was absent for carbamazepine, lamotrigine, levetiracetam, or topiramate in monotherapy exposures.[70–77] However, these ASMs without apoptosis in monotherapy can enhance the apoptosis produced by phenytoin when given in combination, except for levetiracetam, which did not enhance apoptosis. In addition to neuronal apoptosis, there is cell death in developing white matter,[78] synaptic changes,[79,80] and behavioral deficits.[81–83] Unfortunately, most ASMs have not been tested in this model (**Table 3**).

FUTURE DIRECTIONS

Despite advances in knowledge over the past two decades, information is lacking for most ASMs on risks for malformations, neuropsychological outcomes, and animal models. Recommendations to improve the situation have been made including a national reporting system for congenital malformations, routine meta-analyses of cohort studies to detect teratogenic signals, monitoring of ASM prescription practices for women, routine preclinical testing of all new ASMs for neurodevelopmental effects, and improved funding of basic and clinical research to fully delineate risks and underlying mechanisms for ASM-induced anatomic and behavioral teratogenesis.[10] With

Table 3
ASMs tested in the apoptotic model

Data on Risks	Unknown Risks	
Higher Risks	Acetazolamide	Lorazepam
Clonazepam	Brivaracetam	Midazolam
Diazepam	Cannabidiol	Oxcarbazepine
Phenobarbital	Cenobamate	Perampanel
Phenytoin	Clobazam	Pregabalin
Valproate	Diazepam	Primidone
Vigabatrin	Eslicarbazepine	Rufinamide
	Ethosuximide	Stiripentol
Lower Risks	Everolimus	Sultiame
Carbamazepine	Felbamate	Tiagabine
Lamotrigine	Fenfluramine	Zonisamide
Levetiracetam	Gabapentin	
Topiramate	Lacosamide	

Note that the model is predictive of effects in humans, but does not explore all possible mechanisms.

such actions, future care in women requiring ASMs could be evidence-based and achieve precision medicine that focuses on early detection, prediction (eg, via susceptible genotype), and targeted therapies.[84]

SUMMARY

ASMs pose anatomic and behavioral teratogenetic risks to the developing immature brain. These risks vary across ASMs, but remain unknown for many ASMs. Based on present knowledge valproate and phenobarbital pose the greatest risks, whereas lamotrigine and levetiracetam have the lowest risks.

CLINICS CARE POINTS

- Most children born to women with epilepsy are normal but have increased risks for malformations and poor neuropsychological outcomes.
- Women with epilepsy should receive informed consent outlining risks before conception.
- Valproate is a poor first choice ASM for most women with epilepsy of childbearing potential.
- Women with epilepsy of childbearing potential should be taking folic acid.
- Breastfeeding on ASMs seems safe.

DISCLOSURE

K.J. Meador has received research support from the National Institutes of Health, Eisai, and Medtronic Inc. The Epilepsy Study Consortium pays his university for his research consultant time related to Eisai, GW Pharmaceuticals, NeuroPace, Novartis, Supernus, Upsher-Smith Laboratories, UCB Pharma, and Vivus Pharmaceuticals. In addition, K.J. Meador is Co-I and Director of Cognitive Core of the Human Epilepsy Project for the Epilepsy Study Consortium. K.J. Meador is on the editorial boards for Neurology, Cognitive & Behavioral Neurology, Epilepsy & Behavior, and Epilepsy & Behavior Case Reports.

REFERENCES

1. Harden CL, Hopp J, Ting TY, et al. Practice parameter update: management issues for women with epilepsy—focus on pregnancy (an evidence-based review): obstetrical complications and change in seizure frequency: report of the Quality Standards Subcommittee and Therapeutics and Technology Assessment Subcommittee of the American Academy of Neurology and American Epilepsy Society. Neurology 2009;73(2):126–32.
2. The history and stigma of epilepsy. Available at: https://onlinelibrary.wiley.com/doi/pdf/10.1046/j.1528-1157.44.s.6.2.x (accessed 12/26/2021).
3. Friedlander WJ. Who was 'the father of bromide treatment of epilepsy. Arch Neurol 1986;43(5):505–7.
4. Kim JH, Scialli AR. Thalidomide: the tragedy of birth defects and the effective treatment of disease. Toxicol Sci 2011;122(1):1–6.
5. Meadow SR. Anticonvulsant drugs and congenital abnormalities. Lancet 1968; 2(7581):1296.
6. Speidel BD, Meadow SR. Epilepsy, anticonvulsants and congenital malformations. Drugs 1974;8(5):354–65.

7. Tomson T, Battino D, Perucca E. The remarkable story of valproic acid. Lancet Neurol 2016;15(2):141.
8. Centers for Disease Control (CDC). Valproic acid and spina bifida: a preliminary report—France. MMWR Morb Mortal Wkly Rep 1982;31(42):565–6.
9. Tanoshima M, Kobayashi T, Tanoshima R, et al. Risks of congenital malformations in offspring exposed to valproic acid in utero: a systematic review and cumulative meta-analysis. Clin Pharmacol Ther 2015;98(4):417–41.
10. Meador KJ, Loring DW. Developmental effects of antiepileptic drugs and the need for improved regulations. Neurology 2016;86(3):297–306.
11. Meador KJ. Cognitive effects of epilepsy and its treatments, Chapter 93. In: Wyllie E, Cascino GD, Gidal BE, et al, editors. Wyllie's treatment of epilepsy: principles & practice. 7th Edition. Philadelphia: Lippincott Williams & Wilkins; 2020. p. 1058–63.
12. Kellogg MA, Meador KJ. Neurodevelopmental effects of antiepileptic drugs. Neurochem Res 2017;42(7):2065–70.
13. Hernández-Díaz S, Smith CR, Shen A, et al. Comparative safety of antiepileptic drugs during pregnancy. Neurology 2012;78(21):1692–9.
14. Tomson T, Battino D, Bonizzoni E, et al. Comparative risk of major congenital malformations with eight different antiepileptic drugs: a prospective cohort study of the EURAP registry. Lancet Neurol 2018;17(6):530–8.
15. Hunt S, Russell A, Smithson WH, et al. Topiramate in pregnancy: preliminary experience from the UK Epilepsy and Pregnancy Register. Neurology 2008;71(4):272–6.
16. Mawhinney E, Craig J, Morrow J, et al. Levetiracetam in pregnancy: results from the UK and Ireland epilepsy and pregnancy registers. Neurology 2013;80(4):400–5.
17. Campbell E, Kennedy F, Russell A, et al. Malformation risks of antiepileptic drug monotherapies in pregnancy: updated results from the UK and Ireland Epilepsy and Pregnancy Registers. J Neurol Neurosurg Psychiatry 2014;85(9):1029–34.
18. Jentink J, Loane MA, Dolk H, et al. Valproic acid monotherapy in pregnancy and major congenital malformations. N Engl J Med 2010;362(23):2185–93.
19. Jentink J, Dolk H, Loane MA, et al. Intrauterine exposure to carbamazepine and specific congenital malformations: systematic review and case-control study. BMJ 2010;341:c6581.
20. Blotière PO, Raguideau F, Weill A, et al. Risks of 23 specific malformations associated with prenatal exposure to 10 antiepileptic drugs. Neurology 2019;93(2):e167–80.
21. Christensen J, Trabjerg BB, Sun Y, et al. Prenatal exposure to valproate and risk of congenital malformations-Could we have known earlier? A population-based cohort study. Epilepsia 2021;62(12):2981–93.
22. Patorno E, Hernandez-Diaz S, Huybrechts KF, et al. Gabapentin in pregnancy and the risk of adverse neonatal and maternal outcomes: a population-based cohort study nested in the US Medicaid Analytic eXtract dataset. PLoS Med 2020;17(9):e1003322.
23. Adab N, Kini U, Vinten J, et al. The longer term outcome of children born to mothers with epilepsy. J Neurol Neurosurg Psychiatry 2004;75:1575–83.
24. Vinten J, Adab N, Kini U, et al. Neuropsychological effects of exposure to anticonvulsant medication in utero. Neurology 2005;64:949–54.
25. Bromley RL, Mawer G, Clayton-Smith J, et al, Liverpool and Manchester Neurodevelopment Group. Autism spectrum disorders following in utero exposure to antiepileptic drugs. Neurology 2008;71(23):1923–4.

26. Meador KJ, Baker GA, Browning N, et al. Cognitive function at 3 years of age after fetal exposure to antiepileptic drugs. N Engl J Med 2009;360:1597–605.
27. Bromley RL, Mawer G, Love J, et al. Early cognitive development in children born to women with epilepsy: a prospective report. Epilepsia 2010;51:2058–65.
28. Nadebaum C, Anderson VA, Vajda F, et al. Language skills of school-aged children prenatally exposed to antiepileptic drugs. Neurology 2011;76:719–26.
29. Nadebaum C, Anderson V, Vajda F, et al. The Australian brain and cognition and antiepileptic drugs study: IQ in school-aged children exposed to sodium valproate and polytherapy. J Int Neuropsychol Soc 2011;17(1):133–42.
30. Meador KJ, Baker GA, Browning N, et al. Fetal antiepileptic drug exposure and cognitive outcomes at age 6 years (NEAD study): a prospective observational study. Lancet Neurol 2013;12:244–52.
31. Christensen J, Gronborg TK, Sorensen MJ, et al. Prenatal valproate exposure and risk of autism spectrum disorders and childhood autism. JAMA 2013;309:1696–703.
32. Cohen MJ, Meador KJ, Browning N, et al. Fetal antiepileptic drug exposure: adaptive and emotional/behavioral functioning at age 6 years. Epilepsy Behav 2013;29:308–15.
33. Veiby G, Daltveit AK, Schjolberg S, et al. Exposure to antiepileptic drugs in utero and child development: a prospective population-based study. Epilepsia 2013;54:1462–72.
34. Bromley RL, Mawer GE, Briggs M, et al. The prevalence of neurodevelopmental disorders in children prenatally exposed to antiepileptic drugs. J Neurol Neurosurg Psychiatry 2013;84:637–43.
35. Bromley R, Weston J, Adab N, et al. Treatment for epilepsy in pregnancy: neurodevelopmental outcomes in the child. Cochrane Database Syst Rev 2014;CD010236.
36. Baker GA, Bromley RL, Briggs M, et al. IQ at 6 years after in utero exposure to antiepileptic drugs: a controlled cohort study. Neurology 2015;84:382–90.
37. Deshmukh U, Adams J, Macklin EA, et al. Behavioral outcomes in children exposed prenatally to lamotrigine, valproate, or carbamazepine. Neurotoxicol Teratol 2016;54:5–14.
38. Barton S, Nadebaum C, Anderson VA, et al. Memory dysfunction in school-aged children exposed prenatally to antiepileptic drugs. Neuropsychology 2018;32(7):784–96.
39. Elkjaer LS, Bech BH, Sun Y, et al. Association between prenatal valproate exposure and performance on standardized language and mathematics tests in school-aged children. JAMA Neurol 2018;75:663.
40. Unnikrishnan G, Jacob NS, Salim S, et al. Enduring language deficits in children of women with epilepsy and the potential role of intrauterine exposure to antiepileptic drugs. Epilepsia 2020;61(11):2442–51.
41. Christensen J, Grønborg TK, Sørensen MJ, et al. Prenatal valproate exposure and risk of autism spectrum disorders and childhood autism. JAMA 2013;309(16):1696–703.
42. Christensen J, Pedersen L, Sun Y, et al. Association of prenatal exposure to valproate and other antiepileptic drugs with risk for attention-deficit/hyperactivity disorder in offspring. JAMA Netw Open 2019;2(1):e186606.
43. Daugaard CA, Pedersen L, Sun Y, et al. Association of prenatal exposure to valproate and other antiepileptic drugs with intellectual disability and delayed childhood milestones. JAMA Netw Open 2020;3(11):e2025570.

44. Blotière PO, Miranda S, Weill A, et al. Risk of early neurodevelopmental outcomes associated with prenatal exposure to the antiepileptic drugs most commonly used during pregnancy: a French nationwide population-based cohort study. BMJ Open 2020;10(6):e034829.
45. Coste J, Blotiere PO, Miranda S, et al. Risk of early neurodevelopmental disorders associated with in utero exposure to valproate and other antiepileptic drugs: a nationwide cohort study in France. Sci Rep 2020;10(1):17362.
46. Husebye ESN, Gilhus NE, Spigset O, et al. Language impairment in children aged 5 and 8 years after antiepileptic drug exposure in utero: the Norwegian Mother and Child Cohort Study. Eur J Neurol 2020;27(4):667–75.
47. Shallcross R, Bromley RL, Irwin B, et al. Child development following in utero exposure: levetiracetam vs sodium valproate. Neurology 2011;76:383–9.
48. Shallcross R, Bromley RL, Cheyne CP, et al. In utero exposure to levetiracetam vs valproate: development and language at 3 years of age. Neurology 2014;82:213–21.
49. Bromley RL, Calderbank R, Cheyne CP, et al. Cognition in school-age children exposed to levetiracetam, topiramate, or sodium valproate. Neurology 2016;87:1943–53.
50. Meador KJ, Cohen MJ, Loring DW, et al. Two-year-old cognitive outcomes in children of pregnant women with epilepsy in the Maternal Outcomes and Neurodevelopmental Effects of Antiepileptic Drugs Study. JAMA Neurol 2021;78(8):927–36.
51. Cummings C, Stewart M, Stevenson M, et al. Neurodevelopment of children exposed in utero to lamotrigine, sodium valproate and carbamazepine. Arch Dis Child 2011;96(7):643–7.
52. Scolnik D, Nulman I, Rovet J, et al. Neurodevelopment of children exposed in utero to phenytoin and carbamazepine monotherapy. JAMA 1994;271(10):767–70.
53. Verrotti A, Scaparrotta A, Cofini M, et al. Developmental neurotoxicity and anticonvulsant drugs: a possible link. Reprod Toxicol 2014;48:72–80.
54. Reinisch JM, Sanders SA, Mortensen EL, et al. In utero exposure to phenobarbital and intelligence deficits in adult men. JAMA 1995;274:1518–25.
55. Gopinath N, Muneer AK, Unnikrishnan S, et al. Children (10-12 years age) of women with epilepsy have lower intelligence, attention and memory: observations from a prospective cohort case control study. Epilepsy Res 2015;117:58–62.
56. Rihtman T, Parush S, Ornoy A. Preliminary findings of the developmental effects of in utero exposure to topiramate. Reprod Toxicol 2012;34:308–11.
57. Veroniki AA, Rios P, Cogo E, et al. Comparative safety of antiepileptic drugs for neurological development in children exposed during pregnancy and breast feeding: a systematic review and network meta-analysis. BMJ Open 2017;7(7):e017248.
58. Husebye ESN, Gilhus NE, Riedel B, et al. Verbal abilities in children of mothers with epilepsy: association to maternal folate status. Neurology 2018;91(9):e811–21.
59. Bjørk M, Riedel B, Spigset O, et al. Association of folic acid supplementation during pregnancy with the risk of autistic traits in children exposed to antiepileptic drugs in utero. JAMA Neurol 2018;75(2):160–8.
60. Husebye ESN, Gilhus NE, Spigset O, et al. Language impairment in children aged 5 and 8 years after antiepileptic drug exposure in utero: the Norwegian Mother and Child Cohort Study. Eur J Neurol 2020;27(4):667–75.

61. Husebye ESN, Riedel B, Bjørke-Monsen AL, et al. Vitamin B status and association with antiseizure medication in pregnant women with epilepsy. Epilepsia 2021; 62(12):2968–80.
62. Ip S, Chung M, Raman G, et al. A summary of the Agency for Healthcare Research and Quality's evidence report on breastfeeding in developed countries. Breastfeed Med 2009;4(suppl 1):S17–30.
63. Meador KJ, Baker GA, Browning N, et al. Effects of breastfeeding in children of women taking antiepileptic drugs. Neurology 2010;75(22):1954–60.
64. Veiby G, Engelsen BA, Gilhus NE. Early child development and exposure to antiepileptic drugs prenatally and through breastfeeding: a prospective cohort study on children of women with epilepsy. JAMA Neurol 2013;70(11):1367–74.
65. Meador KJ, Baker GA, Browning N, et al. Breastfeeding in children of women taking antiepileptic drugs: cognitive outcomes at age 6 years. JAMA Pediatr 2014; 168(8):729–36.
66. Birnbaum AK, Meador KJ, Karanam A, et al. Antiepileptic drug exposure in infants of breastfeeding mothers with epilepsy. JAMA Neurol 2020;77(4):441–50.
67. Campbell E, Devenney E, Morrow J, et al. Recurrence risk of congenital malformations in infants exposed to antiepileptic drugs in utero. Epilepsia 2013;54(1): 165–71.
68. Vajda FJ, O'Brien TJ, Lander CM, et al. Teratogenesis in repeated pregnancies in antiepileptic drug-treated women. Epilepsia 2013;54(1):181–6.
69. Ikonomidou C, Bittigau P, Ishimaru MJ, et al. Ethanol-induced apoptotic neurodegeneration and fetal alcohol syndrome. Science 2000;287(5455):1056–60.
70. Bittigau P, Sifringer M, Genz K, et al. Antiepileptic drugs and apoptotic neurodegeneration in the developing brain. Proc Natl Acad Sci U S A 2002;99(23): 15089–94.
71. Bittigau P, Sifringer M, Ikonomidou C. Antiepileptic drugs and apoptosis in the developing brain. Ann N Y Acad Sci 2003;993:103–14.
72. Glier C, Dzietko M, Bittigau P, et al. Therapeutic doses of topiramate are not toxic to the developing rat brain. Exp Neurol 2004;187(2):403–9.
73. Manthey D, Asimiadou S, Stefovska V, et al. Sulthiame but not levetiracetam exerts neurotoxic effect in the developing rat brain. Exp Neurol 2005;193(2): 497–503.
74. Katz I, Kim J, Gale K, et al. Effects of lamotrigine alone and in combination with MK-801, phenobarbital, or phenytoin on cell death in the neonatal rat brain. J Pharmacol Exp Ther 2007;322(2):494–500.
75. Kim J, Kondratyev A, Gale K. Antiepileptic drug-induced neuronal cell death in the immature brain: effects of carbamazepine, topiramate, and levetiracetam as monotherapy versus polytherapy. J Pharmacol Exp Ther 2007;323(1):165–73.
76. Kim JS, Kondratyev A, Tomita Y, et al. Neurodevelopmental impact of antiepileptic drugs and seizures in the immature brain. Epilepsia 2007;48(Suppl 5): 19–26.
77. Forcelli PA, Kim J, Kondratyev A, et al. Pattern of antiepileptic drug-induced cell death in limbic regions of the neonatal rat brain. Epilepsia 2011;52(12):e207–11.
78. Kaushal S, Tamer Z, Opoku F, et al. Anticonvulsant drug-induced cell death in the developing white matter of the rodent brain. Epilepsia 2016;57(5):727–34.
79. Forcelli PA, Janssen MJ, Vicini S, et al. Neonatal exposure to antiepileptic drugs disrupts striatal synaptic development. Ann Neurol 2012;72(3):363–72.
80. Al-Muhtasib N, Sepulveda-Rodriguez A, Vicini S, et al. Neonatal phenobarbital exposure disrupts GABAergic synaptic maturation in rat CA1 neurons. Epilepsia 2018;59(2):333–44.

81. Vorhees CV. Developmental neurotoxicity induced by therapeutic and illicit drugs. Environ Health Perspect 1994;102(Suppl 2):145–53.
82. Forcelli PA, Kozlowski R, Snyder C, et al. Effects of neonatal antiepileptic drug exposure on cognitive, emotional, and motor function in adult rats. J Pharmacol Exp Ther 2012;340(3):558–66.
83. Gutherz SB, Kulick CV, Soper C, et al. Brief postnatal exposure to phenobarbital impairs passive avoidance learning and sensorimotor gating in rats. Epilepsy Behav 2014;37:265–9.
84. Li Y, Zhang S, Snyder MP, et al. Precision medicine in women with epilepsy: the challenge, systematic review, and future direction. Epilepsy Behav 2021;118: 107928.

Sleep and Epilepsy
Practical Implications

Madeleine M. Grigg-Damberger, MD[a],
Nancy Foldvary-Schaefer, DO, MS[b],*

KEYWORDS

- Sleep disorders • Sleep • Epilepsy • Antiseizure medications • Daytime sleepiness
- Insomnia • Obstructive sleep apnea

KEY POINTS

- Bidirectional relationships between sleep and epilepsy have significant implications on sleep health and epilepsy outcomes including quality of life in people with epilepsy.
- Insomnia and excessive daytime sleepiness are highly prevalent in people with epilepsy and may signify the presence of primary sleep disorders.
- Sleep–wake states and circadian timing have important implications on seizure occurrence and localizing the epileptogenic zone in epilepsy surgery candidates.
- Sleep deprivation is a key seizure trigger in genetic generalized epilepsies more so than in focal epilepsies.
- Sleep and impaired arousal play key roles in the pathophysiology of SUDEP and patients with epilepsy should not sleep in the prone position.

INTRODUCTION
Key Practical Relationships Between Sleep and Epilepsy

Sleep is a restorative balm for many, often less so for people with epilepsy. Complex bidirectional interactions between sleep and epilepsy can be detrimental to sleep, epilepsy and those affected.

Sleep-related seizures and epilepsy syndromes

Seizures in 10% to 15% of all epilepsies occur primarily or exclusively in sleep. Sleep and/or arousal from sleep are the sole triggers for seizures if awakening epilepsies included. Sleep-related epilepsies are currently classified as sleep-associated, sleep-accentuated or arousal epilepsies (**Table 1**). *Sleep-associated epilepsies*

---

[a] Department of Neurology, University of New Mexico, MSC10 5620, Albuquerque, NM 87131-0001, USA; [b] Sleep Disorders Center, Cleveland Clinic Neurological Institute, 9500 Euclid Avenue, S73, Cleveland, OH 44196, USA
* Corresponding author.
E-mail address: foldvan@ccf.org

Neurol Clin 40 (2022) 769–783
https://doi.org/10.1016/j.ncl.2022.03.008
0733-8619/22/© 2022 Elsevier Inc. All rights reserved.

Table 1		
Epilepsies associated with the sleep–wake cycle		
Sleep-Related	**Sleep-Accentuated**	**Awakening-Related**
• Benign focal epilepsy of childhood with centro-temporal spikes • Panayiotopoulos syndrome • Sleep-related hypermotor epilepsy	• Lennox–Gastaut syndrome • Landau–Kleffner syndrome • Epilepsy with continuous spike waves in sleep • West syndrome	• Juvenile myoclonic epilepsy • Epilepsy with grand mal seizures on awakening

(pure sleep epilepsies) are those in which seizures occur exclusively or primarily during sleep. Most pure sleep epilepsies are focal onset and typically begin in childhood. These include the most frequent syndromes of self-limited focal epilepsy in children: epilepsy with centrotemporal spikes (ECTS) and Panayiotopoulos syndrome (PS) which account for 20% and 13% of childhood epilepsies, respectively.[1] Seizures occur from NREM sleep, and remit before or during adolescence. Sleep-related hypermotor epilepsy (SHE) also most often begins in childhood but usually does not remit.[2] A longitudinal study of 139 patients with SHE followed a median of 16 years found only 22% achieved seizure remission, 28% followed for 30 years.[2] The estimated prevalence of SHE is 1.8/100,000 persons but SHE accounts for 10% of patients referred to epilepsy surgery evaluation.[3]

Sleep-accentuated epilepsies are those in which seizures occur both awake and asleep but interictal epileptiform discharges (IEDs) and sometimes particular types of seizure preferentially occur during sleep.[4] Most sleep-accentuated epilepsies again begin in childhood and are often epileptic encephalopathies: electrical status epilepticus of sleep (ESES), Landau–Kleffner syndrome (LKS), West syndrome (WS) and Lennox–Gastaut syndrome (LGS). The particular sleep-related seizure type often confirms the epilepsy syndrome diagnosis: 1) epileptic spasms in WS typically occur in clusters shortly after awakening from sleep and hypsarrhythmia is most evident during early NREM sleep[5–7]; 2) tonic seizures and/or paroxysmal fast activity (PFA) in NREM sleep help confirm LGS[8]; and 3) ESES warrants neuroimaging revealing perinatal thalamic lesions present in more than half.[9,10]

The most common arousal (awakening) epilepsies are juvenile myoclonic epilepsy (JME) and epilepsy with generalized tonic-clonic (GTC) seizures alone. The diagnosis of JME is missed if a history of myoclonic jerks upon awakening is omitted when taking a seizure history. JME accounts for 5% to 10% of all epilepsies.[11] Seizures in awakening epilepsies are triggered by sleep deprivation and forced early awakening.

Prevalence and impact of sleep disorder symptoms in people with epilepsy

More than 2 dozen studies across more than 3 decades have repeatedly found that sleep/wake disorders (SWDs) in AWE are 2 to 3 times more common than in the general population.[12–22] Using a variety of questionnaires, a 2020 case-control study found insomnia, sleep-disordered breathing (SDB) and restless legs syndrome (RLS) were much more common in 175 AWE than controls: 46% versus 25% for insomnia; 24% versus 5% SDB, and 21% versus 6% for RLS, respectively.[22]

SWDs cast long shadows on the lives of people with epilepsy. SWDs are associated with even lower quality of life (QoL) than in people with epilepsy without SWDs.[23–26] A 2019 case-control study of 122 outpatient AWE (half of whom had their last seizure more than 1 year earlier) found that those with SWDs had the lowest scores on nearly all domains of the Short Form Health Survey (SF-36).[26]

SWDs such as poor sleep quality or insomnia in AWE are also associated with poorer seizure control and more frequent seizures.[27–30] A 2021 cross-sectional population-based study found 22% of AWE who had poorer seizure control reported insomnia (vs 6% in whom epilepsy was controlled).[30] A 2020 prospective cross-sectional study found 53% of 123 AWE had poor sleep quality (based on the validated subjective sleep measure of the Pittsburgh Sleep Quality Index [PSQI scores $\geq$ 5), 50% insomnia symptoms (insomnia severity index [ISI] score $\geq$10), and 32% excessive daytime sleepiness (EDS) with an Epworth Sleepiness Score $\geq$10/24 [27]. Using multivariate analysis, the risk for poor seizure control was 2.8-fold higher in those who reported poor sleep quality, insomnia 1.9-fold.

Another 2020 study found that 43% of 75 consecutive AWE reported poor sleep quality and 24% EDS and patients with poor sleep quality had more frequent seizures.[28] A 2018 study found a PSQI score of $\geq$ 5 and/or an ESS $\geq$10 significantly increased the risk of seizure recurrence in 62 patients with JME followed for 6 months.[29]

Excessive daytime sleepiness is among the most common sleep/wake complaints reported by adults with epilepsy Prospective case-control questionnaire-based studies have found 11%-32% of AWE versus 5%-22% of healthy controls have an ESS score greater than 10 indicative of subjective EDS.[18–20,31–33] A case-control study comparing 180 AWE and 2836 healthy controls found EDS, poor sleep quality, and insomnia were significantly associated with epilepsy with odds ratio of 2.1, 3.5, and 5.9, respectively.[20]

When systematically assessed, subjective and objective hypersomnia is highly prevalent in AWE[34,35]. We systematically investigated subjective and objective sleepiness in 127 AWE using a battery of subjective and objective measures. Pathologic sleepiness with mean sleep latency (MSL) on the multiple sleep latency test (MSLT) < 8 min was present in half of AWE. Nearly one-third of AWE unselected for sleep/wake complaints had MSL $\leq$5 min, a range typical of narcolepsy. Hypersomnia was not explained by seizure frequency, ASM burden, symptoms of insomnia or depression, or PSG findings, although those with MSL less than 5 min were more likely to have OSA.

We recently used the maintenance of wakefulness (MWT) to evaluate the ability of adults with focal epilepsy to stay awake and alert in soporific settings. We found 45% of 41 AWE had abnormal mean sleep latency (<19.4 min), 16% had MSL in the range seen in narcolepsy (<8 min).[34] Only 2 variables predicted shorter MSL on the MWT: a history of focal bilateral tonic-clonic seizures and younger age. The lack of association between MWT parameters and ASMs is an important finding because various aspects of sleepiness are often misattributed to medications. This finding may be due in part to the high utilization of second-generation ASMs (67%) which are less likely to disrupt nocturnal sleep and cause EDS compared with first-generation agents.[21,36–38] Some have hypothesized that difficulty staying awake, alert, and vigilant in AWE may be due to abnormal connectivity of resting state and alertness networks, damaged by recurring seizures?[39–41] No clinical trials aimed at treating this debilitating complaint in AWE yet exist.

A 2021 multicenter cross-sectional study evaluated cognitive performance in 150 people with epilepsy $\geq$12 years of age and taking $\geq$1 ASM (mean age 41 $\pm$ 15 years).[42] They found: 44% reported poor quality sleep (PSQI $\geq$5); 20% reported EDS (ESS >12), and 33% had mild cognitive impairment (MCI) with Montreal Cognitive Assessment Test [MoCA] scores less than 26. Using multivariate regression analysis, they found older age and use of sleep medications, but not poor sleep quality, were independently associated with lower MoCA scores. Poor sleep quality was associated with symptoms of anxiety and depression, and directly correlated with

QoL. Sleep quality was worse in people with focal-onset compared with those with generalized-onset epilepsies.

Obstructive sleep apnea and its treatment in people with epilepsy

A 2017 meta-analysis found obstructive sleep apnea (OSA) was 2.4 times more common in AWE than in age-matched healthy controls and 3-fold more likely to occur in men with epilepsy than women.[43,44] We found OSA in 30% of 134 consecutive AWE neither selected nor referred for sleep disorder symptoms; moderate/severe (apnea–hypopnea index, AHI ≥15) in 16%.[45] Multivariate analysis showed male gender, age greater than 50 years, obesity, and hypertension were associated with higher apnea–hypopnea index (AHI) but only age and ASM burden predicted OSA based on an AHI ≥10.

Smaller studies have shown late-onset epilepsy, status epilepticus, or worsening epilepsy in middle-aged adults warrants consideration of often found untreated OSA.[43,46,47] One study found the onset of OSA symptoms coincided with the first episode of status epilepticus or a clear increase in seizure frequency in middle-aged individuals.[48] OSA was most likely to be found on polysomnography (PSG) in AWE who are older, sleepier, heavier and had their first seizure when older[49]

Positive airway pressure (PAP) therapy is the only OSA treatment extensively studied in AWE, yet still without randomized controlled trials (RCTs). A 2017 meta-analysis found AWE with OSA who were treated with CPAP had 5.3-fold better seizure control than those untreated and were 4-times more likely to be seizure-free.[44] We found among 132 AWE who had adherent use of CPAP significantly more likely to have ≥50% seizure reduction (74% CPAP-treated vs 14% untreated, respectively) and greater mean percentage of seizure reduction (59% vs 17%).[50] After adjusting for age, gender, body mass index, AHI, and epilepsy duration, the odds of successful outcomes in the PAP-treated AWE group were 9.9 and 3.9 times those of the groups with untreated OSA and no OSA, respectively. The group with PAP-treated OSA had 32.3 times the odds of having a ≥50% seizure reduction compared with the group with untreated OSA and 6.1 times compared with the group with no OSA.

Adherent use of PAP therapy can be challenging. A 2021 study examined factors contributing to long-term CPAP adherence in 58 AWE; 19% refused treatment outright, 58% adherent, and 22% showed irregular use.[51] Females with a lower number of total seizures and lower seizure frequency were more likely to be compliant.[51] Motivational interviewing and cognitive-behavioral therapy techniques to improve PAP compliance (including addressing fears and concerns) and engaging support of family and caregivers are associated with greater likelihood of adherence.[52] Adherent PAP use can be achieved in people with intellectual disabilities in whom the expectation that PAP would not be tolerated was the main reason for not trying it.[53] Alternatives to PAP therapy including oral appliances, upper airway surgery, weight loss, and hypoglossal nerve stimulation have not been studied in epilepsy populations.

Risk for sleep deprivation triggering seizures in generalized and focal epilepsies

The risk for sleep deprivation (SD) triggering seizures is greatest for genetic generalized epilepsies, especially JME.[54,55] A study found 77% of 75 patients with JME reported SD as their second most common seizure trigger (after stress).[56] Seizures in JME are facilitated by both sleep loss and sudden arousal.[57] The mean number and duration of seizures during sleep and on an awakening increase in JME following SD.[58] SD (often coupled with acute drug withdrawal and/or alcohol use) was a particularly common cause for recurrence of seizures after a long period of remission in 105 patients with JME.[55] Cautioning patients with JME (especially when adolescent) to maintain regular sleep/wake schedules and sufficient nighttime sleep often goes unheeded resulting in "activation by celebration." Impulsivity, difficulty making decisions, and other frontal executive dysfunctions in some patients with JME (especially when younger) may predispose them to SD.[59,60]

SD may play a weaker role for triggering seizures in focal epilepsies. A study of 19 patients with focal epilepsy who kept electronic diaries for 12–14 weeks found SD did not predict a seizure would occur 12–24 hours later.[61] Whereas, feeling emotional/tired/weary and/or difficulty with thought predicted a seizure likely to occur within 12 hours by odds ratios ranging from 2.0 to 3.4. Improvements in mood reduced the risk for seizures by 25%. A recent study using RNS data from 10 patients with medically refractory focal epilepsies found seizure probability changed with day-to-day variation in sleep duration.[62] An increase in sleep duration by 1.7 ± 0.5 h lowered the odds of seizure recurrence by 27% in the following 48 h. Patients slept longer after a seizure. If the seizure occurred in sleep, sleep quality was also reduced with increased time spent aroused from sleep and reduced REM sleep. The National Sleep Foundation recommends 7–9 h of sleep per night for adults. AWE should be routinely queried about sleep habits and educated on the hazards of chronic sleep deprivation that extends well beyond seizure control and includes cardiovascular, metabolic, and brain health and psychosocial functioning.[63]

Advances in the elucidation of semiology of sleep-related hypermotor epilepsy?

An international consensus conference in 2016 recommended changing the name of nocturnal frontal lobe epilepsy to SHE because: 1) 30% of cases emanate from extra-frontal foci (most often from the temporal or insular-opercular, occasionally from the posterior parietal or posterior cingulate regions)[64,65]; 2) seizures can occur from daytime naps; and 3) hypermotor features better characterize the seizure type.[66]

SHE is characterized by brief relatively stereotyped seizures with asymmetric tonic/dystonic posturing and/or complex hyperkinetic features such as bimanual and bipedal automatisms, kicking, cycling of limbs, and rocking body movements usually associated with explosive vocalizations.[66] Seizures most often occur from NREM 2 sleep.[3] Most patients with SHE also have subtle minor motor seizures characterized by abrupt movements of trunk and upper limbs accompanied by brief arousals which often occur in a quasiperiodic pattern throughout the night.[67]

Thirty percent of drug-resistant SHE epilepsies emanate from extra-frontal epileptic foci. Elegant work analyzing seizure characteristics in 43 patients with drug-resistant frontal and 15 with extra-frontal SHE who underwent stereo-EEG evaluation found: 1) median electrographic duration of frontal SHE seizures was 28 sec; extra-frontal 62 sec; 2) a clinical SHE seizure which lasted greater than 40 sec was more likely extra-frontal onset (sensitivity 55%, specificity 90%); 3) median time for the first video-detectable movement after electrographic seizure onset was significantly shorter for frontal onset seizures (5 sec) versus extra-frontal (18 sec); 4) hypermotor behaviors emerged at a mean of 1.6 sec in frontal seizures versus 9.8 sec in extra-frontal and those beginning greater than 5 sec after electrographic onset had a sensitivity of 75% and a specificity of 90% of extra-frontal onset.[68]

A 2019 retrospective analysis of SEEG recordings in 91 patients with frontal and 44 with extra-frontal SHE undergoing epilepsy surgery evaluation further identified 4 semiology patterns (SPs) of SHE seizure organized in a postero-anterior gradient (SP1-SP4).[69] They found integrated hypermotor movements (SP3) or gestural behaviors with high emotional content (SP4) were frequent, postictal confusion common, but elementary motor signs (SP1) rare in temporal SHE. Frontal SHE, particularly arising from the ventromesial frontal lobe also manifested with SP3 and SP4, however, were more likely to include SP1. In contrast, SP4 was absent in operculoinsular and posterior SHE. Operculoinsular seizures had more diverse semiology (SP1-SP3), while posterior SHE most commonly featured SP1. Last mentioned, searching for nonmotor manifestations (eg, sensory or cognitive auras) present in 70% often provided valuable localizing information.

A 2019 study found emotional facial expressions (fear, laughing, or anger), bilateral facial contraction, bilateral forceful elbow flexion or grasping, or facial flushing were more often observed in frontal onset SHE; oroalimentary automatisms, salivation, seizures awake, salivation, and the chapeau du gendarme sign in temporal onset SHE.[70] A 2020 study confirmed SHE seizures in patients with focal cortical dysplasia type 2 (FCD2) which occur following arousal from sleep are more likely to be extra-frontal onset.[71] Collectively, these features can improve the diagnostic accuracy of SHE and help differentiate it from arousal disorders.

Recently published studies have examined how to distinguish NREM arousal disorders (DOA) from SHE. A study comparing video-PSG recordings of 59 patients with a definite diagnosis of DOA and 30 with SHE found patients with SHE had a greater number of motor events (7 ± 8 per night) than those with DOA (3 ± 2).[72] DOA motor events occurred mostly in NREM 3, SHE in NREM 2. At least one *major* motor event occurring outside NREM 3 suggested SHE (sensitivity 79%, specificity 95%); at least one *minor* event during N3 DOA (73% sensitivity, 72% specificity).

Sleep and identification of the epileptogenic zone in epilepsy surgery evaluations

Pathologic high-frequency oscillations (HFOs, ripples >80 Hz) seem to be a promising biomarker for identifying the epileptogenic zone (EZ) in the epilepsy surgery evaluation.[73] HFOs have their maximal rate in the same sleep stages as IEDs. HFOs in all the brain regions except the frontal lobe are modulated by sleep. HFO rates are highest in NREM sleep (NREM 3 > 2 >1), lowest in wakefulness and REM sleep. Pathologic HFOs are most frequent inside the seizure onset zone (SOZ) than outside it.

A recent study found: 1) 79% of IEDs and 65% of HFOs were phase coupled with slow oscillations; 2) IEDs and pathogenic HFOs were preferentially coupled during the up-to-down transition of the slow oscillation waveform; and 3) nonpathogenic HFOs phase couple with the up phase of the slow oscillation waveform.[74] Neuronal hypersynchronization leading to IEDs and synchronization rather than hyperexcitability would then explain enhanced epileptic activity during sleep.[73]

These findings suggest NREM sleep is the best state to identify the EZ.[75,76] IEDs, HFOs, univariate and bivariate features in the interictal SEEG during the first 10 minutes of NREM 2 and NREM 3 sleep were not different from results achieved by analysis of the SOZ over 12.7 days of monitoring.[77] Use of this algorithm in NREM sleep might lead to more time-efficient invasive presurgical investigations.

Vagal nerve stimulation effects vocal cord, tongue and respiratory function in sleep

A systematic review addressed the effects of vagus nerve stimulation (VNS) and other surgical interventions on sleep.[78] VNS therapy can produce central apneas, obstructive hypopneas, and obstructive apneas in both adults and children.[79,80] One of the largest reports including 22 subjects found OSA after VNS implantation in 86%, severe in 36%, and hypoventilation in 27% of cases.[81] Respiratory events did not decrease significantly with CPAP or bilevel PAP therapy. VNS can also cause an increase in respiratory rate and a decrease in respiratory amplitude, tidal volume, and oxygen saturation during activation.[80] Recent studies confirmed laryngeal dysfunction and glossoptosis, "trap door" of the epiglottis, during VNS stimulation.[82,83] The manufacturer recommends screening for OSA and to consider performing PSG prior and following VNS implantation.[80,84,85] A left lateral cervical EMG electrode placed over the VNS wire is required to correlate VNS activation with airflow and effort signals (**Fig. 1**).

Circadian effects on epilepsy

More than 90% of people with epilepsy have circadian rhythmicity of seizure expression, and many also experience multiday, weekly or longer cycles.[86] Some of these cycles and rhythms are related to sleep itself. The Epilepsy Phenome/Genome Project (EPGP) assessed sleep/wake timing of seizures in 1395 subjects and 546 families and found: 1) seizures in nonacquired focal epilepsy were more likely to occur during sleep than generalized epilepsies with an odds ratio (OR) of 5.2 for convulsive and 4.2 for nonconvulsive seizures; 2) seizures occurring within 1 hour of awakening were more likely to occur in patients with generalized than nonacquired focal epilepsy for both convulsive and nonconvulsive seizures (with OR of 2.3 and 1.7, respectively); 3) frontal onset seizures were more likely than temporal onset seizures to occur during sleep; and 4) seep/wake timing of seizures in first degree relatives predicted timing of seizures in the proband.[87]

Inpatient video-EEG monitoring and seizure diary studies have shown that: 1) frontal lobe seizures occur most often in sleep with an early morning peak; 2) mesial temporal lobe seizures have 2 circadian peaks in morning and late afternoon; and 3) occipital seizures peak in early evening and rarely occur in sleep.[88-91]

Data from neuromodulation devices are providing insight into relationships between seizures, sleep/wake states, and biological rhythm timing. A 2018 study using data from 37 patients with drug-resistant focal onset epilepsy implanted with Neuropace RNS neuromodulatory system found IEDs exhibited multidien rhythms (most often 20–30 days) and seizures occurred preferentially in the rising phase of multidien rhythm.[92] All seizure detections in 134 adults treated with NeuroPace studied over a continuous 84-day period showed a strongly circadian and uniform pattern irrespective of the region of onset that peaked during normal sleep hours.[93] However, long detections varied by region with a monophasic, nocturnally dominant rhythm in neocortical seizures and a more complex pattern and diurnal peak in limbic seizures. These findings have important implications for treatment and safety for patients and caregivers.

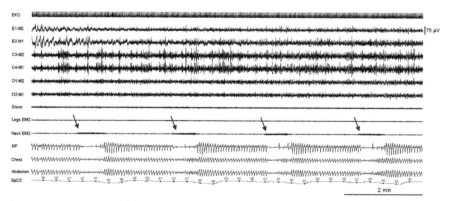

Fig. 1. Vagus nerve stimulation-induced respiratory events illustrated is a 10-min PSG epoch demonstrating reduced flow and respiratory effort coinciding with device activation recorded by a surface electrode over the left lateral neck region.

Roles of sleep and sleep apnea in sudden unexpected death in epilepsy?

Sudden unexpected death in epilepsy (SUDEP) accounts for 15% of epilepsy-related deaths with an incidence of 1.2 per 1000 person years in AWE[94] and lifetime risk of 4.6% to 8%.[95,96] AWE have a 2.5-fold higher mortality rate and 27-fold higher rate of sudden death than the general population.[97]

SUDEP occurs more frequently at night and in the prone position A 2017 systematic review and meta-analysis found that 69% of 880 SUDEP cases occurred in sleep, 31% awake, $P < .001$.[98] A large case-control study found nocturnal seizures increased the risk for SUDEP 2.6-fold after controlling for other risk factors.[99] Seizures from sleep are associated with more severe and longer oxygen desaturations, and are more frequently followed by postictal generalized EEG suppression compared with seizures during wakefulness.[99,100]

Moderate/severe OSA may increase SUDEP risk. We recently found that AWE who had PSG-confirmed moderate/severe OSA had significantly higher rSUDEP-7 inventory scores.[101] Severe OSA (AHI >30) increases the risk for sudden cardiac death during sleep 2.6-fold.[102] Sleep impacts on airway patency, arousal and ventilatory responses to hypoxia and hypercapnia: 1) airway patency is decreased in sleep increasing the likelihood of airway occlusion; 2) inspiratory drive is lower in NREM and lowest in REM sleep; 3) hypoxic and hypercapnic ventilatory responses show circadian rhythms and are higher in the morning and afternoon, lower at night and during sleep leading to lower oxygen saturation and higher CO2 values.[103–106] The QT interval is longer in sleep and later in the night which could lower the threshold for ventricular fibrillation.[107] Cardiac responses to vagal stimuli (eg, ocular compression) show a circadian rhythm with greatest responses occurring in the late night and early hours of the morning.[108]

SUDEP may represent a perfect storm of respiratory, cardiac, arousal, and serotonergic neuronal dysfunction.[109] Caudal brain serotonergic neurons play crucial roles in coordinating control of breathing, arousal, respiratory rhythm generation, blood pressure regulation, thermoregulation, upper airway reflexes, chemosensitivity, and synaptic plasticity. Neuronal activity in these serotonergic neurons in raphe nucleus is highest in wakefulness, reduced in NREM and nearly silent in REM sleep.[110] Impaired serotonergic function following nocturnal seizures may predispose to SUDEP. 5-HT neurons seem to mediate the life-preserving arousal responses to hypercapnia by stimulating arousal.[111,112]

SUMMARY

A variety of bidirectional relationships between sleep and epilepsy have significant clinical implications. At least 10% to 15% of all epilepsies are sleep-related and semiology characteristics are important in diagnosing these. Sleep/wake disorders are more common in AWE than the general population and associated with lower health-related QoL and poorer seizure control. Sleep maybe the best state in people with epilepsy to identify the epileptogenic zone for successful epilepsy surgery and/or neuromodulation and is a state of vulnerability for SUDEP. Identifying and treating SWDs in people with epilepsy and education about sleep position can improve seizure control and QoL and potentially reduce SUDEP.

CLINICS CARE POINTS

- Ten to 15% of all epilepsies are sleep-related. A clinical history of seizures types by sleep–wake state can help confirm certain epilepsy syndromes.

- Obstructive sleep apnea is highly prevalent in AWE of both genders and all ages and is not associated with all the typical risks factors and signs of symptoms, thus necessitating a low index of suspicion. Treatment of OSA reduces seizures in observational series.

- Sleep deprivation triggers seizures in only some people with epilepsy. The risk is greatest for genetic generalized epilepsies and much weaker in focal epilepsies.

- Pathologic HFOs are a promising biomarker for identifying the epileptogenic zone in the epilepsy surgery evaluation. Like IEDs in focal epilepsies, HFO rates are highest in NREM sleep (NREM 3 > 2 >1), lowest in wakefulness and REM sleep.

- Poor sleep quality and insomnia are associated with poorer seizure control. Cognitive-behavioral therapy for insomnia has demonstrated effectiveness in AWE.

- Subjective and objective hypersomnia is highly prevalent in AWE and is associated with poorer QoL but not consistently with ASMs. Sleep laboratory evaluation should be considered in these cases.

- Approximately 70% of SUDEP cases occur in sleep and patients with nocturnal seizures are significantly more likely to die in a prone position than those with diurnal seizures. A lateral decubitus sleep position or supine sleep position in the absence of OSA is recommended in people with epilepsy.

DISCLOSURE

The authors have nothing to disclose.

REFERENCES

1. Pal DK, Ferrie C, Addis L, et al. Idiopathic focal epilepsies: the "lost tribe. Epileptic Disord 2016;18(3):252–88.
2. Licchetta L, Bisulli F, Vignatelli L, et al. Sleep-related hypermotor epilepsy: Long-term outcome in a large cohort. Neurology 2017;88(1):70–7.
3. Menghi V, Bisulli F, Tinuper P, et al. Sleep-related hypermotor epilepsy: prevalence, impact and management strategies. Nat Sci Sleep 2018;10:317–26.
4. Gardella E, Cantalupo G, Larsson PG, et al. EEG features in encephalopathy related to status epilepticus during slow sleep. Epileptic Disord 2019;21(S1): 22–30.
5. Guerrini R, Pellock JM. Age-related epileptic encephalopathies. Handb Clin Neurol 2012;107:179–93.
6. Watanabe K, Negoro T, Aso K, et al. Reappraisal of interictal electroencephalograms in infantile spasms. Epilepsia 1993;34(4):679–85.
7. Koutroumanidis M, Arzimanoglou A, Caraballo R, et al. The role of EEG in the diagnosis and classification of the epilepsy syndromes: a tool for clinical practice by the ILAE Neurophysiology Task Force (Part 2). Epileptic Disord 2017; 19(4):385–437.
8. Arzimanoglou A, French J, Blume WT, et al. Lennox-Gastaut syndrome: a consensus approach on diagnosis, assessment, management, and trial methodology. Lancet Neurol 2009;8(1):82–93.
9. Gibbs SA, Nobili L, Halász P. Interictal epileptiform discharges in sleep and the role of the thalamus in encephalopathy related to status epilepticus during slow sleep. Epileptic Disord 2019;21(S1):54–61.
10. van den Munckhof B, Zwart AF, Weeke LC, et al. Perinatal thalamic injury: MRI predictors of electrical status epilepticus in sleep and long-term neurodevelopment. NeuroImage Clin 2020;26:102227.

11. Camfield CS, Striano P, Camfield PR. Epidemiology of juvenile myoclonic epilepsy. Epilepsy Behav 2013;28(Suppl 1):S15–7.
12. Giorelli AS, Neves GS, Venturi M, et al. Excessive daytime sleepiness in patients with epilepsy: a subjective evaluation. Epilepsy Behav 2011;21(4):449–52.
13. Krishnan P, Sinha S, Taly AB, et al. Sleep disturbances in juvenile myoclonic epilepsy: a sleep questionnaire-based study. Epilepsy Behav 2012;23(3):305–9.
14. Chen NC, Tsai MH, Chang CC, et al. Sleep quality and daytime sleepiness in patients with epilepsy. Acta Neurol Taiwan 2011;20(4):249–56.
15. Maestri M, Giorgi FS, Pizzanelli C, et al. Daytime sleepiness in de novo untreated patients with epilepsy. Epilepsy Behav 2013;29(2):344–8.
16. Ruangkana P, Chinvarun Y, Udommongkol C, et al. Excessive daytime sleepiness and obstructive sleep apnea in Thai epileptic patients. J Med Assoc Thai 2014;97(Suppl 2):S175–80.
17. Yazdi Z, Sadeghniiat-Haghighi K, Naimian S, et al. Prevalence of sleep disorders and their effects on sleep quality in epileptic patients. Basic Clin Neurosci 2013;4(1):36–41.
18. Piperidou C, Karlovasitou A, Triantafyllou N, et al. Influence of sleep disturbance on quality of life of patients with epilepsy. Seizure 2008;17(7):588–94.
19. Gammino M, Zummo L, Bue AL, et al. Excessive daytime sleepiness and sleep disorders in a population of patients with epilepsy: a case-control study. J Epilepsy Res 2016;6(2):79–86.
20. Im HJ, Park SH, Baek SH, et al. Associations of impaired sleep quality, insomnia, and sleepiness with epilepsy: A questionnaire-based case-control study. Epilepsy Behav 2016;57(Pt A):55–9.
21. Foldvary-Schaefer N, Neme-Mercante S, Andrews N, et al. Wake up to sleep: the effects of lacosamide on daytime sleepiness in adults with epilepsy. Epilepsy Behav 2017;75:176–82.
22. Khachatryan SG, Ghahramanyan L, Tavadyan Z, et al. Sleep-related movement disorders in a population of patients with epilepsy: prevalence and impact of restless legs syndrome and sleep bruxism. J Clin Sleep Med 2020;16(3):409–14.
23. Xu X, Brandenburg NA, McDermott AM, et al. Sleep disturbances reported by refractory partial-onset epilepsy patients receiving polytherapy. Epilepsia 2006;47(7):1176–83.
24. Manni R, Tartara A. Evaluation of sleepiness in epilepsy. Clin Neurophysiol 2000;111(Suppl 2):S111–4.
25. Khatami R, Zutter D, Siegel A, et al. Sleep-wake habits and disorders in a series of 100 adult epilepsy patients–a prospective study. Seizure 2006;15(5):299–306.
26. Gutter T, Callenbach PMC, Brouwer OF, et al. Prevalence of sleep disturbances in people with epilepsy and the impact on quality of life: a survey in secondary care. Seizure 2019;69:298–303.
27. Planas-Ballve A, Grau-Lopez L, Jimenez M, et al. Insomnia and poor sleep quality are associated with poor seizure control in patients with epilepsy. Neurologia 2020;11:S0213-4853(19)30139-2.
28. Çilliler AE, Güven B. Sleep quality and related clinical features in patients with epilepsy: A preliminary report. Epilepsy Behav 2020;102:106661.
29. Buratti L, Natanti A, Viticchi G, et al. Impact of sleep disorders on the risk of seizure recurrence in juvenile myoclonic epilepsy. Epilepsy Behav 2018;80:21–4.

30. Tian N, Wheaton AG, Zack M, et al. Sleep duration and quality among U.S. adults with epilepsy: National Health Interview Survey 2013, 2015, and 2017. Epilepsy Behav 2021;122:108194.
31. Malow BA, Bowes RJ, Lin X. Predictors of sleepiness in epilepsy patients. Sleep 1997;20(12):1105–10.
32. Pizzatto R, Lin K, Watanabe N, et al. Excessive sleepiness and sleep patterns in patients with epilepsy: a case-control study. Epilepsy Behav 2013;29(1):63–6.
33. Ismayilova V, Demir AU, Tezer FI. Subjective sleep disturbance in epilepsy patients at an outpatient clinic: a questionnaire-based study on prevalence. Epilepsy Res 2015;115:119–25.
34. Gorantla S, Foldvary-Schaefer N, Andrews N, et al. High prevalence of pathological alertness and wakefulness on maintenance of wakefulness test in adults with focal-onset epilepsy. Epilepsy Behav 2021;125:108400.
35. Grigg-Damberger M, Andrews N, Wang L, et al. Subjective and objective hypersomnia highly prevalent in adults with epilepsy. Epilepsy Behav 2020;106:107023.
36. Foldvary-Schaefer N, De Leon Sanchez I, Karafa M, et al. Gabapentin increases slow-wave sleep in normal adults. Epilepsia 2002;43(12):1493–7.
37. Foldvary N, Perry M, Lee J, et al. The effects of lamotrigine on sleep in patients with epilepsy. Epilepsia 2001;42(12):1569–73.
38. Shvarts V, Chung S. Epilepsy, antiseizure therapy, and sleep cycle parameters. Epilepsy Res Treat 2013;2013:670682.
39. Gao YJ, Wang X, Xiong PG, et al. Abnormalities of the default-mode network homogeneity and executive dysfunction in people with first-episode, treatment-naive left temporal lobe epilepsy. Eur Rev Med Pharmacol Sci 2021;25(4):2039–49.
40. Gao Y, Zheng J, Li Y, et al. Decreased functional connectivity and structural deficit in alertness network with right-sided temporal lobe epilepsy. Medicine (Baltimore) 2018;97(14):e0134.
41. Zheng J, Qin B, Dang C, et al. Alertness network in patients with temporal lobe epilepsy: a fMRI study. Epilepsy Res 2012;100(1–2):67–73.
42. Fonseca E, Campos Blanco DM, Castro Vilanova MD, et al. Relationship between sleep quality and cognitive performance in patients with epilepsy. Epilepsy Behav 2021;122:108127.
43. Maurousset A, De Toffol B, Praline J, et al. High incidence of obstructive sleep apnea syndrome in patients with late-onset epilepsy. Neurophysiol Clin 2017;47(1):55–61.
44. Lin Z, Si Q, Xiaoyi Z. Obstructive sleep apnoea in patients with epilepsy: a meta-analysis. Sleep Breath 2017;21(2):263–70.
45. Foldvary-Schaefer N, Andrews ND, Pornsriniyom D, et al. Sleep apnea and epilepsy: who's at risk? Epilepsy Behav 2012;25(3):363–7.
46. Chihorek AM, Abou-Khalil B, Malow BA. Obstructive sleep apnea is associated with seizure occurrence in older adults with epilepsy. Neurology 2007;69(19):1823–7.
47. Haut SR, Katz M, Masur J, et al. Seizures in the elderly: impact on mental status, mood, and sleep. Epilepsy Behav 2009;14(3):540–4.
48. Hollinger P, Khatami R, Gugger M, et al. Epilepsy and obstructive sleep apnea. Eur Neurol 2006;55(2):74–9.
49. Manni R, Terzaghi M, Arbasino C, et al. Obstructive sleep apnea in a clinical series of adult epilepsy patients: frequency and features of the comorbidity. Epilepsia 2003;44(6):836–40.

50. Pornsriniyom D, Kim H, Bena J, et al. Effect of positive airway pressure therapy on seizure control in patients with epilepsy and obstructive sleep apnea. Epilepsy Behav 2014;37:270–5.

51. Şenel GB, Karadeniz D. Factors determining the long-term compliance with PAP therapy in patients with sleep-related epilepsy. Clin Neurol Neurosurg 2021;202: 106498.

52. Rapelli G, Pietrabissa G, Manzoni GM, et al. Improving CPAP adherence in adults with obstructive sleep apnea syndrome: a scoping review of motivational interventions. Front Psychol 2021;12:705364.

53. van den Broek N, Broer L, Vandenbussche N, et al. Obstructive sleep apnea in people with intellectual disabilities: adherence to and effect of CPAP. Sleep Breath 2021;25(3):1257–65.

54. Serafini A, Rubboli G, Gigli GL, et al. Neurophysiology of juvenile myoclonic epilepsy. Epilepsy Behav 2013;28(Suppl 1):S30–9.

55. Sokic D, Ristic AJ, Vojvodic N, et al. Frequency, causes and phenomenology of late seizure recurrence in patients with juvenile myoclonic epilepsy after a long period of remission. Seizure 2007;16(6):533–7.

56. da Silva Sousa P, Lin K, Garzon E, et al. Self-perception of factors that precipitate or inhibit seizures in juvenile myoclonic epilepsy. Seizure : J Br Epilepsy Assoc 2005;14(5):340–6.

57. Genton P, Thomas P, Kasteleijn-Nolst Trenite DG, et al. Clinical aspects of juvenile myoclonic epilepsy. Epilepsy Behav 2013;28(Suppl 1):S8–14.

58. Sousa NA, Sousa Pda S, Garzon E, et al. [EEG recording after sleep deprivation in a series of patients with juvenile myoclonic epilepsy]. Arq Neuropsiquiatr 2005;63(2B):383–8.

59. Zamarian L, Hofler J, Kuchukhidze G, et al. Decision making in juvenile myoclonic epilepsy. J Neurol 2013;260(3):839–46.

60. Pung T, Schmitz B. Circadian rhythm and personality profile in juvenile myoclonic epilepsy. Epilepsia 2006;47(Suppl 2):111–4.

61. Haut SR, Hall CB, Borkowski T, et al. Clinical features of the pre-ictal state: mood changes and premonitory symptoms. Epilepsy Behav 2012;23(4):415–21.

62. Dell KL, Payne DE, Kremen V, et al. Seizure likelihood varies with day-to-day variations in sleep duration in patients with refractory focal epilepsy: a longitudinal electroencephalography investigation. EClinicalMedicine 2021;37:100934.

63. Hirshkowitz M, Whiton K, Albert SM, et al. National Sleep Foundation's sleep time duration recommendations: methodology and results summary. Sleep Health 2015;1(1):40–3.

64. Proserpio P, Cossu M, Francione S, et al. Insular-opercular seizures manifesting with sleep-related paroxysmal motor behaviors: a stereo-EEG study. Epilepsia 2011;52(10):1781–91.

65. Gibbs SA, Proserpio P, Terzaghi M, et al. Sleep-related epileptic behaviors and non-REM-related parasomnias: Insights from stereo-EEG. Sleep Med Rev 2016; 25:4–20.

66. Tinuper P, Bisulli F, Cross JH, et al. Definition and diagnostic criteria of sleep-related hypermotor epilepsy. Neurology 2016;86(19):1834–42.

67. Tinuper P, Bisulli F. From nocturnal frontal lobe epilepsy to sleep-related hypermotor epilepsy: a 35-year diagnostic challenge. Seizure 2017;44:87–92.

68. Gibbs SA, Proserpio P, Francione S, et al. Seizure duration and latency of hypermotor manifestations distinguish frontal from extrafrontal onset in sleep-related hypermotor epilepsy. Epilepsia 2018;59(9):e130–4.

69. Gibbs SA, Proserpio P, Francione S, et al. Clinical features of sleep-related hypermotor epilepsy in relation to the seizure-onset zone: a review of 135 surgically treated cases. Epilepsia 2019;60(4):707–17.
70. Nitta N, Usui N, Kondo A, et al. Semiology of hyperkinetic seizures of frontal versus temporal lobe origin. Epileptic Disord 2019;21(2):154–65.
71. Eltze CM, Landre E, Soufflet C, et al. Sleep related epilepsy in focal cortical dysplasia type 2: insights from sleep recordings in presurgical evaluation. Clin Neurophysiol 2020;131(3):609–15.
72. Proserpio P, Loddo G, Zubler F, et al. Polysomnographic features differentiating disorder of arousals from sleep-related hypermotor epilepsy. Sleep 2019;42(12).
73. Frauscher B, Gotman J. Sleep, oscillations, interictal discharges, and seizures in human focal epilepsy. Neurobiol Dis 2019;127:545–53.
74. Weiss SA, Song I, Leng M, et al. Ripples have distinct spectral properties and phase-amplitude coupling with slow waves, but indistinct unit firing, in human epileptogenic hippocampus. Front Neurol 2020;11:174.
75. Frauscher B. Localizing the epileptogenic zone. Curr Opin Neurol 2020;33(2): 198–206.
76. Li J, Grinenko O, Mosher JC, et al. Learning to define an electrical biomarker of the epileptogenic zone. Hum Brain Mapp 2020;41(2):429–41.
77. Klimes P, Cimbalnik J, Brazdil M, et al. NREM sleep is the state of vigilance that best identifies the epileptogenic zone in the interictal electroencephalogram. Epilepsia 2019;60(12):2404–15.
78. Romero-Osorio Ó, Gil-Tamayo S, Nariño D, et al. Changes in sleep patterns after vagus nerve stimulation, deep brain stimulation or epilepsy surgery: Systematic review of the literature. Seizure 2018;56:4–8.
79. Nagarajan L, Walsh P, Gregory P, et al. Respiratory pattern changes in sleep in children on vagal nerve stimulation for refractory epilepsy. Can J Neurol Sci 2003;30(3):224–7.
80. Parhizgar F, Nugent K, Raj R. Obstructive sleep apnea and respiratory complications associated with vagus nerve stimulators. J Clin Sleep Med 2011;7(4): 401–7.
81. Dye TJ, Hantragool S, Carosella C, et al. Sleep disordered breathing in children receiving vagus nerve stimulation therapy. Sleep Med 2021;79:101–6.
82. Oliveira Santos M, Bentes C, Teodoro T, et al. Complex sleep-disordered breathing after vagus nerve stimulation: broadening the spectrum of adverse events of special interest. Epileptic Disord 2020;22(6):790–6.
83. Zambrelli E, Saibene AM, Furia F, et al. Laryngeal motility alteration: A missing link between sleep apnea and vagus nerve stimulation for epilepsy. Epilepsia 2016;57(1):e24–7.
84. Oh DM, Johnson J, Shah B, et al. Treatment of vagus nerve stimulator-induced sleep-disordered breathing: A case series. Epilepsy Behav Rep 2019;12: 100325.
85. Available at: https://www.livanova.com/epilepsy-vnstherapy/en-gb/safety-information
86. Stirling RE, Cook MJ, Grayden DB, et al. Seizure forecasting and cyclic control of seizures. Epilepsia 2021;62(Suppl 1): S2–s14.
87. Winawer MR, Shih J, Beck ES, et al. Genetic effects on sleep/wake variation of seizures. Epilepsia 2016;57(4):557–65.
88. Herman ST, Walczak TS, Bazil CW. Distribution of partial seizures during the sleep–wake cycle: differences by seizure onset site. Neurology 2001;56(11): 1453–9.

89. Durazzo TS, Spencer SS, Duckrow RB, et al. Temporal distributions of seizure occurrence from various epileptogenic regions. Neurology 2008;70(15): 1265–71.

90. Nzwalo H, Menezes Cordeiro I, Santos AC, et al. 24-hour rhythmicity of seizures in refractory focal epilepsy. Epilepsy Behav 2016;55:75–8.

91. Karafin M, St Louis EK, Zimmerman MB, et al. Bimodal ultradian seizure periodicity in human mesial temporal lobe epilepsy. Seizure 2010;19(6):347–51.

92. Baud MO, Kleen JK, Mirro EA, et al. Multi-day rhythms modulate seizure risk in epilepsy. Nat Commun 2018;9(1):88.

93. Spencer DC, Sun FT, Brown SN, et al. Circadian and ultradian patterns of epileptiform discharges differ by seizure-onset location during long-term ambulatory intracranial monitoring. Epilepsia 2016;57(9):1495–502.

94. DeGiorgio CM, Curtis A, Hertling D, et al. Sudden unexpected death in epilepsy: Risk factors, biomarkers, and prevention. Acta Neurol Scand 2019;139(3): 220–30.

95. Shorvon S, Tomson T. Sudden unexpected death in epilepsy. Lancet 2011; 378(9808):2028–38.

96. Thurman DJ, Hesdorffer DC, French JA. Sudden unexpected death in epilepsy: assessing the public health burden. Epilepsia 2014;55(10):1479–85.

97. Holst AG, Winkel BG, Risgaard B, et al. Epilepsy and risk of death and sudden unexpected death in the young: a nationwide study. Epilepsia 2013;54(9): 1613–20.

98. Ali A, Wu S, Issa NP, et al. Association of sleep with sudden unexpected death in epilepsy. Epilepsy Behav 2017;76:1–6.

99. Lamberts RJ, Thijs RD, Laffan A, et al. Sudden unexpected death in epilepsy: people with nocturnal seizures may be at highest risk. Epilepsia 2012;53(2): 253–7.

100. Latreille V, Abdennadher M, Dworetzky BA, et al. Nocturnal seizures are associated with more severe hypoxemia and increased risk of postictal generalized EEG suppression. Epilepsia 2017;58(9):e127–31.

101. Soontornpun AAN, Bena J, Grigg-Damberger M, et al. Obstructive sleep apnea is a risk factor for sudden unexplained death in epilepsy (SUDEP). Sleep 2021; 43:A310.

102. Gami AS, Howard DE, Olson EJ, et al. Day-night pattern of sudden death in obstructive sleep apnea. N Engl J Med 2005;352(12):1206–14.

103. Sowho M, Amatoury J, Kirkness JP, et al. Sleep and respiratory physiology in adults. Clin Chest Med 2014;35(3):469–81.

104. Abbott SBG, Souza G. Chemoreceptor mechanisms regulating CO_2 -induced arousal from sleep. J Physiol 2021;599(10):2559–71.

105. Kaur S, Saper CB. Neural Circuitry Underlying Waking Up to Hypercapnia. Front Neurosci 2019;13:401.

106. Haxhiu MA, Mack SO, Wilson CG, et al. Sleep networks and the anatomic and physiologic connections with respiratory control. Front Biosci 2003;8: d946–62.

107. Gula LJ, Krahn AD, Skanes AC, et al. Clinical relevance of arrhythmias during sleep: guidance for clinicians. Heart 2004;90(3):347–52.

108. Ramet J, Hauser B, Waldura J, et al. Circadian rhythm of cardiac responses to vagal stimulation tests. Pediatr Neurol 1992;8(2):91–6.

109. Bozorgi A, Lhatoo SD. Seizures, cerebral shutdown, and SUDEP: SUDEP – a perfect storm. Epilepsy Currents 2013;13(5):236–40.

110. Trulson ME, Jacobs BL. Raphe unit activity in freely moving cats: correlation with level of behavioral arousal. Brain Res 1979;163(1):135–50.
111. Buchanan GF, Richerson GB. Central serotonin neurons are required for arousal to CO2. Proc Natl Acad Sci U S A 2010;107(37):16354–9.
112. Buchanan GF, Richerson GB. Role of chemoreceptors in mediating dyspnea. Respir Physiol Neurobiol 2009;167(1):9–19.

Dietary Treatments for Epilepsy

Babitha Haridas, MBBS*, Eric H. Kossoff, MD

KEYWORDS

• Ketogenic diet • Ketosis • Refractory • Epilepsy • Glut1 deficiency

KEY POINTS

- The ketogenic diet therapy is a useful and effective therapy for epilepsy.
- It is the treatment of choice for certain metabolic conditions, such as Glut1 deficiency and pyruvate dehydrogenase deficiency.
- It has been recently found to be an effective antiseizure therapy in superrefractory status epilepticus.

INTRODUCTION

The year 2021 marks exactly a century from when the ketogenic diet (KD) was first reported in the medical literature as a useful antiseizure therapy.[1] With the advent of newer antiseizure medications (ASMs), the KD was rarely used in the United States until it caught the public's interest in 1994 when it produced seizure freedom in a child with refractory epilepsy (www.charliefoundation.org).[2] This led to several clinical trials, thus solidifying the role of the KD as one of the four major treatments for epilepsy, along with ASMs, neuromodulation, and surgery. The success of KD therapy (KDT) in children has resulted in its expansion to the adult population and for indications outside of epilepsy.

Although the advantages of the KD were seen at its inception, there have been several alternative diet therapies that have been formulated in the past 20 years to maintain efficacy while maximizing tolerability, hence expanding its use to a larger population. Alternative diet therapies include the medium-chain triglyceride (MCT) diet, low glycemic index treatment (LGIT), and modified Atkins diet (MAD). During the course of this review, we discuss the administration of KDT and highlight its role for specific epilepsy syndromes.

Departments of Neurology and Pediatrics, Johns Hopkins University, Johns Hopkins Hospital, Suite 2158, 200 North Wolfe Street, Baltimore, MD 21287, USA
* Corresponding author.
E-mail address: bharida1@jh.edu

Neurol Clin 40 (2022) 785–797
https://doi.org/10.1016/j.ncl.2022.03.009

KETOGENIC DIET OPTIONS
Classic Ketogenic Diet

The classic KD (CKD) is a high fat, adequate protein, low-carbohydrate diet that has been in use since 1921. It is administered using a ratio of fats to carbohydrates and proteins, typically at 4:1, using a gram scale to weigh food portions. In patients reporting poor tolerability, those having fat-related side effects, infants, and adolescents, a ratio of 3:1 or lower is used.[3] Studies have shown that 4:1 has better efficacy in children with Lennox-Gastaut syndrome, with seizure freedom in 55% of patients, compared with 31% of patients in the 3:1 KD group at 3 months.[4] At the CKD's creation, the total amount of calories and fluids were restricted to 75% to 80% of typical recommendations for age.[5] These parameters are no longer restricted, although they are measured by an experienced ketogenic dietician to gain a complete assessment of the ratio of the diet.

Medium-Chain Triglyceride Diet

Although the CKD uses mostly long-chain triglycerides, the MCT diet focuses on MCTs, which yield more ketones per kilocalorie of energy.[6] The higher ketogenic potential of MCT provides more allowance for carbohydrates and protein in this modification, thus potentially improving tolerability. Because the traditional MCT diet was associated with gastrointestinal side effects, most centers today use a modified MCT diet wherein 30% of energy is derived from MCT and 30% is derived from long-chain fatty acids.[3] A randomized controlled trial (RCT) comparing the CKD and MCT diet found both to be of equal efficacy.[7]

Low Glycemic Index Treatment

The LGIT was formulated to optimize the tolerability of the KD using more carbohydrates, but with permitted carbohydrates having a low glycemic index (typically <50).[8] In this diet therapy, patients are typically not producing ketones in their urine. Pfeifer and Thiele[8] noted that 8/11 patients treated solely with LGIT demonstrated greater than 50% reduction in seizures with four of these patients becoming seizure free. Additional studies with a larger group of patients found that there was greater than 50% reduction from baseline seizure frequency in 42% to 66% of the population with follow-up at 1 to 12 months.[9] An RCT found that at 3 months, 6 out of 20 (30%) patients achieved more than 50% seizure reduction from baseline. Two of these six patients had more than 90% seizure reduction.[10] These studies have also noted that although an increase in efficacy was seen with lower glucose levels at some time points, there was no correlation with β-hydroxybutyrate levels.[9]

Modified Atkins Diet

MAD is a high-fat, low-carbohydrate therapy that provides approximately 1:1 to 2:1 ketogenic ratio.[3] A ketogenic ratio is not tabulated/followed because of significant daily variability. Carbohydrates are restricted to 20 g/day, fats are strongly encouraged to maintain ketosis, and protein is not measured.[5] Efficacy trials have revealed 65% had greater than 50% seizure reduction at 6 months, including 35% with greater than 90% improvement.[11] An RCT comparing MAD with the CKD revealed comparable efficacy, although the MAD was better tolerated.[12] There was a significantly higher reduction in seizures in children younger than 2 years of age who were treated with the KD, compared with the MAD.[12]

A recent multicenter RCT compared CKD with the MAD and LGIT in 158 children and found there was a reduction in median daily seizures from nine to three per day with CKD and four with the MAD and LGIT. MAD and LGIT were not inferior in comparison with KD. There was a rapid reduction in seizures by 40% to 50% in the first 4 weeks of CKD and MAD initiation, whereas the benefit with LGIT was gradual with a 50% reduction by 10 to 12 weeks.[13]

INITIATION OF THE KETOGENIC DIET
Preinitiation

The International Ketogenic Diet Study Group (IKDSG) consensus statement from 2018 has strongly advised a clinic visit before initiation of KDT to ensure safety and maximize efficacy while discussing goals and expectations (**Box 1**).[3] In patients in whom a cause has not been identified, it is also recommended that there should be more comprehensive evaluation to identify potential surgical candidates. The group has recommended that KDT be provided for at least 3 months before considering it nonefficacious; families should be counseled to give KDT that period of time as a minimum.[3]

Inpatient Versus Outpatient Initiation

Eighty percent of the centers involved in the IKDSG reported initiating the CKD as an inpatient.[3] Primary goals with an inpatient admission are to closely monitor the patient and to provide teaching for caregivers.[3] Studies have demonstrated three-patient admission groups had significantly longer CKD durations compared with one-child

---

Box 1
Recommendations for pre-KDT evaluation

Counseling
- Discuss seizure reduction, medication, and cognitive expectations
- Potential psychosocial and financial barriers to the use of KDT
- Review antiseizure drugs and other medications for carbohydrate content
- Recommend family read parent-oriented KDT information
- Child life specialist contact in advance of admission if available

Nutritional evaluation
- Baseline weight, height, and ideal weight for stature
- Head circumference in infants
- Body mass index when appropriate
- Nutrition intake history: 3-day food record, food preferences, allergies, aversions, and intolerances
- Establish diet formulation: infant, oral, enteral, or a combination
- Decision on which diet to begin (CKD, MCT, MAD, and LGIT)
- Calculation of calories, fluid, and ketogenic ratio (or percentage of MCT oil or carbohydrates per day)
- Establish vitamin and mineral supplementation based on dietary reference intake

Laboratory evaluation
- Complete blood count with platelets
- Electrolytes to include serum bicarbonate, total protein, calcium
- Serum liver and kidney tests (including albumin, blood urea nitrogen, and creatinine)
- Fasting lipid profile
- Vitamin D level
- Urinalysis
- Antiseizure drug levels (if applicable)

Ancillary testing (optional)
- Electrocardiogram
- MRI of brain
- Echocardiogram, strongly consider if history of heart disease
- Urine organic acids (if diagnosis unclear)
- Serum amino acids (if diagnosis unclear)

admission groups (P = .001), possibly because of the development of a solid support system and more caregiver interactions.[14]

Studies have demonstrated that outpatient initiation is also successful.[15] This confers the advantage of reduced health care costs and stress to the patient and caregivers.[3,15] Both the MAD and LGIT are typically started as an outpatient, usually without a fasting period.

Gradual Initiation Versus Fasting Period

The traditional method of initiation of the CKD involves fasting for 12 to 24 hours with carbohydrate-free fluids.[3] However, studies have shown that gradual initiation maintains seizure efficacy with fewer side effects.[16] Most epilepsy centers that were part of the IKDSG opined that fasting was optional but could be useful in situations where a more rapid benefit was desired, such as in status epilepticus. However, it should be avoided in children younger than 2 years of age.[3]

INDICATIONS FOR THE KETOGENIC DIET

Eighty-eight percent of the members of the IKDSG believed that dietary therapies should be strongly considered early on in the treatment of 12 conditions as listed alphabetically in **Box 2**. Several other indications for the KDT were also suggested where KD is helpful, but not necessarily an indication (**Box 3**). Even in patients with an underlying genetic cause, KDT has been found to produce a responder rate of 63% and 61% at 1 and 3 months, respectively.[17]

Angelman Syndrome

Angelman syndrome is characterized by severe developmental delay, speech impairment, ataxia, hyperactivity, seizures, and a characteristic happy disposition. This

---

Box 2
Epilepsy syndromes and conditions for which KDT has been consistently reported as more beneficial (>70%) than the average 50% KDT response (defined as >50% seizure reduction)

Angelman syndrome

Complex I mitochondrial disorders

Dravet syndrome

Epilepsy with myoclonic atonic seizures (Doose syndrome)

Febrile infection-related epilepsy syndromes

Formula fed (solely) children or infants

Glucose transporter protein I deficiency syndrome

Infantile spasms

Ohtahara syndrome

Pyruvate dehydrogenase deficiency

Superrefractory status epilepticus

Tuberous sclerosis complex

From Kossoff EH, Zupec-Kania BA, Auvin S, et al. Optimal clinical management of children receiving dietary therapies for epilepsy: Updated recommendations of the International Ketogenic Diet Study Group. Epilepsia Open. 2018;3(2):175–192. Published 2018 May 21. https://doi.org/10.1002/epi4.12225; with permission

---

Box 3
Conditions for which KDT has been consistently reported as moderately beneficial (not better than the average dietary therapy response, or in limited single-center case reports)

Adenylosuccinate lyase deficiency

CDKL5 encephalopathy

Childhood absence epilepsy

Cortical malformations

Epilepsy of infancy with migrating focal seizures

Epileptic encephalopathy with continuous spike-and-wave during sleep

Glycogenosis type V

Juvenile myoclonic epilepsy

Lafora body disease

Landau-Kleffner syndrome

Lennox-Gastaut syndrome

Phosphofructokinase deficiency

Rett syndrome

Subacute sclerosing panencephalitis

From Kossoff EH, Zupec-Kania BA, Auvin S, et al. Optimal clinical management of children receiving dietary therapies for epilepsy: Updated recommendations of the International Ketogenic Diet Study Group. Epilepsia Open. 2018;3(2):175–192. Published 2018 May 21. https://doi.org/10.1002/epi4.12225; with permission

---

neurogenetic disorder is typically caused by genetic abnormalities involving chromosome 15q11-q13.[18] Studies showed that 11/31 patients placed on the CKD reported it to be the best overall treatment.[19] LGIT produced seizure freedom in 6/23 patients with seizure freedom apart from intercurrent infection/illness or excessive carbohydrate intake in 7/23 patients. The average time on the diet was 3 years.[20] Case reports have also indicated a dramatic response in status epilepticus following the initiation of KDT.[21]

Complex I Mitochondrial Disorders

Complex I deficiency is one of the most commonly identified biochemical mitochondrial defects and is associated with epilepsy. The use of ketone bodies in patients with respiratory chain complex defects has been shown to cause heteroplasmic shifting between and within cells. KDT is useful in heteroplasmic mitochondrial DNA disorders because of the possibility that ketone bodies can differentiate between respiration compromised and normal cells.[22] Because of the risk of acute decompensation with fasting, these patients would benefit from close monitoring if an initial fasting period is used. Ten of 14 patients with intractable childhood epilepsy with respiratory chain complex defects had a reduction in seizure frequency.[23] Eighty percent of these patients were able to reduce or discontinue their ASMs following initiation of KDT.[23]

Dravet Syndrome

Dravet syndrome is typically associated with drug-resistant epilepsy with multiple seizure types, recurrent status epilepticus, developmental delay, and cognitive impairment because of mutations in the SCN1a gene.[24] Studies have indicated that ASMs, such as valproic acid (VPA), topiramate, and levetiracetam, are typically associated with 30% to 40% responder rate.[25] KD showed a 70% responder rate and was found to be equally effective when compared with combination therapy with stiripentol, VPA, and clobazam.[25]

Epilepsy with Myoclonic-Atonic Seizures (Doose Syndrome)

Seizures associated with epilepsy with myoclonic-atonic seizures are typically of multiple semiologies, although primarily "drop" seizures, and are associated with a risk of epileptic encephalopathy.[26] A retrospective review demonstrated that 83% experienced seizure reduction by greater than 50% and 47% were seizure-free following 2 years of the MAD.[26] In another cohort of 23 children, there was a favorable response to the KD in five patients despite an average of five ASMs and a median of 17 months having had passed since the onset of seizures.[27] A multicenter retrospective chart review of 166 children with epilepsy with myoclonic-atonic seizures found that KDT was the most effective treatment.[28]

Febrile Infection-Related Epilepsy Syndrome

Febrile infection-related epilepsy syndrome is considered a subcategory of new-onset refractory status epilepticus (RSE) wherein RSE develops following a febrile infection with fever starting between 2 weeks and 24 hours before onset of RSE in an otherwise healthy patient.[29] Studies have demonstrated that KDT can dramatically control seizures that were not responsive to ASM and immunotherapy.[30,31] An early initiation of KDT was noted to improve outcomes.[30] Six of seven diet responders were continued on the KDT for a mean of 1 year with rare seizures on its discontinuation.[31]

Formula-Fed Infants

KDT is initiated with relative ease in formula-fed infants, especially those with an existing gastrostomy tube. Studies have indicated that patients who were given ketogenic formula were more likely to continue the diet and that the use of a feeding tube was not associated with early KDT withdrawal.[32] In a center where 61/226 patients were formula-fed while on the KDT, all 61 were found to have better seizure control than the typical solid food–fed child.[33] Formula has been found to be palatable, easy to calculate components of, and is frequently covered by insurance companies because it is considered medical therapy.[33]

Glucose Transporter Type 1 Deficiency Syndrome

Glut-1 is normally expressed in the endothelial cells forming the blood-brain barrier. Its deficiency results in suboptimal glucose transport across the blood-brain barrier. This manifests as early onset absence epilepsy, paroxysmal eye-head movements, developmental delays, ataxia, and paroxysmal exertion-induced dystonia.[34] Ninety-six percent of the IKDSG believed that KDT should be first line for Glut1 deficiency syndrome (Glut1DS) over triheptanoin or any other product, even if the patient does not have seizures.[3] A survey of families with Glut1DS reported that 80% of patients had greater than 90% reduction in seizures with the KD.[34]

Infantile Spasms (West Syndrome)

West syndrome consists of the triad of infantile spasms (IS), hypsarrhythmia, and developmental delay/regression. A meta-analysis revealed that patients with IS may benefit from the KD with a median rate of seizure freedom in around one-third of patients. More than a 50% seizure reduction was seen in 60% of patients.[35] The KD is well-established as a therapy for refractory IS, but what about new-onset? A retrospective, case-control chart review found 8/13 infants with IS started on the KD as initial therapy were spasm-free within 18 days. Those who do not respond to the KD can then be treated with hormonal therapy.[36] In studies that have compared the KD with corticotropin, 10/16 patients achieved electroclinical remission at Day 28 with the KD compared with 11/16 on corticotropin with better tolerability with the KD.[37]

Ohtahara Syndrome

Ohtahara syndrome is a form of early infantile epileptic encephalopathy characterized by frequent tonic spasms, drug-resistant epilepsy, poor psychomotor development, and burst-suppression pattern on electrocardiogram (EEG).[38] Although numerous ASMs have been used with inconsistent response, several centers have reported an electroclinical improvement with implementation of the KD.[39,40]

Pyruvate Dehydrogenase Deficiency

Pyruvate dehydrogenase deficiency (PDHD) is typically characterized by neurodevelopmental delay, seizures, hypotonia, and congenital lactic acidosis.[41] KDT was found to be effective and safe for most patients with improvement across motor, cognitive, social, and epilepsy domains.[42] A less restrictive form of the KD has been tried to improve tolerability in patients with dihydrolipoamide dehydrogenase deficiency, a subtype of PDHD, and has demonstrated an improvement in survival.[43]

Superrefractory Status Epilepticus

RSE is associated with up to 32% mortality; long-lasting effects, such as developmental deterioration in 34% patients; and new-onset epilepsy (in 36% of pediatric patients).[44,45] A prospective multicenter study demonstrated ketosis in a median of 2 days with EEG resolution of seizures in 7 days of initiation in 71.4%. Seventy-nine percent were weaned off continuous infusions within 2 weeks of initiation of the KD. Seven of 12 patients with 3-month follow-up continued to have seizure freedom/reduction. The KD was typically started with enteral preparations following a 12- to 24-hour period of fasting.[46] Some centers have reported using a parenteral formulation.[47] Similar response has been found in the adult population.[48,49] Concomitant use of propofol with the KD can raise the risk of propofol infusion syndrome and should be avoided.[3] The overall relative safety of the KD, paucity of hemodynamic instability, and ease of administration in the critically ill population makes it a good treatment option for this high-mortality condition.

Tuberous Sclerosis Complex

Tuberous sclerosis complex (TSC) is associated with multiorgan involvement with intractable, early onset epilepsy. In a multicenter case series of children with TSC and epilepsy, 11/12 had greater than 50% reduction in seizures.[50] Studies have shown that decanoic acid can selectively inhibit AMPA receptors, bind to PPAR-γ, and inhibit mTORC1 activity, thus possibly contributing to the profound antiseizure effect in this population.[51–53]

CONTRAINDICATIONS

Because of the metabolic adaptation that is required for the transition from carbohydrates to lipids as the primary energy source, an intact fat metabolism pathway is required. Patients should be screened for disorders of fatty acid oxidation and transport if there is clinical concern, especially in the setting of epilepsy with unclear cause (**Box 4**).[3]

ADVERSE EFFECTS

The most common side effects involve the gastrointestinal tract and include constipation, emesis, and abdominal pain in up to 50% of children, which are usually mild and reversible.[3,54] During CKD initiation, 28% had hypoglycemia with 16% had two or more episodes of hypoglycemia. These immediate side effects were not linked to later seizure control inefficacy.[54]

There have been reports of a significant increase in plasma cholesterol, low-density lipoprotein, very low-density lipoprotein, triglycerides, and total apolipoprotein B levels with a reduction in high-density lipoprotein at 6 to 24 months with the KD.[55] Acute pancreatitis has been reported in the presence of elevated triglyceride levels, but is rare.[56] Those receiving solely formula-based KDT were less likely to have hypercholesterolemia. This hypercholesteremia improved spontaneously in approximately 50%.[57] Strategies to reduce hyperlipidemia include increasing MCT oils, olive oil, carnitine, and omega-3-fatty acid supplementation. Reducing the KD ratio and excluding all fatty meats, egg yolk, cream, butter, animal fat, palm oil, and coconut oil may also be helpful.[3]

Cardiomyopathy and prolonged QT interval have been reported in case series.[58] Other studies have reported no disturbing effects on ventricular functions in children with epilepsy.[59] Although no definitive information is gleaned regarding long-term vascular outcomes, the IKDSG made note of studies that noted an increase in arterial stiffness in children, whereas other studies demonstrated no change in carotid intima-media thickness.[3]

Renal calculi may occur in 3% to 7% of patients on KDT and rarely require surgical intervention.[3] Oral potassium citrate is an effective preventative measure.[60] Weight loss is common at the initiation of the diet. Most patients successfully regain the weight.[61] Studies have indicated negative effects on growth with the CKD, with younger children at a higher risk.[3]

Box 4
Contraindications to the use of the KDT

Absolute
- Primary carnitine deficiency
- Carnitine palmitoyltransferase I or II deficiency
- Carnitine translocase deficiency
- β-Oxidation defects
- Medium-chain acyl dehydrogenase deficiency
- Long-chain acyl dehydrogenase deficiency
- Short-chain acyl dehydrogenase deficiency
- Long-chain 3-hydroxyacyl-CoA deficiency
- Medium-chain 3-hydroxyacyl-CoA deficiency
- Pyruvate carboxylase deficiency
- Porphyria

Relative
- Inability to maintain adequate nutrition
- Surgical focus identified by neuroimaging and video-EEG monitoring
- Parent or caregiver noncompliance
- Propofol concurrent use (risk of propofol infusion syndrome may be higher)

CONCOMITANT ANTISEIZURE THERAPY

Patients are typically on numerous ASMs at the time of initiation of KDT, hence a few points of importance are highlighted here. VPA is a short-chain fatty acid, which could increase fatty acid oxidation and can cause a theoretic risk of hepatotoxicity. Studies have indicated that adverse events with the combination of KDT and VPA are similar to those on KDT without VPA.[62,63] Supplemental carnitine may be required in children on KDT with VPA. The addition of a carbonic anhydrase inhibitor (eg, topiramate, zonisamide) to the KD may cause a worsening of preexisting metabolic acidosis. Exact timing of ASM reduction is unclear, reductions are usually not made in the first month on KDT.[3] In a group of 232 patients, 18.5% were able to stop ASMs while on KDT with 14% being able to remain off ASMs for extended periods.[64]

DISCONTINUATION OF KETOGENIC DIET THERAPY

Discontinuation of KDT should be based on the patient's response and underlying diagnosis. A mean of 3.2 months on KDT is required to assess efficacy (before discontinuing for inefficacy). Typically, it is continued for 1 to 2 years when successful.[3] In Glut1DS it is recommended that KDT is maintained for as long as tolerated by the patient.[34] In IS, 46% were found to be spasm-free within 2 weeks and had a normal EEG within 2 months of treatment. Those who were spasm free were continued on the diet for 6 months and did not have a recurrence of spasms on its discontinuation.[65]

Although the CKD can be discontinued abruptly in an emergency, it is more often reduced gradually over 1 to 2 months by a ratio of 1:1 every 2 weeks (eg, 4:1–3:1–2:1), with ongoing nutritional supplementation and reintroduction of regular foods.[3] Children with 50% to 99% seizure reduction have a three times higher risk of increased seizures during discontinuation.[66] Risk of recurrence is higher in those with EEG abnormalities, structural lesions, and TSC. Before discontinuation of KDT, a routine EEG may be helpful in counseling patients/families. If seizures recur, the KDT ratio should revert to the previously effective ratio, if the parents and physician wish.[3]

DIET THERAPY IN ADULTS

Although one of the earliest case series of 100 adolescents and adults reported a 56% reduction in seizures with the KD, there was a lull in the use of KDT in adults from the 1930s until more recently.[67] In a pooled analysis of 20 studies conducted on adults, 34% with focal epilepsy were responders compared with 48% with generalized epilepsy.[68] A significant challenge with KDT in adults has been compliance. A meta-analysis with data from 270 adults revealed a compliance rate of 45% (38% for CKD and 56% for MAD).[69] The use of a ketogenic formula at initiation of KDT has been shown to improve diet adherence (>50%) at 6 months.[70]

SUMMARY

KDT has been in use for more than a century. It is a safe and effective treatment of those with refractory epilepsy and is the favored first-line agent in such conditions as Glut1DS and PDHD. KDT has also been shown to be a safe and effective way to terminate superrefractory status epilepticus. The wide reach of dietary therapies and its global usage has resulted in the formation of the International Neurologic Ketogenic Society, a professional organization devoted to the advancement of broad-spectrum metabolism-based therapies in neurology (www.neuroketo.org/).

CLINICS CARE POINTS

- Ketogenic diet therapy is a safe and effective method to treat epilepsy in both adults and children. It is the favored first line agent in Glut-1 deficiency syndrome and pyruvate dehydrogenase deficiency.

- The main contraindication to bear in mind is that the ketogenic diet therapies require an intact fat metabolism pathway. Most common side effects include constipation, emesis, abdominal pain, hypoglycemia, and weight loss. An average of 3.2 months is required to assess the efficacy of ketogenic diet therapy (prior to discontinuing for inefficacy).

DISCLOSURE

B. Haridas: Nothing to disclose. E.H. Kossoff: Consultant to Atkins Nutritionals, Nutricia, Cerecin, and Bloom Science. Royalties from Oxford Press, Springer Publishing, and UpToDate.

REFERENCES

1. Wilder RM. The effects of ketonemia on the course of epilepsy. Mayo Clin Proc 1921;2:307–8.
2. Kossoff EH. More fat and fewer seizures: dietary therapies for epilepsy. Lancet Neurol 2004;3(7):415–20.
3. Kossoff EH, Zupec-Kania BA, Auvin S, et al. Optimal clinical management of children receiving dietary therapies for epilepsy: updated recommendations of the International Ketogenic Diet Study Group. Epilepsia Open 2018;3(2):175–92.
4. Seo JH, Lee YM, Lee JS, et al. Efficacy and tolerability of the ketogenic diet according to lipid:nonlipid ratios: comparison of 3:1 with 4:1 diet. Epilepsia 2007; 48(4):801–5.
5. Kossoff EH. Dietary therapies for epilepsy. In: Wyllie E, Gidal B, editors. Wyllie's the treatment of epilepsy: principles and practice. 7th edition. Philadelphia: Wolters Kluwer; 2021. p. 772–8.
6. Huttenlocher PR, Wilbourne AJ, Sigmore JM. Medium chain triglycerides as a therapy for intractable childhood epilepsy. Neurology 1971;1:1097–103.
7. Neal EG, Chaffe H, Schwartz RH, et al. The ketogenic diet for the treatment of childhood epilepsy: a randomised controlled trial. Lancet Neurol 2008;7(6): 500–6.
8. Pfeifer HH, Thiele EA. Low-glycemic-index treatment: a liberalized ketogenic diet for treatment of intractable epilepsy. Neurology 2005;65(11):1810–2.
9. Muzykewicz DA, Lyczkowski DA, Memon N, et al. Efficacy, safety, and tolerability of the low glycemic index treatment in pediatric epilepsy. Epilepsia 2009;50(5): 1118–26.
10. Lakshminarayanan K, Agarawal A, Panda PK, et al. Efficacy of low glycemic index diet therapy (LGIT) in children aged 2-8 years with drug-resistant epilepsy: a randomized controlled trial. Epilepsy Res 2021;171:106574.
11. Kossoff EH, McGrogan JR, Bluml RM, et al. A modified Atkins diet is effective for the treatment of intractable pediatric epilepsy. Epilepsia 2006;47(2):421–4.
12. Kim JA, Yoon JR, Lee EJ, et al. Efficacy of the classic ketogenic and the modified Atkins diets in refractory childhood epilepsy. Epilepsia 2016;57(1):51–8.
13. Sondhi V, Agarwala A, Pandey RM, et al. Efficacy of ketogenic diet, modified Atkins diet, and low glycemic index therapy diet among children with drug-resistant epilepsy: a randomized clinical trial. JAMA Pediatr 2020;174(10):944–51.

14. Alem D, Jager L, Turner Z, et al. Does the size of a ketogenic diet admission group influence outcomes? Epilepsy Behav 2021;121(Pt A):108059.

15. van der Louw E, Olieman J, Poley MJ, et al. Outpatient initiation of the ketogenic diet in children with pharmacoresistant epilepsy: an effectiveness, safety and economic perspective. Eur J Paediatr Neurol 2019;23(5):740–8.

16. Bergqvist AG, Schall JI, Gallagher PR, et al. Fasting versus gradual initiation of the ketogenic diet: a prospective, randomized clinical trial of efficacy. Epilepsia 2005;46(11):1810–9.

17. Jagadish S, Payne ET, Wong-Kisiel L, et al. The ketogenic and modified Atkins diet therapy for children with refractory epilepsy of genetic etiology. Pediatr Neurol 2019;94:32–7.

18. Kishino T, Lalande M, Wagstaff J. UBE3A/E6-AP mutations cause Angelman syndrome. Nat Genet 1997;15(1):70–3.

19. Thibert RL, Conant KD, Braun EK, et al. Epilepsy in Angelman syndrome: a questionnaire-based assessment of the natural history and current treatment options. Epilepsia 2009;50(11):2369–76.

20. Grocott OR, Herrington KS, Pfeifer HH, et al. Low glycemic index treatment for seizure control in Angelman syndrome: a case series from the Center for Dietary Therapy of Epilepsy at the Massachusetts General Hospital. Epilepsy Behav 2017;68:45–50.

21. Stein D, Chetty M, Rho JM. A "happy" toddler presenting with sudden, life-threatening seizures. Semin Pediatr Neurol 2010;17(1):35–8.

22. Santra S, Gilkerson RW, Davidson M, et al. Ketogenic treatment reduces deleted mitochondrial DNAs in cultured human cells. Ann Neurol 2004;56(5):662–9.

23. Kang HC, Lee YM, Kim HD, et al. Safe and effective use of the ketogenic diet in children with epilepsy and mitochondrial respiratory chain complex defects. Epilepsia 2007;48(1):82–8.

24. Ragona F, Granata T, Dalla Bernardina B, et al. Cognitive development in Dravet syndrome: a retrospective, multicenter study of 26 patients. Epilepsia 2011;52(2):386–92.

25. Dressler A, Trimmel-Schwahofer P, Reithofer E, et al. Efficacy and tolerability of the ketogenic diet in Dravet syndrome: comparison with various standard antiepileptic drug regimen. Epilepsy Res 2015;109:81–9.

26. Wiemer-Kruel A, Haberlandt E, Hartmann H, et al. Modified Atkins diet is an effective treatment for children with Doose syndrome. Epilepsia 2017;58(4):657–62.

27. Kilaru S, Bergqvist AGC. Current treatment of myoclonic astatic epilepsy: clinical experience at the Children's Hospital of Philadelphia. Epilepsia 2007;48(9):1703–7.

28. Nickels K, Kossoff EH, Eschbach K, et al. Epilepsy with myoclonic-atonic seizures (Doose syndrome): clarification of diagnosis and treatment options through a large retrospective multicenter cohort. Epilepsia 2021;62(1):120–7.

29. Hirsch LJ, Gaspard N, van Baalen A, et al. Proposed consensus definitions for new-onset refractory status epilepticus (NORSE), febrile infection-related epilepsy syndrome (FIRES), and related conditions. Epilepsia 2018;59(4):739–44.

30. Peng P, Peng J, Yin F, et al. Ketogenic diet as a treatment for super-refractory status epilepticus in febrile infection-related epilepsy syndrome. Front Neurol 2019;10:423.

31. Nabbout R, Mazzuca M, Hubert P, et al. Efficacy of ketogenic diet in severe refractory status epilepticus initiating fever induced refractory epileptic encephalopathy in school age children (FIRES). Epilepsia 2010;51(10):2033–7.

32. Kim SH, Shaw A, Blackford R, et al. The ketogenic diet in children 3 years of age or younger: a 10-year single-center experience. Sci Rep 2019;9(1):8736.

33. Kossoff EH, McGrogan JR, Freeman JM. Benefits of an all-liquid ketogenic diet. Epilepsia 2004;45(9):1163.

34. Klepper J, Akman C, Armeno M, et al. Glut1 deficiency syndrome (Glut1DS): state of the art in 2020 and recommendations of the International Glut1DS Study Group. Epilepsia Open 2020;5(3):354–65.

35. Prezioso G, Carlone G, Zaccara G, et al. Efficacy of ketogenic diet for infantile spasms: a systematic review. Acta Neurol Scand 2018;137(1):4–11.

36. Kossoff EH, Hedderick EF, Turner Z, et al. A case-control evaluation of the ketogenic diet versus ACTH for new-onset infantile spasms. Epilepsia 2008;49(9):1504–9.

37. Dressler A, Benninger F, Trimmel-Schwahofer P, et al. Efficacy and tolerability of the ketogenic diet versus high-dose adrenocorticotropic hormone for infantile spasms: a single-center parallel-cohort randomized controlled trial. Epilepsia 2019;60(3):441–51.

38. Ohtahara S, Yamatogi Y. Epileptic encephalopathies in early infancy with suppression-burst. J Clin Neurophysiol 2003;20(6):398–407.

39. Sivaraju A, Nussbaum I, Cardoza CS, et al. Substantial and sustained seizure reduction with ketogenic diet in a patient with Ohtahara syndrome. Epilepsy Behav Case Rep 2015;3:43–5.

40. Ishii M, Shimono M, Senju A, et al. No To Hattatsu 2011;43(1):47–50.

41. Patel KP, O'Brien TW, Subramony SH, et al. The spectrum of pyruvate dehydrogenase complex deficiency: clinical, biochemical and genetic features in 371 patients. Mol Genet Metab 2012;106(3):385–94.

42. Sofou K, Dahlin M, Hallböök T, et al. Ketogenic diet in pyruvate dehydrogenase complex deficiency: short- and long-term outcomes. J Inherit Metab Dis 2017;40(2):237–45.

43. Staretz-Chacham O, Pode-Shakked B, Kristal E, et al. The effects of a ketogenic diet on patients with dihydrolipoamide dehydrogenase deficiency. Nutrients 2021;13(10):3523.

44. Sahin M, Menache CC, Holmes GL, et al. Outcome of severe refractory status epilepticus in children. Epilepsia 2001;42(11):1461–7.

45. Barnard C, Wirrell E. Does status epilepticus in children cause developmental deterioration and exacerbation of epilepsy? J Child Neurol 1999;14(12):787–94.

46. Arya R, Peariso K, Gaínza-Lein M, et al. Efficacy and safety of ketogenic diet for treatment of pediatric convulsive refractory status epilepticus. Epilepsy Res 2018;144:1–6.

47. Lin JJ, Lin KL, Chan OW, et al. Intravenous ketogenic diet therapy for treatment of the acute stage of super-refractory status epilepticus in a pediatric patient. Pediatr Neurol 2015;52(4):442–5.

48. Cervenka MC, Hocker S, Koenig M, et al. Phase I/II multicenter ketogenic diet study for adult superrefractory status epilepticus. Neurology 2017;88(10):938–43.

49. Francis BA, Fillenworth J, Gorelick P, et al. The feasibility, safety and effectiveness of a ketogenic diet for refractory status epilepticus in adults in the intensive care unit. Neurocrit Care 2019;30(3):652–7.

50. Kossoff EH, Thiele EA, Pfeifer HH, et al. Tuberous sclerosis complex and the ketogenic diet. Epilepsia 2005;46(10):1684–6.

51. Chang P, Augustin K, Boddum K, et al. Seizure control by decanoic acid through direct AMPA receptor inhibition. Brain 2016;139(Pt 2):431–43.

52. Simeone TA, Matthews SA, Samson KK, et al. Regulation of brain PPARgamma2 contributes to ketogenic diet anti-seizure efficacy. Exp Neurol 2017;287(Pt 1): 54–64.

53. Warren EC, Dooves S, Lugarà E, et al. Decanoic acid inhibits mTORC1 activity independent of glucose and insulin signaling. Proc Natl Acad Sci U S A 2020; 117(38):23617–25.

54. Lin A, Turner Z, Doerrer SC, et al. Complications during ketogenic diet initiation: prevalence, treatment, and influence on seizure outcomes. Pediatr Neurol 2017; 68:35–9.

55. Kwiterovich PO Jr, Vining EP, Pyzik P, et al. Effect of a high-fat ketogenic diet on plasma levels of lipids, lipoproteins, and apolipoproteins in children. JAMA 2003; 290(7):912–20.

56. Stewart WA, Gordon K, Camfield P. Acute pancreatitis causing death in a child on the ketogenic diet. J Child Neurol 2001;16(9):682.

57. Nizamuddin J, Turner Z, Rubenstein JE, et al. Management and risk factors for dyslipidemia with the ketogenic diet. J Child Neurol 2008;23(7):758–61.

58. Best TH, Franz DN, Gilbert DL, et al. Cardiac complications in pediatric patients on the ketogenic diet. Neurology 2000;54(12):2328–30.

59. Özdemir R, Güzel O, Küçük M, et al. The effect of the ketogenic diet on the vascular structure and functions in children with intractable epilepsy. Pediatr Neurol 2016;56:30–4.

60. McNally MA, Pyzik PL, Rubenstein JE, et al. Empiric use of potassium citrate reduces kidney-stone incidence with the ketogenic diet. Pediatrics 2009;124(2): e300–4.

61. Wibisono C, Rowe N, Beavis E, et al. Ten-year single-center experience of the ketogenic diet: factors influencing efficacy, tolerability, and compliance. J Pediatr 2015;166(4):1030–6.e1.

62. Lyczkowski DA, Pfeifer HH, Ghosh S, et al. Safety and tolerability of the ketogenic diet in pediatric epilepsy: effects of valproate combination therapy. Epilepsia 2005;46(9):1533–8.

63. Spilioti M, Pavlou E, Gogou M, et al. Valproate effect on ketosis in children under ketogenic diet. Eur J Paediatr Neurol 2016;20(4):555–9.

64. Shah LM, Turner Z, Bessone SK, et al. How often is antiseizure drug-free ketogenic diet therapy achieved? Epilepsy Behav 2019;93:29–31.

65. Hong AM, Turner Z, Hamdy RF, et al. Infantile spasms treated with the ketogenic diet: prospective single-center experience in 104 consecutive infants. Epilepsia 2010;51(8):1403–7.

66. Worden LT, Turner Z, Pyzik PL, et al. Is there an ideal way to discontinue the ketogenic diet? Epilepsy Res 2011;95(3):232–6.

67. Barborka CJ. Epilepsy in adults. Arch Neurol Psychiatry 1930;23(5):904.

68. Husari KS, Cervenka MC. The ketogenic diet all grown up: ketogenic diet therapies for adults. Epilepsy Res 2020;162:106319.

69. Ye F, Li XJ, Jiang WL, et al. Efficacy of and patient compliance with a ketogenic diet in adults with intractable epilepsy: a meta-analysis. J Clin Neurol 2015;11(1): 26–31.

70. McDonald TJW, Henry-Barron BJ, Felton EA, et al. Improving compliance in adults with epilepsy on a modified Atkins diet: a randomized trial. Seizure 2018;60:132–8.

Evaluation and Treatment of Psychogenic Nonepileptic Seizures

Nicholas J. Beimer, MD[a,b,*], William Curt LaFrance Jr, MD, MPH[c]

KEYWORDS

- Psychogenic • Nonepileptic • Functional • Seizures • Multidisciplinary • Behavioral
- Therapy • Treatment

KEY POINTS

- Psychogenic nonepileptic seizures (PNES) cause debilitating symptoms and negatively impact function, quality of life, and health care utilization; however, there are multiple evidence-based treatments available.
- Because of the complex symptoms and comorbidities of PNES, a comprehensive neuropsychiatric evaluation is necessary, and a multidisciplinary team of clinicians is important for evaluation and treatment.
- An integrated, multidisciplinary team approach is the best means of addressing the cross-disciplinary diagnostic and treatment challenges that exist for PNES and should be implemented in any neurology clinic where possible.

 Video content accompanies this article at http://www.neurologic.theclinics. com.

INTRODUCTION

Psychogenic nonepileptic seizures (PNES) are episodes characterized by abnormal motor, sensory, and/or cognitive changes that resemble epileptic seizures (ES). PNES are not due to abnormal neuronal epileptiform activity and are instead associated with underlying psychological conflict or conflicts, and often with comorbidities, such as anxiety, depression, traumatic life events, and personality disorders.[1] The term PNES is presently the most commonly used and accepted terminology; however,

[a] Department of Neurology, Michigan Medicine, University of Michigan, F2593 UH South, 1500 East Medical Center Drive, Ann Arbor, MI 48109-5223, USA; [b] Department of Psychiatry, Michigan Medicine, University of Michigan, F2593 UH South, 1500 East Medical Center Drive, Ann Arbor, MI 48109-5223, USA; [c] Alpert Medical School, Brown University, Rhode Island Hospital, 593 Eddy Street, Potter 3, Providence, RI 02903-4923, USA
* Corresponding author. Department of Neurology, Michigan Medicine, University of Michigan, F2593 UH South, 1500 East Medical Center Drive, Ann Arbor, MI 48109-5223.
E-mail address: Nbeimer@med.umich.edu

Neurol Clin 40 (2022) 799–820
https://doi.org/10.1016/j.ncl.2022.03.017   neurologic.theclinics.com

alternatives, such as functional seizures or dissociative seizures, are used.[2] PNES are classified in the *Diagnostic and Statistical Manual of Mental Disorders* (Fifth Edition) as a type of functional neurologic symptom disorder (FND) or conversion disorder.[3]

PNES are estimated to have a prevalence of up to 33/100,000 and an annual incidence of 1.4/100,000.[4,5] Although PNES is less common than epilepsy, the presence of PNES among outpatient epilepsy clinics and inpatient seizure monitoring units (SMUs) is disproportionately higher and can be seen as frequently as 10% and 40%, respectively.[6–8] This high proportion of PNES seen in epilepsy centers likely represents the overall negative impact that PNES have on function; quality of life, disability rates, refractoriness of symptoms, and psychiatric comorbidities, such as anxiety and depression, which are more severe, when compared with epilepsy.[9–11]

The impact of PNES extends well beyond the individual with seizures, contributing significantly to health care cost and utilization.[12] Studies have shown a promising reduction in health resource utilization after PNES diagnosis, with significant decreases in diagnostic testing, antiseizure medication (ASM) use, as well as both outpatient and emergency department visits.[13,14] Another study did not show significant improvement during the 3-year interval following diagnosis of PNES.[15] Not only does PNES impact the United States, but also there is significant burden and difficulty with access to treatment in both developed and undeveloped countries.[16] Thus, there is a clear need to further improve PNES evaluation and treatment. The evidence base for PNES treatments is growing, including conventional cognitive behavioral therapy,[17] neurobehavioral therapy (NBT),[18,19] mindfulness-based intervention,[20] and prolonged exposure therapy.[21]

DISCUSSION
Importance of Multidisciplinary Approach for Diagnosis and Treatment

The first step in treatment is accurate diagnosis. Increasing evidence for PNES treatments exists; however, there is not a singular method to evaluate and treat patients with PNES. The American Neuropsychiatric Association Committee on Research recently published a review of evidence-based practice of evaluation of PNES.[22] This review highlights that a detailed account of seizure semiology has the highest yield for diagnosis of PNES along with additional support clinical factors, such as history of traumatic experiences, posttraumatic stress disorder (PTSD), personality disorders, and medical comorbidities, such as numerous allergies, chronic pain, mild traumatic brain injury, neurologic comorbidities, and other conversion disorder/functional neurologic symptoms or somatic symptom disorders. Furthermore, assessing psychological traits, such as avoidance, somatization, and dissociation, is also helpful, and their identification can inform the treatment plan. The gold-standard diagnostic test remains video electroencephalographic (EEG) capture of a typical episode, with consistent history. Overall, a comprehensive neuropsychiatric evaluation is necessary for evaluation of patients with PNES, and thus, a multidisciplinary approach is naturally the most practical model of evaluating and treating PNES.

Team-based multidisciplinary approaches to care are becoming more readily implemented for complex medical, neurologic, and psychological conditions, and there is evidence that this approach improves outcomes in disease, such as amyotrophic lateral sclerosis and somatoform disorder.[23,24] Because of the nature of neuropsychiatric symptoms and psychosocial problems that are prevalent in patients with PNES, evaluation and treatment can be challenging owing to the overlap of problems transcending multiple disciplines, including, but not limited to neurology, psychiatry, psychology, physiatry, and social work. Thus, an integrated, multidisciplinary team is one approach toward addressing the cross-disciplinary diagnostic and treatment challenges that exist for PNES. Integration of the team encourages the practice of communication between clinicians, including both the multidisciplinary team and the referring clinicians, as well as with patients and families, and facilitates a consistent message from all clinicians in the process, which is a critical step in helping patients understand and accept the diagnosis. This team process, when integrated into existing health care systems, allows for a seamless transition that bridges evaluation to treatment (**Fig. 1**). There is limited, but growing, evidence to support the multidisciplinary approach in evaluation and treatment of PNES.[25,26] Therefore, when able to be coordinated, multidisciplinary approaches to evaluation and treatment of PNES should be considered in any neurology clinic where possible.

The Neurology Clinic

Evaluation for PNES often begins in the outpatient neurology clinic. Although new-onset seizures are likely to be assessed acutely in the emergency department, many of these patients will ultimately be referred to neurologists for expert consultation. Whether the neurology consultation occurs in the emergency department or in the neurology clinic, an evaluation for a first seizure of life should be undertaken, which is focused on distinguishing the cause of seizures among multiple possibilities, including new-onset epilepsy, acute symptomatic seizures, provoked seizures, and PNES.[27] Furthermore, syncope should also be considered among the top differential diagnoses, as it represents a common mimic of new-onset seizures.[28] Because results of initial diagnostic evaluation are not always available immediately, and because a normal evaluation cannot exclude epilepsy, a judgment about beginning empiric treatment with an ASM must also be decided at the first visit. This is not to say that new-onset epilepsy should be assumed to be the default among all possible diagnoses, rather the history and physical examination should shape the judgment about the likelihood of new-onset epilepsy, syncope, PNES, versus other paroxysmal conditions and dictate the appropriate initial evaluation and treatment.[29] For example, if the event concerning for a seizure is characterized by abrupt loss of consciousness, brief convulsions, followed by a quick return to consciousness and the patient has a significant

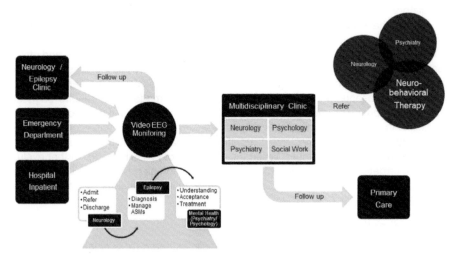

Fig. 1. Flow chart of the evaluation and treatment of PNES.

cardiac history with a documented arrhythmia on cardiac telemetry, it would be reasonable to assume convulsive cardiogenic syncope to be the most likely explanation, prompting appropriate evaluation and treatment. Likewise, if the semiology of the event is characterized by flailing, thrashing, and asynchronous movements with side-to-side head shaking and weeping that lasts several minutes with preserved consciousness, it would be reasonable to approach the event as most likely to be PNES. It is important to remember that PNES should not be considered a diagnosis of exclusion, with appropriate workup to establish a definitive diagnosis to mitigate diagnostic delays; early, accurate diagnosis of PNES portends a better prognosis.[30]

Among types of epilepsy, frontal lobe onset ES are often considered unusual in their presentation, owing to intense behavioral and/or affect signs and symptoms that could raise suspicion for the possibility of PNES.[29] For example, frontal lobe ES may lack a significant postictal phase and have preserved consciousness, like PNES. Furthermore, ES arising from the prefrontal cortex can have variable manifestations and include odd gestural movements, laughing, shouting, and thrashing of extremities, similar to PNES. In contrast, frontal lobe ES tend to be shorter in duration (seconds) and occur out of physiologic sleep.[31]

Because of the importance of making a diagnosis of PNES as early as possible, yet also balancing the risk of missing a diagnosis of epilepsy, formal criteria have been established for defining the levels of diagnostic certainty.[1,32] Ideally, the patient history should be consistent with PNES; an event with typical semiology of PNES should be witnessed on video by a clinician experienced in the diagnosis of epilepsy, and there should not be any associated epileptiform abnormalities on coregistered EEG immediately before, during, or after the captured event. Video EEG monitoring ideally occurs in the inpatient setting, during which any currently prescribed ASMs have been weaned off. As noted, long-term monitoring (LTM) video EEG is the gold standard for definitive diagnosis; however, there are situations when inpatient LTM may not be available or practical. Examples of these situations include infrequent events (eg, less than once every 2 weeks), environmentally bound events (eg, "my seizures only happen when I'm up and up and moving around a lot"), distance (eg, no SMU center close enough for patient to access), and undermanaged comorbidities (eg, patient reporting severe nicotine dependence or severe anxiety that limits their ability to remain inpatient for LTM). In order of decreasing level of diagnostic rigor, ambulatory EEG with video,[33] home video recordings,[34] and other home-monitoring devices[35,36] have been evaluated for the purpose of ictal capture outside the monitoring unit.

The neurology clinic evaluation often involves referral for additional testing and other consultants. Depending on the suspected diagnosis, whether this involves setting up video EEG monitoring, obtaining brain imaging, tilt-table testing, or cardiac event monitoring, subsequent referrals are also commonly made when results suggest that events might be physiologic (eg, cardiogenic or metabolic), or if psychogenic/psychological in origin. For syncopal events with evidence of abnormalities on tilt-table testing, autonomic, or cardiac event monitors, referral to cardiology is indicated for further evaluation and treatment. When the diagnosis of PNES is made, further evaluation and targeted treatment should be initiated as soon as possible, which will likely include a multidisciplinary team of clinicians, including mental health clinician evaluation.

The Multidisciplinary Team

The composition of the ideal multidisciplinary clinical team for evaluation and treatment of PNES could include a neurologist/epileptologist, psychiatrist, psychologist, social worker, and dedicated administrative support staff (**Table 1**). Examples of multi-disciplinary team models exist for child and adult patients.[25,37,38] For a discussion of one example of a Multidisciplinary Clinic for PNES, the authors reference a clinical program offered within the Comprehensive Epilepsy Program at Michigan Medicine, Ann Arbor, Michigan.[39] This is just one model that exists and could include, but does not have to be limited to, other allied health professionals to further enhance the depth and breadth of the team, such as advanced practice providers (eg, nurse practitioners and physician assistants), registered nurses, physical and occupational therapy, speech-language pathology, and neuropsychology.[40]

Although each member of the multidisciplinary team has unique expertise and responsibilities, there are also universal skills and knowledge that team members should possess, which include an ability to gauge patient and family understanding and acceptance of the diagnosis, the importance of addressing social determinants of health that commonly affect those living with PNES, the need to thoroughly evaluate for neurologic and psychiatric comorbidities, and the basic tenets of treating PNES. Team members with a clinical role should have an understanding between epilepsy, physiologic nonepileptic events, and PNES and be able to discuss the differences with patients and family. Members should be able to evaluate patient understanding and acceptance of the PNES diagnosis, hear patient goals, collect a thorough social and mental health history, assess for past and ongoing risk of abuse, violence, or neglect, assess substance use patterns, identify social and community supports, assess current living situation, recognize the role of culture, religion, and spirituality, and be aware of the financial and insurance limitations on patients being able to appropriately get evaluation and treatment.

For the neurologist evaluating seizures, the ideal training background is that of a comprehensive and solid foundation in general neurology, in addition to fellowship training in clinical neurophysiology and/or epilepsy, which equips the neurologist to be comfortable in the diagnosis of PNES, in terms of both diagnostic certainty and ability to communicate the diagnosis of PNES to the patient. In addition, there should also be a thorough assessment for that of possible comorbid epilepsy, which occurs in about 10% of patients with seizures.[41] Common among patients with PNES are other neurologic symptoms, and the neurologist should be prepared to evaluate, treat, or refer patients for expert evaluation and treatment of other symptoms and conditions, such as headache, movement and gait disorders, disturbances of sensation, pain, cognitive dysfunction, obstructive sleep apnea, and vascular disease. When indicated, patients should also be referred for indicated physical, occupational, and speech therapy and for outpatient neuropsychological evaluation for patients who report significant cognitive complaints that interfere with functioning. The neurologist should lead care coordination of the treatment team, communicating the diagnosis and management plan with co-treaters, and schedule follow-up appointments for patients with PNES at regular intervals, as indicated, based on the nature and severity of symptoms. A common follow-up timeframe with neurology after multidisciplinary evaluation could be within 3 to 6 months.

For the psychiatrist assessing seizures, the ideal training background would be that of broad exposure to general psychiatry, with additional training in a neuropsychiatry fellowship, or in consultation-liaison psychiatry, also known as psychosomatic medicine. The neuropsychiatry-trained or the consultation-liaison psychiatrist is able to focus on the interplay of comorbid psychiatric and general neurology and medical conditions, which often occur in patients with PNES. In addition, the psychiatrist should be able to evaluate, treat, or refer for expert evaluation and treatment of anxiety, depression, suicidal ideation, psychosis, PTSD, obsessive compulsive disorder

Table 1
Multidisciplinary team members

Discipline	Neurologist	Psychiatrist	Psychologist	Social Worker	Administrative Support
Training background and/or expertise	Neurology and epilepsy	Neuropsychiatry/ consultation liaison psychiatry	Health psychology	Licensed master social worker	Patient services associate

Role	• Classify diagnostic certainty of PNES
	• Communicate diagnosis of PNES
	• Evaluate for risk of comorbid epilepsy and perform additional diagnostic testing and treat as indicated
	• Assess developmental history
	• Evaluate and treat for
	  o Headache
	  o Movement disorders
	  o Sensory disturbances and pain
	  o Cognitive impairment
	  o Stroke
	  o Obstructive sleep apnea
	• Refer as indicated for
	  o Physical therapy
	  o Occupational therapy
		• Evaluate and treat/ refer for
		  o Developmental and psychosocial history
		  o Anxiety
		  o Depression
		  o Suicidal ideation
		  o Psychosis
		  o PTSD/trauma/abuse history
		  o OCD
		  o Substance use disorders
		  o Nightmares
		  o Insomnia
		  o Personality disorders
			• Evaluate
			  o Social history
			  o Mental health history
			  o Trauma/abuse/neglect history
			  o Safety
			  o Substance use/abuse
			  o Coping strategies
			  o Strengths
			  o Social support/living situation
			  o Culture
			  o Religion/spirituality
			  o Financial/insurance
			Treat or refer
			  o Psychotherapy
			    ■ Individual
			    ■ Group
			    ■ Family/couple's therapy
			    ■ Trauma focused
			    ■ Dialectical behavior therapy
			    ■ Other specific therapies (Eye movement desensitization and reprocessing, prolonged exposure, mindfulness, and other)
			    ■ Pastoral care/religious community support
			• Recommend
			  o Follow-up with current therapist and provide information about PNES
				• Obtain treatment team and referral releases of information
				• Schedule
				• Multidisciplinary evaluation
				• Therapy appointments
				• Facilitate communication
				  o Evaluation and treatment recommendations
				    ■ Patient
				    ■ Family
				    ■ Referring clinician
				    ■ Primary care

	○ Speech-language pathology evaluation and treatment ○ Neuropsychology testing	diagnosis and provide treatment recommendations

Universal skills and knowledge of all team members	• Understand differences between epilepsy, physiologic nonepileptic events, and psychogenic nonepileptic seizures
	• Evaluate patient/family understanding and acceptance of PNES diagnosis
	• Recognize the importance of evaluating, treating, and addressing neurology, psychiatric, and psychological diagnoses, as well as social determinants of health
	• Understand and address patient goals
	• Provide the following:
	  ○ Specific treatment recommendations for PNES
	  ○ Additional evaluation or treatment of neurologic and psychiatric comorbidities
	  ○ Resources to address social determinants of health	

(OCD), substance use disorders, nightmares, insomnia, abuse/trauma history, other somatic, and personality disorders. Follow-up with psychiatry should be scheduled to foster best-practice, evidence-based psychiatric care of any comorbid disorder listed above that is actively being treated (eg, using a trauma-focused therapy for comorbid PTSD). In some cases, patients with PNES have significant comorbid psychiatric disorders and may already be established with a mental health clinician, and continuation of ongoing follow-up with psychiatry should be encouraged. Treatment approach and recommendations from the psychiatrist serving as a multidisciplinary PNES team member can be very helpful for other treating psychiatrists who may have an established relationship with the patient but may not be as knowledgeable or experienced in evaluating or treating PNES or other somatic symptom disorders (eg, psychogenic/functional movement disorder), and its psychiatric comorbidities. Patients who have controlled and managed psychiatric comorbidities may not necessarily require any additional evaluation or treatment with the PNES team psychiatry consultant, following multidisciplinary evaluation, and follow-up can be on an as needed basis.

The psychologist and social worker have some similar responsibilities as part of the multidisciplinary team, although each has unique strengths and skillsets in caring for patients with PNES. For the psychologist, a training background in health psychology is particularly beneficial, which at its core recognizes the importance of the biological, psychological, and social contributions to both wellness and illness.[42,43] In a complementary way, social workers interpret the medical and social diagnoses for patients and other agencies, collaborate between the individual patient and broader hospital organization, perform discharge planning, secure provisions for patients to adjust to a complex and potentially disabling condition, and provide health education.[44] More specifically, the core responsibilities served by both psychology and social work in the multidisciplinary clinic include review of elements collected in the history gathered by the neurologist and psychiatrist, which include the following: social and mental health history, trauma, abuse, neglect, safety, substance abuse, coping strategies, strengths, social supports and living situation, culture, military service, legal history, religion and spirituality practices, and financial/insurance barriers. Although some multidisciplinary teams divide these "nonmedical" elements to nonphysicians, these elements are important for all multidisciplinary team clinicians to assess, including psychiatry and neurology, because patients sometimes divulge different information to different clinicians. Likewise, although disciplines of psychiatry, psychology, social work, and other licensed professional counselors and therapists might be considered the traditional providers of psychotherapy, all multidisciplinary team members have the potential to treat patients with PNES, including neurologists.[45,46] Indeed, there is a growing number of neurologists/epileptologists taking on this responsibility in personally delivering NBT for treatment of PNES.[47]

Last, but certainly not least, effective administrative support is critical for efficient functioning of the multidisciplinary team. This support staff schedules outpatient appointments, such as new patient evaluations, as well as therapy appointments. In addition, collecting releases of information for sharing the summary of impressions and recommendations from the multidisciplinary team, and delivering to the patient, family, referring clinicians, and primary care are critical aspects of communication from the multidisciplinary team.

The Multidisciplinary Clinic

As an example of an active multidisciplinary clinic for PNES, a program offered within the Comprehensive Epilepsy Program at Michigan Medicine, is highlighted,[39] which is directed by one of the authors (N.B.). In this model, the patient's first point of contact with the multidisciplinary team occurs via an inpatient consultation with health psychology after a diagnosis of PNES is confirmed and communicated to the patient by the neurology and/or epilepsy services during the inpatient admission for video EEG LTM (see **Fig. 1**). The health psychologist of the multidisciplinary team is consulted by the primary neurology service for an initial inpatient evaluation before discharge from the SMU. This initial assessment focuses on patient understanding and acceptance of the PNES diagnosis and ideally occurs with a warm handoff from the neurology and/or epilepsy inpatient services to a mental health clinician. Information is provided about any recommended additional evaluation and the treatment plan. Upon discharge from the SMU, the patient is scheduled by inpatient unit administrative staff for follow-up in the outpatient neurology or epilepsy clinic, ideally with the referring clinician who ordered the video EEG LTM. This outpatient neurologist is responsible for routine follow-up after admission to provide the standard of care for evaluation and management of PNES. Also, upon discharge, a discharge referral order is placed by the primary inpatient service to the multidisciplinary clinic for PNES in the outpatient Neurology Clinic at Michigan Medicine.

The Multidisciplinary Clinic for PNES at Michigan Medicine is an outpatient, coordinated evaluation that offers 3 hour-long visits for 3 new patients per clinic half-day with a neurologist (N.B.), psychiatrist, and either a social worker or a health psychologist (**Fig. 2**). The social worker and health psychologist in this design have similar responsibilities, primarily representing the role of the therapist; the interchangeability of this

Time	Patient 1	Patient 2	Patient 3
8:00 AM	Neurology	Psychiatry	Psychosocial
9:00 AM	Psychiatry	Psychosocial	Neurology
10:00 AM	Psychosocial	Neurology	Psychiatry
11:00 AM	Team Discussion		
11:15 AM	Team + Patient Group Discussion		
11:30 AM		Team + Patient Group Discussion	
11:45 AM			Team + Patient Group Discussion

Fig. 2. Sample Multidisciplinary PNES Clinic schedule.

position allows for scheduling flexibility of the clinic, as well as the ability for the health psychologist to perform consultations in the hospital for patients with newly diagnosed PNES. Each of the multidisciplinary team members has unique but overlapping roles and responsibilities (see **Table 1**) during the individual, one-on-one appointments of the evaluation. Family and friends who often accompany patients to the clinic are asked to give privacy to the patient during sensitive portions of the history, such as discussions about trauma, abuse, or neglect, but are later encouraged to attend and provide input when their perspective is helpful, such as when describing the semiology of seizures.

After finishing the 3 initial evaluations with neurology, psychiatry, and social worker or health psychologist, all patients are given a break of variable duration, between 15 and 45 minutes, which allows the multidisciplinary team to discuss each patient's case individually, coming to a consensus for recommendations, and then inviting each patient one at a time into a group discussion with all multidisciplinary team members (**Fig. 3**), to relay an integrative model, holistic, biopsychosocial-spiritual formulation.[48] Family and friends whom the patient wishes to be present are encouraged to attend at this point. Each clinician takes a turn relaying their portion of recommendations, starting with neurology, followed by psychiatry, and finishing with social work or health psychology. For example, the neurologist will discuss the diagnosis of PNES, the certainty of the diagnosis, and any recommended additional testing or changes to medications, such as stopping unnecessary ASMs (when a patient has lone PNES and no indication for the ASM, eg, migraine prophylaxis, neuropathic pain, bipolar disorder). The psychiatrist may address recommendations to start an antidepressant/anxiety medication, if indicated, and tapering off chronic and as-needed benzodiazepines and opiates if prescribed in the community. Last, the social worker or health psychologist will recommend the type of psychotherapy and provide information on resources and scheduling. The meeting concludes with the patient and family/friends asking any remaining questions. This process is repeated for all patients seen during the half-day clinic.

Follow-up planning after the visit is coordinated for all disciplines evaluating the patient in the Multidisciplinary PNES Clinic. All patients are recommended to follow up in

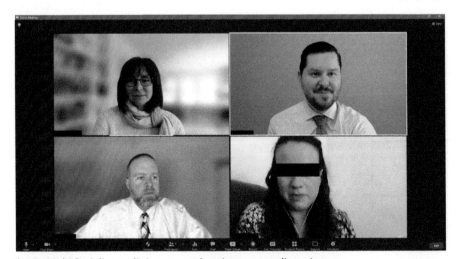

Fig. 3. Multidisciplinary clinic team and patient group discussion.

Michigan Medicine either with the referring neurologist or in the epilepsy or general neurology clinics, no longer than 6 months from the evaluation. Patients who are referred from a significant distance will make a follow-up visit with their referring local neurologist. Routine follow-up with psychiatry, either within Michigan Medicine or locally, is recommended for patients already being cared for by a mental health clinician before multidisciplinary evaluation. When indicated, patients are scheduled by neurology clinic scheduling staff within 3 to 4 months with the multidisciplinary team psychiatrist to follow up for medication management for conditions such as anxiety or depression. In other cases, patients are recommended to establish care with a local psychiatrist, and referrals are recommended to a psychiatrist geographically convenient for the patient, via community mental health, or internally within Michigan Medicine. A similar process occurs for follow-up scheduling for psychotherapy. Patients are offered an appointment for manualized NBT with one of the Michigan Medicine multidisciplinary team members, all of which have seizure therapy training and the capability of fulfilling the role of seizure counselor (Video 1). If patients already have a current outside therapist, incorporating the NBT seizure treatment workbook[49] into present therapy sessions is recommended, using the accompanying therapist guide,[50] and an offer is extended to verbally communicate with local therapists about the recommended treatment approach. After the multidisciplinary clinic evaluation is complete, a summary of impressions and treatment recommendations is collated

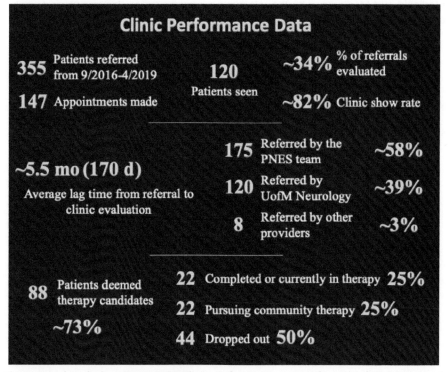

Clinic Performance Data

355 Patients referred from 9/2016-4/2019

120 Patients seen

~34% % of referrals evaluated

147 Appointments made

~82% Clinic show rate

~5.5 mo (170 d) Average lag time from referral to clinic evaluation

175 Referred by the PNES team **~58%**

120 Referred by UofM Neurology **~39%**

8 Referred by other providers **~3%**

88 Patients deemed therapy candidates **~73%**

22 Completed or currently in therapy **25%**

22 Pursuing community therapy **25%**

44 Dropped out **50%**

Fig. 4. Initial Multidisciplinary PNES Clinic performance metrics from the first 2.5 years of clinic operation from 9/2016 through 4/2019.[73] The top section displays the population size and clinic throughput. The middle section displays referral patterns. The bottom section displays psychotherapy treatment information. University of Michigan.

into a single document, which is visible to the patient and copied to the referring neurologist, primary care physician, and any relevant treating clinicians, including from psychiatry and therapists.

Regarding the performance and effectiveness of the multidisciplinary clinic for PNES within the Comprehensive Epilepsy Program at Michigan Medicine, initial data suggest that patients receiving the evaluation report satisfaction with the comprehensive approach, and that those receiving NBT show a reduction in seizures and improvement in comorbidities and quality of life, similar to the pilot multicenter randomized controlled trial in civilians[18] and in veterans,[19] on which the treatment is based. From an administrative perspective, the clinic is successful from an operational and fiscal standpoint. Administrative areas that need improvement include addressing wait times before first evaluation given the prevalence and need and increasing the psychotherapy bandwidth (**Fig. 4**). An unpublished analysis of the financial and billing metrics for the clinic from January 2019 through March 2021 showed several promising characteristics. For example, the actual reimbursement for professional charges was between 34% and 37% of that billed, similar to other outpatient clinics within Michigan Medicine. In addition, bundled denials occurred in only 48/395 (12%) of hospital administration records, which is also on par with other clinics, although it should be noted that this is not the final denial rate owing to ongoing insurance and billing processes at the time of data collection. As expected, the professional billing payer mix showed that most patients were covered by government insurance programs, such as Medicaid and Medicare, with the minority covered by private insurance, and rarely, automobile insurance coverage.

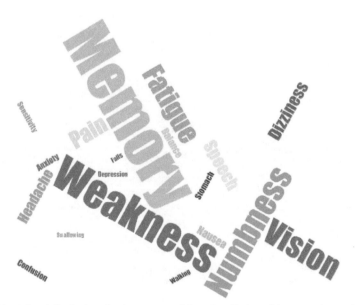

Fig. 5. Word cloud displaying the frequency of functionally impairing symptoms other than seizures described by patients evaluated in the Multidisciplinary PNES Clinic at Michigan Medicine.[39] Font size is proportional to the frequency of reported symptoms: larger = more frequent; smaller = less frequent.

Regarding the demographics and outcomes of patients referred to the Multidisciplinary Clinic at Michigan Medicine, there is an institutional review board–approved registry at the University of Michigan (Registration and Evaluation of Patients with Psychogenic Non-Epileptic Seizures, HUM00135099) to further study the sample and evaluate the effectiveness of the clinic, from which preliminary data are becoming available (**Fig. 5**, **Tables 2** and **3**).[39] The clinic also will incorporate NES REDCap Database variables, used by sites that have trained in the intervention, for systematic collection of outcome measures.[51] In the clinical experience of one of the authors (N.B.), most patients who have been evaluated in the multidisciplinary clinic and

Table 2
Multidisciplinary PNES Clinic demographic characteristics within the Comprehensive Epilepsy Program at Michigan Medicine (collected by Beimer NJ, January 25, 2021, unpublished data)[39]

Multidisciplinary PNES Clinic Demographics	
	N (%)
Age	
18–30	143 (26%)
31–45	206 (38%)
46–60	148 (27%)
61–75	41 (7%)
>75	9 (2%)
Oldest age	91
Youngest age	18
Average age	41
Gender	
Female	423 (77%)
Male	123 (23%)
Race	
American Indian and Alaska Native	4 (0.7%)
Asian	3 (0.6%)
Black or African American	52 (10%)
Native Hawaiian and Other Pacific Islander	2 (0.4%)
Other	15 (3%)
White or caucasian	460 (86%)
Ethnicity	
Hispanic	20 (4%)
Non-Hispanic	515 (96%)
Marital status	
Divorced	31 (8%)
Legally separated	5 (1%)
Married	157 (39%)
Significant other	11 (3%)
Single	191 (47%)
Widowed	7 (2%)
Vital status	
Alive	541 (99%)
Deceased	6 (1%)

Table 3
Multidisciplinary PNES Clinic at Michigan Medicine demographic variables (provided with incomplete data) (collected by Beimer NJ, January 25, 2021, unpublished data)[39]

Multidisciplinary PNES Clinic Demographics	
	N (%)
Sex/Gender Identity	
Female	29 (59%)
Genderqueer	1 (2%)
Male	11 (22%)
Transgender female	2 (4%)
Transgender male	5 (10%)
Two-spirit	1 (2%)
Sexual orientation	
Asexual	1 (2%)
Bisexual	6 (15%)
Gay	1 (2%)
Lesbian	2 (5%)
Pansexual	1 (2%)
Something else	1 (2%)
Straight	29 (70%)
Years of education completed	
8	1 (1%)
10	1 (1%)
11	2 (2%)
12	40 (37%)
13	10 (9%)
13.5	2 (2%)
14	24 (22%)
15	4 (4%)
16	15 (14%)
17	1 (1%)
18	3 (3%)
19	3 (3%)
20	3 (3%)
Employment status	
Active military duty	1 (<1%)
Disabled	17 (9%)
Full time	53 (29%)
Not employed	95 (52%)
Part time	11 (6%)
Retired	4 (2%)
Self-employed	2 (1%)

completed manualized NBT[49] have found improvement in social functioning and reduction in seizure frequency, burden, and/or other somatic symptoms.

Professionals in the Community

Although the National Association of Epilepsy Centers (NAEC) requires level 4 centers to have a mental health member for the center (NAEC Web site or levels publication

Table 4

Centers offering multidisciplinary clinics and/or clinicians with interdisciplinary expertise for evaluation and treatment of psychogenic nonepileptic seizures in the United States

Health Care Institution	Primary Location	Epilepsy Center Accreditation		Clinicians Within Each Institution with Special Interest in the Evaluation and Treatment of PNES			
		NAEC Level 4	ECoE	Neurology/ Epilepsy	Psychiatry	Psychotherapy	PT, OT, or SLP
Banner Health	Phoenix, AZ			X	X	X	c
Baylor University	Houston, TX	X		X	X	X	X
Brown University/Rhode Island Hospital	Providence, RI	X		X	X	X	X
Brigham & Women's Hospital	Boston, MA	X		X	X	X	
Cleveland Clinic	Cleveland, OH	X		X	X	X	
Emory University	Atlanta, GA	X		X	X	X	X
Johns Hopkins University	Baltimore, MD	X		X		X	X
Massachusetts General Hospital	Boston, MA	X		X	X	X	X
Mayo Clinic	Rochester, MN	X				X	
Michigan Medicine	Ann Arbor, MI	X		X	X	X	X
Minnesota Epilepsy Group	St. Paul, MN	X				X	
Northeast Regional Epilepsy Group	New York, NY	X		X	X	X	
Northwestern Medicine	Chicago, IL	X				X	
University of Colorado	Aurora, CO	X		X	X	X	
Spectrum Health	Grand Rapids, MI	X		X	X	X	
Stanford University	Stanford, CA	X		X	X	X	
University of California San Francisco	San Francisco, CA	X		X	X		

(continued on next page)

Table 4
(continued)

Health Care Institution	Primary Location	Epilepsy Center Accreditation		Clinicians Within Each Institution with Special Interest in the Evaluation and Treatment of PNES			
		NAEC Level 4	ECoE	Neurology/ Epilepsy	Psychiatry	Psychotherapy	PT, OT, or SLP
Veterans Health Administration	Baltimore, MD	X	X	X		X	
	Boston, MA	X	X	b		X	
	Durham, NC	X	X	X		X	
	Houston, TX	X	X	X	X	X	X
	Madison, WI	X	X	X	X		
	Miami, FL	X	X	X			
	Providence, RI	X	a	X		X	
	San Francisco, CA	X	X	X	X	X	
	Seattle, WA	X	X	X			
	Portland, OR	X	X	X	X	X	
	West Haven, CT	X	X	X		X	
Yale University	New Haven, CT	X		X	X	X	

Abbreviations: OT, occupational therapy; PT, physical therapy; SLP, speech-language pathology.

a ECOE affiliate.
b Neurology/epilepsy specialists available to evaluate for PNES, but none with special interest. Compiled from online, publicly available sources.[66,67]
c available by referral in the community.

REF), there are relatively few centers capable of diagnosing, neuropsychiatrically evaluating, *and treating* patients with PNES. Although a program may be designated a "comprehensive" epilepsy center, many do not offer services to a large portion of those diagnosed with PNES in their units. To address this treatment gap, the number of programs and specialists addressing PNES is growing, steadily. The need for multidisciplinary expertise in evaluating and treating patients with PNES naturally leads to larger health care institutions being better positioned to support such dedicated programs, although there are examples found among academic, government, and privately owned groups. A list of health care institutions in the United States with multidisciplinary programs and/or clinicians with interdisciplinary expertise for evaluation and treatment of PNES is found in **Table 4**.[39,52–64] Nearly all of these centers are designated either level 4 comprehensive epilepsy centers[65] or Veterans Affairs Epilepsy Centers of Excellence (VA ECoE) affiliated,[66] which can be found via searchable online databases designed to locate programs and individual clinicians with special interest in the evaluation and treatment of PNES and functional neurologic symptom (conversion) disorder.[67,68] Within the VA ECoE, seizure therapy clinics have also been created for the treatment of veterans with PNES using NBT, in collaboration with the VA National TeleMental Health Center.[19,69] In addition, local chapters of the Epilepsy Foundation have developed statewide networks of mental health professionals that have expertise in treating PNES.[70,71]

Future Directions

Although great advances in PNES diagnosis and treatment have been made in the last 20 years, more work is needed, including lessening disparities (cost, access, travel, child and adolescent services), addressing stigma, understanding comorbidities, improving diagnostic tools (video, wearables, serology, imaging, biomarkers), and broadening management tools (psychotherapies, rehabilitation therapies, biologics, and neurostimulation). These needs are outlined and described in articles that address research needs in not only PNES but also other FND/conversion disorder (CD) manifestations.[40,72]

SUMMARY

Patients with PNES represent a distinct, challenging group among those with functional neurologic symptom (conversion) disorders and involve a complex set of symptoms and comorbidities, which are best evaluated and treated by a multidisciplinary team of clinicians. Multidisciplinary, collaborative care is becoming more common, using evidence-based treatment, and the outpatient neurology clinics at sites not currently caring for these patients hold potential for providing such a model of care, with coordination of services. Best practice care for PNES should encourage the integration of neurology and mental health professionals to improve communication among clinicians and with patients, allowing for better care and outcomes. Multidisciplinary clinics hold promise for moving us toward holistic evaluation and treatment of disease and should be used wherever possible as a means of improving the lives of patients living with PNES.

CLINICS CARE POINTS

- Because of the nature of neuropsychiatric symptoms and psychosocial problems in patients with psychogenic nonepileptic seizures, multiple disciplines are necessary for evaluation and treatment, including, but not limited to, neurology, psychiatry, psychology, and social work.

- Multiple evidence-based treatments for psychogenic nonepileptic seizures exist, including cognitive behavioral therapy, neurobehavioral therapy, mindfulness-based intervention, and prolonged exposure therapy.
- Multidisciplinary clinics for evaluation and treatment of psychogenic nonepileptic seizures can aid patients in reducing seizures and improving comorbidities and quality of life and are viable from operational and fiscal perspectives.
- Integration of a multidisciplinary team for patients with psychogenic nonepileptic seizures into existing health care systems and neurology clinics allows for a seamless transition that bridges evaluation to treatment.

ACKNOWLEDGMENTS

Thank you to Dr Craig Hansen and Dr Charles Asbury for their work in contributing to the unpublished data and creation of **Figs. 4** and **5**, respectively. Thank you to Dr Elissa Patterson, Najda Robinson-Mayer, and Dr G. Scott Winder as co-founders of the Multidisciplinary PNES Clinic at Michigan Medicine.

DISCLOSURE

N.J. Beimer has served as an ad hoc reviewer for *Epilepsy & Behavior*; has received honoraria from MedLink LLC and Decker Intellectual Properties; has received research support from the Health Resources and Services Administration (HRSA H98MC30374, co-I), NIH (R01 NS094399-10, co-I), the University of Michigan Department of Neurology, and the Pediatric Epilepsy Research Foundation; serves on the Epilepsy Foundation of Michigan Professional Advisory Board, and has provided medicolegal expert testimony. W.C. LaFrance, Jr. has served on the editorial boards of *Epilepsia*, *Epilepsy & Behavior*, *Journal of Neurology, Neurosurgery and Psychiatry*, and *Journal of Neuropsychiatry and Clinical Neurosciences*; receives editor's royalties from the publication of *Gates and Rowan's Nonepileptic Seizures*, 3rd edition (Cambridge University Press, 2010) and 4th ed (2018); author's royalties for *Taking Control of Your Seizures: Workbook and Therapist Guide* (Oxford University Press, 2015); has received research support from the Department of Defense (DoD WSIXWH-17-0169), NIH (NINDS 5K23NS45902 [PI]), Providence VAMC, Center for Neurorestoration and Neurotechnology, Rhode Island Hospital, the American Epilepsy Society (AES), the Epilepsy Foundation (EF), Brown University, and the Siravo Foundation; serves on the Epilepsy Foundation New England Professional Advisory Board, the Functional Neurological Disorder Society Board of Directors, the American Neuropsychiatric Association Advisory Council; has received honoraria for the American Academy of Neurology and AES Annual Meetings; has served as a clinic development consultant at University of Colorado Denver, Cleveland Clinic, Spectrum Health, Emory University, Oregon Health Sciences University, and Vanderbilt University; and has provided medicolegal expert testimony.

SUPPLEMENTARY DATA

Supplementary data related to this article can be found online at https://doi.org/10.1016/j.ncl.2022.03.017.

REFERENCES

1. LaFrance WC Jr, Baker GA, Duncan R, et al. Minimum requirements for the diagnosis of psychogenic nonepileptic seizures: a staged approach: a report from the

International League Against Epilepsy Nonepileptic Seizures Task Force. Epilepsia 2013;54(11):2005–18.

2. Kerr WT, Stern JM. We need a functioning name for PNES: Consider dissociative seizures. Epilepsy Behav 2020;105:107002.

3. American Psychiatric Association. Diagnostic and statistical manual of mental disorders. 5th edition. Arlington, VA: American Psychiatric Association; 2013. DSM-5.

4. Benbadis SR, Allen Hauser W. An estimate of the prevalence of psychogenic non-epileptic seizures. Seizure 2000;9(4):280–1.

5. Sigurdardottir KR, Olafsson E. Incidence of psychogenic seizures in adults: a population-based study in Iceland. Epilepsia 1998;39(7):749–52.

6. Martin R, Burneo JG, Prasad A, et al. Frequency of epilepsy in patients with psychogenic seizures monitored by video-EEG. Neurology 2003;61(12):1791–2.

7. Alsaadi TM, Marquez AV. Psychogenic nonepileptic seizures. Am Fam Physician 2005;72(5):849–56.

8. Asadi-Pooya AA, Emami Y, Emami M. Psychogenic non-epileptic seizures in Iran. Seizure 2014;23(3):175–7.

9. Abe C, Denney D, Doyle A, et al. Comparison of psychiatric comorbidities and impact on quality of life in patients with epilepsy or psychogenic nonepileptic spells. Epilepsy Behav 2020;102:106649.

10. Avalos JC, Silva BA, Tevés Echazu MF, et al. Quality of life in patients with epilepsy or psychogenic nonepileptic seizures and the contribution of psychiatric comorbidities. Epilepsy Behav 2020;112:107447.

11. Asadi-Pooya AA, Bazrafshan M. Employment and disability status in patients with functional (psychogenic nonepileptic) seizures. Brain Behav 2021;11(3):e02016.

12. Razvi S, Mulhern S, Duncan R. Newly diagnosed psychogenic nonepileptic seizures: health care demand prior to and following diagnosis at a first seizure clinic. Epilepsy Behav 2012;23(1):7–9.

13. Martin RC, Gilliam FG, Kilgore M, et al. Improved health care resource utilization following video-EEG-confirmed diagnosis of nonepileptic psychogenic seizures. Seizure 1998;7(5):385–90.

14. Nunez-Wallace KR, Murphey DK, Proto D, et al. Health resource utilization among US veterans with psychogenic nonepileptic seizures: A comparison before and after video-EEG monitoring. Epilepsy Res 2015;114:114–21.

15. Salinsky M, Storzbach D, Goy E, et al. Health care utilization following diagnosis of psychogenic nonepileptic seizures. Epilepsy Behav 2016;60:107–11.

16. Kanemoto K, LaFrance WC Jr, Duncan R, et al. PNES around the world: Where we are now and how we can close the diagnosis and treatment gaps-an ILAE PNES Task Force report [published correction appears in Epilepsia Open. Epilepsia Open 2017;2(3):307–16.

17. Goldstein LH, Robinson EJ, Mellers JDC, et al. Cognitive behavioural therapy for adults with dissociative seizures (CODES): a pragmatic, multicentre, randomised controlled trial. Lancet Psychiatry 2020;7(6):491–505.

18. LaFrance WC Jr, Baird GL, Barry JJ, et al. Consortium. Multicenter pilot treatment trial for psychogenic nonepileptic seizures: a randomized clinical trial. JAMA Psychiatry 2014;71(9):997–1005.

19. LaFrance WC Jr, Ho WLN, Bhatla A, et al. Treatment of psychogenic nonepileptic seizures (PNES) using video telehealth. Epilepsia 2020;61(11):2572–82.

20. Baslet G, Dworetzky B, Perez DL, et al. Treatment of psychogenic nonepileptic seizures: updated review and findings from a mindfulness-based intervention case series. Clin EEG Neurosci 2015;46(1):54–64.

21. Myers L, Vaidya-Mathur U, Lancman M. Prolonged exposure therapy for the treatment of patients diagnosed with psychogenic non-epileptic seizures (PNES) and post-traumatic stress disorder (PTSD). Epilepsy Behav 2017;66:86–92.

22. Baslet G, Bajestan SN, Aybek S, et al. Evidence-Based Practice for the Clinical Assessment of Psychogenic Nonepileptic Seizures: A Report From the American Neuropsychiatric Association Committee on Research. J Neuropsychiatry Clin Neurosci 2021;33(1):27–42.

23. Rooney J, Byrne S, Heverin M, et al. A multidisciplinary clinic approach improves survival in ALS: a comparative study of ALS in Ireland and Northern Ireland. J Neurol Neurosurg Psychiatry 2015;86(5):496–501.

24. Houtveen JH, van Broeckhuysen-Kloth S, Lintmeijer LL, et al. Intensive multidisciplinary treatment of severe somatoform disorder: a prospective evaluation. J Nerv Ment Dis 2015;203(2):141–8.

25. Libbon R, Gadbaw J, Watson M, et al. The feasibility of a multidisciplinary group therapy clinic for the treatment of nonepileptic seizures. Epilepsy Behav 2019; 98(Pt A):117–23.

26. Fredwall M, Terry D, Enciso L, et al. Outcomes of children and adolescents 1 year after being seen in a multidisciplinary psychogenic nonepileptic seizures clinic. Epilepsia 2021;62(10):2528–38.

27. Gavvala JR, Schuele SU. New-onset seizure in adults and adolescents: a review. JAMA 2016;316(24):2657–68.

28. Maloney EM, Chaila E, O'Reilly ÉJ, et al. Incidence of first seizures, epilepsy, and seizure mimics in a geographically defined area. Neurology 2020;95(5):e576–90.

29. Leibetseder A, Eisermann M, LaFrance WC Jr, et al. How to distinguish seizures from non-epileptic manifestations. Epileptic Disord 2020;22(6):716–38.

30. Lempert T, Schmidt D. Natural history and outcome of psychogenic seizures: a clinical study in 50 patients. J Neurol 1990;237(1):35–8.

31. Lee RW, Worrell GA. Dorsolateral frontal lobe epilepsy. J Clin Neurophysiol 2012; 29(5):379–84.

32. Benbadis SR, LaFrance WC Jr, Papandonatos GD, et al, NES Treatment Workshop. Interrater reliability of EEG-video monitoring. Neurology 2009;73(11): 843–6.

33. Syed TU, LaFrance WC Jr, Loddenkemper T, et al. Outcome of ambulatory video-EEG monitoring in a~10,000 patient nationwide cohort. Seizure 2019;66:104–11.

34. Tatum WO, Hirsch LJ, Gelfand MA, et al. Assessment of the Predictive Value of Outpatient Smartphone Videos for Diagnosis of Epileptic Seizures. JAMA Neurol 2020;77(5):593–600.

35. Regalia G, Onorati F, Lai M, et al. Multimodal wrist-worn devices for seizure detection and advancing research: focus on the Empatica wristbands. Epilepsy Res 2019;153:79–82.

36. Zsom A, Tsekhan S, Hamid T, et al. Ictal autonomic activity recorded via wearable-sensors plus machine learning can discriminate epileptic and psychogenic nonepileptic seizures. Annu Int Conf IEEE Eng Med Biol Soc 2019;2019: 3502–6.

37. Sawchuk T, Buchhalter J. Psychogenic nonepileptic seizures in children - Psychological presentation, treatment, and short-term outcomes. Epilepsy Behav 2015;52(Pt A):49–56.

38. Fenton L, Rothberg B, Strom L, et al. Chapter 19. Integrative care model for neurology and psychiatry: non-epileptic seizures project. In: Connelly JV, Feinstein MS, editors. Integrating behavioral health and primary care: pathways

for integrated care. Feinstein RE. New York: Oxford University Press; 2017. p. 351–66.

39. Comprehensive Epilepsy Program. Department of Neurology, Michigan Medicine. Available at: https://medicine.umich.edu/dept/neurology/clinical-programs/comprehensive-epilepsy-program. Accessed November 17, 2021.

40. LaFaver K, LaFrance WC, Price ME, et al. Treatment of functional neurological disorder: current state, future directions, and a research agenda. CNS Spectrums 2021;26(6):607–13.

41. Benbadis SR, Agrawal V, Tatum WO 4th. How many patients with psychogenic nonepileptic seizures also have epilepsy? Neurology 2001;57(5):915–7.

42. Kaplan RM. Health psychology: where are we and where do we go from here? Mens Sana Monogr 2009;7(1):3–9.

43. Andrasik F, Goodie JL, Peterson AL, editors. Biopsychosocial assessment in clinical health psychology. London: Guilford Press; 2015.

44. Reisch M. The challenges of health care reform for hospital social work in the United States. Soc Work Health Care 2012;51(10):873–93.

45. Chen DK, Maheshwari A, Franks R, et al. Brief group psychoeducation for psychogenic nonepileptic seizures: a neurologist-initiated program in an epilepsy center. Epilepsia 2014;55(1):156–66.

46. Wiseman H, Mousa S, Howlett S, et al. A multicenter evaluation of a brief manualized psychoeducation intervention for psychogenic nonepileptic seizures delivered by health professionals with limited experience in psychological treatment. Epilepsy Behav 2016;63:50–6.

47. Jung Y, Chen DK, Bullock KD, et al. Chapter 33. Training in treatment of psychogenic nonepileptic seizures. In: Gates and Rowan's nonepileptic seizures. Lafrance WC Jr and schachter SC. New York: Cambridge University Press; 2018. p. 344–57.

48. Mack JD, LaFrance WC Jr. Chapter 21. Psychological Treatment of Functional Movement Disorder. In: LaFaver K, Maurer CW, Perez DL, et al, editors. Functional movement disorders: an interdisciplinary case-based approach. Switzerland: Springer Nature; 2022. p. 267–90.

49. Reiter JM, Andrews D, Reiter C, et al. Taking Control of Your Seizures: Workbook (Treatments That Work). New York, NY: Oxford University Press; 2015.

50. LaFrance WC Jr, Wincze JP. Treating nonepileptic seizures: therapist Guide. Treatments that work. New York, NY: Oxford University Press; 2015.

51. Harris PA, Taylor R, Thielke R, et al. Research electronic data capture (REDCap)– a metadata-driven methodology and workflow process for providing translational research informatics support. J Biomed Inform 2009;42(2):377–81.

52. Epilepsy. Baylor College of Medicine, Healthcare: Neurology. Available at: https://www.bcm.edu/healthcare/specialties/neurology/epilepsy. Accessed December 23, 2021.

53. Neuropsychiatry. Department of Neurology, Brown Biology and Medicine. Available at: https://www.brown.edu/academics/medical/neurology/neuropsychiatry. Accessed November 21, 2021.

54. Diagnosis and management of psychogenic non-epileptic seizures. Cleveland Clinic. 2019. Available at: https://my.clevelandclinic.org/podcasts/neuro-pathways/diagnosis-and-management-of-psychogenic-non-epileptic-seizures. Accessed November 21, 2021.

55. Emory comprehensive epilepsy program. Emory University School of Medicine. Available at: https://med.emory.edu/departments/neurology/programs_centers/epilepsy.html. Accessed December 23, 2021.

56. Functional neurological disorders (FND) treatment program. Massachusetts General Hospital. Available at: https://www.massgeneral.org/neurology/treatments-and-services/functional-neurological-disorder. Accessed November 21, 2021.

57. Functional neurologic disorders/conversion disorder. Mayo Clinic; 2019. Available at: https://www.mayoclinic.org/diseases-conditions/conversion-disorder/doctors-departments/ddc-20355203. Accessed November 21, 2021.

58. MN Epilepsy Group. Focused expertise. comprehensive care. Minnesota Epilepsy Group; 2021. Available at: https://mnepilepsy.org/. Accessed November 21, 2021.

59. Psychogenic non-epileptic seizures program. Northeast Regional Epilepsy Group. Available at: https://www.epilepsygroup.com/clinical-detail4-10-12/epilepsy-psychogenic-nonepileptic-NES-PNES.htm. Accessed November 21, 2021.

60. NES treatment. University of Colorado Anschutz Medical Campus. Available at: https://www.nestreatmentucd.org/. Accessed November 21, 2021.

61. Non-epileptic Seizures. Spectrum Health. Available at: https://www.spectrumhealth.org/patient-care/neurosciences/epilepsy-and-seizures/nonepileptic-seizures. Accessed November 21, 2021.

62. Functional neurological disorder program. Stanford Medicine, Department of Psychiatry and Behavioral Sciences. Available at: https://med.stanford.edu/psychiatry/patient_care/fnd.html. Accessed November 21, 2021.

63. Epilepsy Centers of Excellence VA, Altalib H, Cavazos J, et al. Providing Quality Epilepsy Care for Veterans. Fed Pract 2016;33(9):26–32.

64. Epilepsy & Seizures. Yale Medicine. Available at: https://www.yalemedicine.org/departments/epilepsy-and-seizures. Accessed November 21, 2021.

65. National Association of Epilepsy Centers. All epilepsy center locations. 2016. Available at: https://www.naec-epilepsy.org/about-epilepsy-centers/find-an-epilepsy-center/all-epilepsy-center-locations. Accessed November 20, 2021.

66. U.S. Department of Veterans Affairs. Veterans health administration, epilepsy centers of excellence (ECOE), epilepsy centers of excellence near you. 2010. Available at: https://www.epilepsy.va.gov/ecoe.asp. Accessed November 20, 2021.

67. Myers L. Psychogenic non epileptic seizures, PNES referral sites. Available at: https://nonepilepticseizures.com/epilepsy-psychogenic-NES-information-referral-sites.php. Accessed November 20, 2021.

68. FND Hope International. Managing FND, find a provider. 2021. Available at: https://fndhope.org/living-fnd/managing-fnd-find-provider/. Accessed November 20, 2021.

69. LaFrance WC Jr, Altalib H. Veterans with psychogenic nonepileptic seizures (PNES). Veterans Administration Epilepsy Centers of Excellence Epilepsy Basic Training Video Series; 2017. Available at: https://youtu.be/NIX-yNTX86w.

70. Seizure smart mental health professional network. Epilepsy foundation of Michigan. Available at: https://www.epilepsymichigan.org/page.php?id=474. Accessed November 22, 2021.

71. Preferred Provider Network. Epilepsy Foundation of Colorado. Available at: https://www.nestreatmentucd.org/wp-content/uploads/2021/10/PPN-Family-Flyer-2021.pdf. Accessed November 22, 2021.

72. Perez DL, Edwards MJ, Nielsen G, et al. Decade of progress in motor functional neurological disorder: continuing the momentum. J Neurol Neurosurg Psychiatry 2021;92:668–77.

73. Hansen C., Beimer N.J., Winder G.S., et al. Performance metrics of a multidisciplinary clinic for the evaluation and management of patients with psychogenic nonepileptic seizures (PNES). Poster presented at: American Epilepsy Society Annual Meeting; December 2019; Baltimore, MD.

Racialized Inequities in Epilepsy Burden and Treatment

Magdalena Szaflarski, PhD

KEYWORDS

- Race • Ethnicity • Seizures • Racialized minorities • Structural racism • Health care
- Treatment • Epidemiology

KEY POINTS

- Health inequities are unjust and avoidable differences in health across social groups.
- Racialized inequities signify race-based and ethnicity-based disparities due to systemic racism and racialization (racial meaning making).
- Racialized minorities carry a disproportionate burden of epilepsy and receive lower or suboptimal levels of care and treatment, but evidence is still fragmented.
- Little attention has been given to social structures and processes at the roots of racialized inequities in epilepsy, which impedes health equity building in epilepsy.
- Updated conceptual frameworks and further research into social causes of these inequities are needed.

INTRODUCTION

Racial and ethnic minority populations have been known for decades to bear a disproportionate burden of epilepsy. By mid-2000s, black adults aged 20 to 59 years had a higher prevalence of epilepsy than their white and Hispanics/Latinx counterparts.[1–3] In addition, Native Americans[4] and some Hispanic/Latinx groups (eg, elderly men) had a higher prevalence of epilepsy than white or non-Hispanic/Latinx people.[5] Nonwhite groups also showed a higher incidence of status epilepticus across all ages[6] and higher rates of risk factors for epilepsy including diabetes, stroke, and depression.[7,8]

Racial and ethnic differences in epilepsy epidemiology prompted an examination of the role of race/ethnicity in epilepsy treatment.[9] Evidence indicated higher rates of hospitalization and the use of emergency department (ED) services for epilepsy among nonwhite than white groups; low use of neurologists, reliance on primary care, and low or irregular use of antiseizure drugs (ASD) among black persons with epilepsy (PWE); and cultural (eg, language, stigma) barriers to epilepsy care among racial/ethnic

Department of Sociology, University of Alabama at Birmingham, 1720 2nd Avenue South, Birmingham, AL 35294-1152, USA
E-mail address: szaflam@uab.edu
Twitter: @MagdalenaSzafl1 (M.S.)

Neurol Clin 40 (2022) 821–830
https://doi.org/10.1016/j.ncl.2022.03.010
0733-8619/22/© 2022 Elsevier Inc. All rights reserved.

minority and immigrant populations. Black patients with epilepsy also showed lower use of advanced epilepsy treatments, such as epilepsy surgery. Research examining potential explanations of these observed and purported disparities in epilepsy treatment—ranging from socioeconomic factors to the patient–provider relationship and psychosocial factors—was sparse.

The purpose of this article is 3-fold: 1) review current conceptual thinking about race and health, 2) highlight newer evidence about the role of race/ethnicity in epilepsy burden and treatment, and 3) assess how contemporary thinking about racial/ethnic disparities and their roots has (or has not) taken hold in the epilepsy field.

DEFINITIONS

Health inequities are unjust and avoidable (preventable) differences in health across social groups.[10,11]

Racialized health inequities are based on unfair treatment based on race and/or ethnicity. In the United States, race and ethnicity are significant predictors of health and access to and quality of health care *over and beyond* socioeconomic factors.[12]

Race is a social construct. Race is ascribed to and by people based on observed phenotypic differences, or perceived patterns of physical difference, such as skin color or eye shape. The scientific consensus is that race does not exist as a purely biological category—because genetic variation is far greater within than between "racial" groups.[13,14] More critically, skin color has no natural association with group differences in ability or behavior.[15] Still, race has played a key role in structuring social relations.

Ethnicity is a concept that is distinct from but overlapping with race. Ethnicity is a voluntary identity linked to geographic place of birth or national heritage. However, some ethnic groups and individuals from ethnic minority and immigrant backgrounds have become *racialized* because of the color or tone of their skin or other physiologic features. In fact, research shows that darker skin tone is associated with social disadvantage and experiences of discrimination regardless of racial identification.[16]

Racism is a key driver of health/health care disparities.[17] *Racism* is "an ideology of racial domination,"[18] where one group presumes biological or cultural superiority over one or more other groups. Racism is distinct from *racial discrimination*, which means unequal treatment, or *racial inequality*, which means unequal outcomes. In the contemporary United States, racism is widely condemned, and racial inequalities and discrimination are not always the immediate result of racism.[19] There are now new forms of racisms that contribute to health inequities: *implicit bias, racialization,* and *institutional (structural) racism*.

An *implicit bias* is an unconsciously triggered belief in the inferiority of, or negative attitude toward a group or groups. Research has shown that, on average, people more readily associate positive attributes and stereotypes with whites than with other races, particularly black race.[20] Furthermore, health-care professionals exhibit the same levels of implicit bias as the wider population.[21] Specifically, there are complex interactions between patient and provider characteristics that influence clinician–patient interactions. These biases, in turn, affect diagnosis and treatment decisions and levels of care.

Racialization is the process of constructing racial meaning, part of which is categorization based on race, which is then extrapolated to individuals and broader culture, signifying race.[22] Research has shown that system-wide racial inequalities are produced (and reproduced) at multiple levels, from cognitive classification processes to governmental structures and methods (eg, census data). Racialization occurs at the microlevel society through daily human interactions and meaning making. For example, during the COVID-19 pandemic, Asians have been reporting more experiences with discrimination, with some having been directly accused of "spreading and causing COVID-19."[17,23]

Structural racism refers to racial discrimination, inequality, exploitation, and domination in organizational or institutional contexts, such as the labor market, educational institutions, or health care services.[24] Structural racism occurs in systems or organizations where distribution of resources privileges one racial group (mainly white people) over another (nonwhite people) without overt racism. Research has shown that despite antidiscriminatory policies, racial discrimination persists in hiring, credit, and housing markets.[19,25] Black and Hispanic adults are also more likely than white adults to report being treated unfairly in health care.[23] Black patients are also more likely to report that a provider seemed not to believe them or refused a test or treatment (eg, pain medication) that the patients believed they needed. Other research has called attention to the use of race in health care as undermining clinical diagnosis and treatment through disease stereotyping and nomenclature (eg, imprecise labels conflating race and ancestry) or the use of race in clinical calculators and screening metrics (eg, a correction factor) that may contribute to racialized health inequalities.[17]

The COVID-19 pandemic and the Black Life Matters movement have exposed structural racism—from unequal impact of the pandemic on racial/ethnic minorities to violence against people of color—and ignited calls for action.[26–28] An editorial in *Neurology Today* called systemic racism, fueled by white supremacy, a public health crisis and "neurotoxic for Black Americans."[29] Considering the current thinking and engagement, an assessment of the epilepsy field in this area is imperative.

CURRENT EVIDENCE
Epidemiology

Prevalence. Some of the most important research on epilepsy epidemiology in the United States comes from the Centers of Disease Control and Prevention Epilepsy Program.[30] Early adult data from the National Health Interview Survey (NHIS) indicated prevalence of lifetime seizure to be highest for non-Hispanic black vis-à-vis other racial/ethnic groups.[31] However, the age-adjusted rates were similar for non-Hispanic white (1.2%) and black (1.4%) respondents.[32] Other surveillance studies of adults have shown active epilepsy prevalence to be lowest in Hispanics (0.5%).[33]

The NHIS data for children/adolescents showed the highest prevalence for American Indian (1.3%) and black (0.9%) followed by white and multiracial (each 0.7%) and Asian (0.5%) children/adolescents.[34] The rate for Hispanics (0.5%) was lower than for non-Hispanics (0.8%). The racial differences were explained after adjusting for age, sex, insurance, ethnicity, and poverty status. However, Hispanic children/adolescents continued to have lower rates than non-Hispanic whites after all adjustments. Furthermore, in a household-based study of adults and children in the Washington, DC area, lifetime prevalence of epilepsy was 2.1% among black residents, compared with 0.8% for whites and 1% for each Hispanics and "other" race.[35] Even after adjusting for age and education, lifetime prevalence was 1.9 higher and prevalence of active epilepsy was 2.2 higher for black versus white persons. Among children in a clinical study, Hispanics/Latinx, especially in low-income areas, were more likely to have ongoing seizures that worsened over time.[36] Epidemiologic research on American Native groups is still fragmented, but evidence suggests a higher prevalence.[3]

Incidence. Early surveillance in the United States indicated the epilepsy incidence rate to vary by race/ethnicity: 65 per 100,000 persons in white non-Hispanic compared with 72 in white Hispanics, 131 in black non-Hispanics, and 162 in black Hispanics.[3] These differences persisted after adjusting for age and sex. The incidence of status epilepticus has also been higher in nonwhites with the largest gap observed in infants and the elderly.[6] In the Washington, DC study,[35] the incidence rate was 3 times higher for black than white persons (102 vs 33) and lower for Hispanic than other non-Hispanic people (22 vs 68), but the latter subsamples were small. Notably, a diagnosis validation process indicated that epilepsy was more often overreported in Hispanics than in other racial/ethnic groups, even though Hispanics had relatively low rates of epilepsy, possibly due to the "healthy migrant" effect.

Evidence is mixed for new-onset epilepsy in health care utilization records. The majority (61%) of new-onset epilepsy in Medicare claims have been reported to be black.[37] However, fewer (22%) of incident epilepsy cases in the Medicaid data were black.[38]

Classification of epilepsy. Racial/ethnic differences in the prevalence of generalized and focal epilepsy among patients with nonacquired epilepsies was examined using data from the Epilepsy Genome/Phenome Project, a multisite/multicountry study.[39] The study found a higher proportion of generalized epilepsy among whites than among black patients and among Hispanics compared with non-Hispanics, although the latter difference was explained after adjusting for race. However, those findings were limited due the underrepresentation of black patients and unclassifiable epilepsy being more common for black patients.

In a large cohort study of patients in the epilepsy-monitoring unit, black patients were more likely to have temporal lobe epilepsy (TLE) than their white counterparts.[40] TLE is difficult to control with medications, and epilepsy surgery is often warranted. Further investigation revealed that black patients with TLE were more likely to have seizure onset in adulthood and have normal magnetic resonance imaging (MRI) results.

Posttraumatic seizures. A population-based study[41] using electronic medical records (EMR) found a higher proportion of black patients (31.1%) to have traumatic brain injury (TBI) with posttraumatic seizures than TBI without seizures (27.9%). In a multivariable analysis, cases with seizures were 1.3 times more likely to be black than white, adjusting for other factors. It is likely that high rates of childhood trauma and infections related to poor living conditions and overall higher rates of risk factors for epilepsy in the South contribute to these inequities.

Health Care

Findings about health care utilization are also variable, but racial/ethnic inequities are noted. Research shows disproportionately high ED use and low ASD adherence among black PWE. A study based on EMRs found a third of the patients with ED visit for epilepsy to be black.[42] Compared with white patients, black patients were more likely to have public insurance and visit ED multiple times within 1 year and were less likely to have a regular source of care. Black patients were also more likely to have missed or ran out of ASD before visiting ED.

Research has also found follow-up neurology care to be more common among white than black patients,[43] but, among Medicare beneficiaries, American Indians/American Natives (AIAN) had the lowest rate (62%) of neurology follow-up and the largest proportion (29%), who had to pay deductible for medical visits, compared with 11% to 19% for other racial groups. In another study, black and Hispanic PWE in California were less likely to receive video electroencephalogram (VEEG), after accounting for various individual-level and contextual factors.[44] Race/ethnicity did not affect access to specialized epilepsy care in veterans, as indicated by years to referral and number of computerized tomography (CTs), MRIs, and electroencephalogram (EEGs).[45]

Having insurance is essential for accessing epilepsy care. Insurance coverage significantly increased for PWE in the United States, but the racial/ethnic distribution of insurance coverage is unclear.[46] Another study showed insurance to be predictive of a neurologist visit, but race/ethnicity was not.[47] Even among people who are insured, epilepsy care can accrue high costs and distribution of those costs may vary by race/ethnicity. Among Medicare beneficiaries, 27% of black PWE had high cost of epilepsy care compared with whites (19%).[48]

Treatment Trajectories and Quality of Care

Additional research has documented racialized inequities in epilepsy care pathways. Among PWE on Medicaid, white and black patients were more likely than other racial groups to follow pathway 1: seizure–epilepsy diagnosis–ASD, whereas American Natives/Pacific Islanders were more likely to follow pathway 3: seizure–seizure–epilepsy diagnosis–ASD.[49] Racial/ethnic groups also differed within and across pathways in time between initial seizure to epilepsy diagnosis with Native Americans/Pacific Islanders having some of the longest trajectories.

Another Medicaid study[38] has examined 5 markers of quality of care for newly diagnosed PWE: seeing a neurologist, diagnostic evaluation (VEEG, imaging tests), ASD medication adherence, having serum drug levels checked, and being in the top quartile of negative health events. In that study, 37% of patients saw a neurologist within 1 year of index epilepsy date, but there were no racial/ethnic differences in seeing a neurologist except Native Hawaiians/Other Pacific Islanders were less likely, whereas black persons were more likely than white persons, to see a neurologist. On other markers, AIAN and persons of Hispanic/Hispanic-mixed race were more likely to receive diagnostic evaluation, and black and persons of Hispanic/Hispanic-mixed race were less likely to adhere to ASDs.

Other research has either confirmed or disagreed with those findings. In the NHIS data, no racial/ethnic differences were noted in a neurology visit or ASD use among adults, after adjusting for other factors.[32,47] However, Hispanic/Latinx children with new-onset epilepsy in a clinical setting had more ED visits, experienced reduced likelihood of drug-responsive epilepsy, and had longer time to seizure control (8 years) compared with white non-Hispanics (5.6 years).[50] In the Hispanic group, higher health-care costs were associated with reduced likelihood of drug-responsiveness.

Among elderly, ASD use varied from 78% among whites to 89% among AIAN.[37] The most commonly used ASDs varied by racial group. For example, levetiracetam was the most commonly prescribed ASD in all groups except AIAN who were more commonly prescribed phenytoin. In addition, blacks had the longest time from the index event to initial ASD (61 days) and Asians had the shortest (56 days). New-onset cases with ASD starting within 30 days of the index event varied from 50% among whites to 54% among AIAN. However, among cases taking more than one ASD, the average time to first ASD was longest for AIAN (93 days) compared shorter time among whites (31 days), Hispanics (39 days), Asians (45 days), and blacks (50 days). These race differences in ASD treatment were fully explained by other sociodemographic and health factors. However, in another Medicare study, early ASD adherence was lower among black and Asian beneficiaries compared with whites, after adjusting for other factors.[51]

Risk of interaction of ASD on nonepileptic drugs (NED) among incident cases among PWE on Medicare was also shown highest (30%) among black and AIAN people than other racial groups.[52] Among prevalent cases, the risk ranged from 33% among Asians to 42% among Hispanics.

Advanced therapies. Disparities in epilepsy surgery have been documented among adults and children with refractory epilepsy using the National Inpatient Sample (NIS) and the Kids Inpatient Database.[53] Among children, 60% of whites, 7% of blacks, 15% Hispanics, and 10% of other races received epilepsy surgery. Among adults, the respective rates by race were as follows: 69%, 7%, 9%, and 8%. However, whites were overrepresented and blacks were underrepresented in the data; the representation effect was not explained by socioeconomic status. These findings confirmed the earlier study from the NIS that showed that white patients were more likely to receive surgery than racial minorities,[54] and smaller proportions of black patients than white patients were discharged for surgery after presurgical evaluation in a longitudinal study.[44] However, in another study, natural language processing algorithm trained on physician notes did not produce varying epilepsy presurgical evaluation scores based on race or socioeconomic status among either children or elderly.[55]

In addition, black patients with refractory epilepsy in the NIS were less likely than whites to use vagal nerve stimulator (VNS).[56] Furthermore, some research indicates that racialized minorities may be underrepresented or take longer to enroll in epilepsy trials.[57,58]

MAIN FINDINGS

The literature on racial inequities in epilepsy burden and treatment has significantly expanded during the last decade. Approaches to investigating the problem have been diverse—from general population studies using survey methods to investigations of federal insurance data and clinical data from EMRs. Current evidence shows or suggests the following:

- *Epidemiology*: Notwithstanding some variations by group and setting, black, Hispanic/Latinx, and Native American PWE carry a disproportionate burden of epilepsy in incidence, deaths from epilepsy, prevalence in some geographic and low-SES areas, and risk factors.
- *Health care use:* Black and Native American PWE are more likely to seek care for seizures in ED, not have a regular source of care, and have public insurance—but that can be a protective factor. Black and white rates of seeing a neurologist are similar, but Native Americans may have less neurology follow-up.
- *Treatment*: Black PWE show low adherence to ASDs and among elderly longer time to initial ASD than other groups, but their treatment pathways and quality of care may be similar to those of white PWE. However, American Natives/Pacific Islanders and younger Hispanic/Latinx groups have longer time to remission than other racial/ethnic groups. Moreover, black, Native American, and possibly Hispanic/Latinx PWE may have relatively high risks of interaction of ASD on NED.
- *Advanced therapies:* Racialized groups (especially children) are significantly less likely to receive epilepsy surgery, and black PWE may be less likely to be discharged for surgery after presurgical evaluation or use VNS than white PWE. Both black and Hispanic/Latinx PWE may need more time to enroll in clinical trials than white PWE.
- *Cost of care:* A few studies indicate that, compared with white PWE, costs of epilepsy care may be higher for black and Native American than white PWE enrolled in public insurance programs.

REMAINING GAPS AND FUTURE DIRECTIONS

Despite growing evidence about racial inequities in epilepsy, knowledge of the underlying mechanisms for these inequities is limited. Notably, little has been done to investigate systemic causes of these inequities, such as contemporary forms of racism: implicit bias, racialization, and structural racism, and their effects on epilepsy care and outcomes in PWE from racialized backgrounds. Thus, to close the existing gaps, the following directions are recommended:

- Many studies of the social determinants of health in epilepsy do not examine race/ethnicity, focusing on socioeconomic factors. This can be corrected in future research.
- Underlying mechanisms for racialized inequities in epilepsy must be conceptualized not only per current thinking about race and health, especially the role of racism and racialization, but also per cultural factors (eg, beliefs about epilepsy, stigma).
- Intersectionality is a powerful framework for understanding health inequities,[59] which has not yet found its way to epilepsy inequity research. Research at the intersection of racialized status and other social positions, as well as epilepsy discrimination intersecting with racialized status, would produce new knowledge regarding points of intervention to eliminate racialized inequities in epilepsy.
- To engage these new conceptual frameworks, diverse research approaches and methodologies are required, including more qualitative, mixed-method, and community engaged and community-participatory research. Epilepsy data at the individual level must be analyzed in relation to relevant data about racialized societal inequities.[11]
- Rethinking of standard racial/ethnic categories would also move the field forward: empirical research on racialized health inequalities "must engage with the profound challenges of conceptualizing, operationalizing, and analyzing the very data deployed–i.e., racialized categories—to document racialized health inequities."[11] Standard racial/ethnic categories, which are commonly used in health disparities research, combine individuals from a variety of backgrounds. Moreover, self-identifications can depend on questions asked and vary across life course or social contexts, whereas mixed racial/ethnic self-identifications increase the difficulty of assessing which race and/or ethnicity is responsible for disparities.[16]
- It is imperative to adopt an antiracist and social justice stance for epilepsy inequity research. Published research on racialized inequities must articulate the underlying mechanisms for inequities such as structural racism, racialization, and implicit bias.

SUMMARY

The growing understanding of racialized inequities in epilepsy is encouraging. However, engagement with contemporary framing of race and health is lacking. Social science insights can complement epidemiologic and health services research to understand the roots of racial inequities. Engaging epilepsy community members from racialized backgrounds is also essential, will strengthen the research, and help to move the field forward.

DISCLOSURE

The author has nothing to disclose.

REFERENCES

1. Centers for Disease C, Prevention. Prevalence of self-reported epilepsy–United States, 1986-1990. MMWR Morb Mortal Wkly Rep 1994;43(44):810–1, 817-818.

2. Hauser WA. Incidence and prevalence. In: Engel J, Pedley TA, editors. Epilepsy: a comprehensive textbook. Philadelphia: Lippincott-Raven; 1998. p. 47–58.
3. Theodore WH, Spencer SS, Wiebe S, et al. Epilepsy in North America: a report prepared under the auspices of the global campaign against epilepsy, the international bureau for epilepsy, the international league against epilepsy, and the World Health Organization. Epilepsia 2006;47(10):1700–22.
4. Levy JE, Neutra R, Parker D. Hand trembling, frenzy witchcraft, and moth madness: a study of Navajo seizure disorders. Tucson, AZ: University of Arizona Press; 1987.
5. Holden EW, Thanh Nguyen H, Grossman E, et al. Estimating prevalence, incidence, and disease-related mortality for patients with epilepsy in managed care organizations. Epilepsia 2005;46(2):311–9.
6. DeLorenzo RJ, Hauser WA, Towne AR, et al. A prospective, population-based epidemiologic study of status epilepticus in Richmond, Virginia. Neurology 1996;46(4):1029–35.
7. Dunlop DD, Song J, Lyons JS, et al. Racial/ethnic differences in rates of depression among preretirement adults. Am J Public Health 2003;93(11):1945–52.
8. Sacco RL, Boden-Albala B, Abel G, et al. Race-ethnic disparities in the impact of stroke risk factors: the northern Manhattan stroke study. Stroke 2001;32(8):1725–31.
9. Szaflarski M, Szaflarski JP, Privitera MD, et al. Racial/ethnic disparities in the treatment of epilepsy: What do we know? What do we need to know? Epilepsy Behav 2006;9(2):243–64.
10. Braveman P, Gruskin S. Defining equity in health. J Epidemiol Community Health 2003;57(4):254–8.
11. Krieger N. Structural Racism, Health Inequities, and the Two-Edged Sword of Data: Structural Problems Require Structural Solutions. Front Public Health 2021;9:655447.
12. Institute of Medicine (IOM). In: Smedley BD, Stith AY, Nelson AR, editors. Unequal treatment: confronting racial and ethnic disparities in health care. Washington, DC: National Academies Press; 2003.
13. Fiske ST. Interpersonal stratification: status, power, and subordination. In: Fiske ST, Gilbert DT, Lindzey D, editors. Handbook of social psychology. 5th edition. New York: Wiley; 2010. p. 941–82.
14. Rosenberg NA, Pritchard JK, Weber JL, et al. Genetic structure of human populations. Science 2002;298(5602):2381–5.
15. Clair M, Denis JS. Racism, Sociology of. In: Wright JD, editor. International encyclopedia of the social & behavioral sciences, vol. 19, 2nd edition. Boston, MA: Elsevier; 2015. p. 857–63.
16. Perreira KM, Wassink J, Harris KM. Beyond race/ethnicity: skin color, gender, and the health of young adults in the United States. Popul Res Policy Rev 2019;38(2): 271–99.
17. Tong M, Artiga S. Use of race in clinical diagnosis and decision making: overview and implications. Kasier Family Foundation. Available at: https://www.kff.org/racial-equity-and-health-policy/issue-brief/use-of-race-in-clinical-diagnosis-and-decision-making-overview-and-implications/. Accessed February 11, 2022.
18. Wilson WJ. The bridge over the racial divide: rising inequality and coalition politics. Berkley, CA: University of California Press; 1999.
19. Pager D, Shepherd H. The sociology of discrimination in employment, housing, credit, and consumer markets. Annu Rev Sociol 2008;34:181–209.
20. Bnaji MR, Grenwald AG. Blindspot: the hidden biases of good people. New York: Delacorte Press; 2013.

21. FitzGerald C, Hurst S. Implicit bias in healthcare professionals: a systematic review. BMC Med Ethics 2017;18(1):19.
22. Murji K, Solomos J. Racialization: studies in theory and practice. New York: Oxford University Press; 2005.
23. Artiga S, Hill L, Corallo B, et al. Asian immigrant experiences with racism, immigration-related fears, and the COVID-19 pandemic. Kasier Family Foundation. Available at: https://www.kff.org/coronavirus-covid-19/issue-brief/asian-immigrant-experiences-with-racism-immigration-related-fears-and-the-covid-19-pandemic/. Accessed February 11, 2022.
24. Stokely C, Hamilton CV. Black power: the politics of liberation in America. New York: Vintage Books; 1967.
25. Quillan L. New approaches to understinding racial prejudice and discrimiantion. Annu Rev Sociol 2006;32:299–328.
26. Bailey ZD, Feldman JM, Bassett MT. How Structural racism works - racist policies as a root cause of U.S. racial health inequities. N Engl J Med 2021;384(8):768–73.
27. Rivara FP, Bradley SM, Catenacci DV, et al. Structural racism and JAMA Network Open. JAMA Netw Open 2021;4(6):e2120269.
28. Churchwell K, Elkind MSV, Benjamin RM, et al. Call to action: structural racism as a fundamental driver of health disparities: a presidential advisory from the american heart association. Circulation 2020;142(24):e454–68.
29. Shaw G. It's a public health crisis: how systemic racism can be neurotoxic for Black Americans. Neurol Today. Available at: https://journals.lww.com/neurotodayonline/blog/breakingnews/pages/post.aspx?PostID=990. Accessed February 11, 2022.
30. Tian N, Croft JB, Kobau R, et al. CDC-supported epilepsy surveillance and epidemiologic studies: A review of progress since 1994. Epilepsy Behav 2020;109:107123.
31. Strine TW, Kobau R, Chapman DP, et al. Psychological distress, comorbidities, and health behaviors among U.S. adults with seizures: results from the 2002 National Health Interview Survey. Epilepsia 2005;46(7):1133–9.
32. Tian N, Boring M, Kobau R, et al. Active epilepsy and seizure control in adults - United States, 2013 and 2015. MMWR Morb Mortal Wkly Rep 2018;67(15):437–42.
33. Kobau R, Luo Y-H, Zach MM, et al. Epilepsy in adults and access to care - United States, 2010. MMWR Morb Mortal Wkly Rep 2012;61(45):909–13.
34. Miller GF, Coffield E, Leroy Z, et al. Prevalence and costs of five chronic conditions in children. J Sch Nurs 2016;32(5):357–64.
35. Kroner BL, Fahimi M, Kenyon A, et al. Racial and socioeconomic disparities in epilepsy in the District of Columbia. Epilepsy Res 2013;103(2–3):279–87.
36. Fitzgerald MP, Kaufman MC, Massey SL, et al. Assessing seizure burden in pediatric epilepsy using an electronic medical record-based tool through a common data element approach. Epilepsia 2021;62(7):1617–28.
37. Martin RC, Faught E, Szaflarski JP, et al. What does the U.S. Medicare administrative claims database tell us about initial antiepileptic drug treatment for older adults with new-onset epilepsy? Epilepsia 2017;58(4):548–57.
38. Bensken WP, Navale SM, Andrew AS, et al. Markers of quality care for newly diagnosed people with epilepsy on medicaid. Med Care 2021;59(7):588–96.
39. Friedman D, Fahlstrom R, Investigators E. Racial and ethnic differences in epilepsy classification among probands in the Epilepsy Phenome/Genome Project (EPGP). Epilepsy Res 2013;107(3):306–10.

40. Allen SE, Limdi NA, Westrick AC, et al. Racial differences in adult-onset MRI-negative temporal lobe epilepsy. Epilepsy Behav 2019;100(Pt A):106501.
41. Wilson DA, Selassie AW. Risk of severe and repetitive traumatic brain injury in persons with epilepsy: a population-based case-control study. Epilepsy Behav 2014;32:42–8.
42. Fantaneanu TA, Hurwitz S, van Meurs K, et al. Racial differences in emergency department visits for seizures. Seizure 2016;40:52–6.
43. Avetisyan R, Cabral H, Montouris G, et al. Evaluating racial/ethnic variations in outpatient epilepsy care. Epilepsy Behav 2013;27(1):95–101.
44. Schiltz NK, Koroukian SM, Lhatoo SD, et al. Temporal trends in pre-surgical evaluations and epilepsy surgery in the U.S. from 1998 to 2009. Epilepsy Res 2013; 103(2–3):270–8.
45. Modiano YA, Karakas C, Haneef Z. Social determinants do not affect access to specialized epilepsy care in veterans. Epilepsy Behav 2021;121(Pt A):108071.
46. Kobau R, Sapkota S, Koh HK, et al. National declines in the percentages of uninsured among adults aged 18-64 years with active epilepsy, 2010 and 2013 to 2015 and 2017-U.S. National Health Interview Survey. Epilepsy Behav 2019;97:316–8.
47. Szaflarski M, Wolfe JD, Tobias JGS, et al. Poverty, insurance, and region as predictors of epilepsy treatment among US adults. Epilepsy Behav 2020;107:107050.
48. Pisu M, Richman J, Szaflarski JP, et al. High health care costs in minority groups of older US Medicare beneficiaries with epilepsy. Epilepsia 2019;60(7):1462–71.
49. Bensken WP, Navale SM, Andrew AS, et al. Delays and disparities in diagnosis for adults with epilepsy: Findings from U.S. Medicaid data. Epilepsy Res 2020;166: 106406.
50. Gregerson CHY, Bakian AV, Wilkes J, et al. Disparities in pediatric epilepsy remission are associated with race and ethnicity. J Child Neurol 2019;34(14):928–36.
51. Terman SW, Kerr WT, Marcum ZA, et al. Antiseizure medication adherence trajectories in Medicare beneficiaries with newly treated epilepsy. Epilepsia 2021; 62(11):2778–89.
52. Faught E, Szaflarski JP, Richman J, et al. Risk of pharmacokinetic interactions between antiepileptic and other drugs in older persons and factors associated with risk. Epilepsia 2018;59(3):715–23.
53. Sanchez Fernandez I, Stephen C, Loddenkemper T. Disparities in epilepsy surgery in the United States of America. J Neurol 2017;264(8):1735–45.
54. Englot DJ, Ouyang D, Garcia PA, et al. Epilepsy surgery trends in the United States, 1990–2008. Neurology 2012;78(16):1200–6.
55. Wissel BD, Greiner HM, Glauser TA, et al. Investigation of bias in an epilepsy machine learning algorithm trained on physician notes. Epilepsia 2019;60(9):e93–8.
56. Fox J, Lekoubou A, Bishu KG, et al. Recent patterns of vagal nerve stimulator use in the United States: Is there a racial disparity? Epilepsia 2019;60(4):756–63.
57. McCann ZH, Szaflarski M, Szaflarski JP. A feasibility study to assess social stress and social support in patients enrolled in a cannabidiol (CBD) compassionate access program. Epilepsy Behav 2021;124:108322.
58. Szaflarski M, Hansen B, Bebin EM, et al. Social correlates of health status, quality of life, and mood states in patients treated with cannabidiol for epilepsy. Epilepsy Behav 2017;70(Pt B):364–9.
59. Homan P, Brown TH, King B. Structural intersectionality as a new direction for health disparities research. J Health Soc Behav 2021;62(3):350–70.

Autism Spectrum Disorder and Epilepsy

Churl-Su Kwon, MD, MPH, FRSPH[a], Elaine C. Wirrell, MD, FRCPC[b],
Nathalie Jetté, MD, MSc, FRCPC[c],*

KEYWORDS

- Seizures • ASD • Genetic • Antiseizure medications • Epilepsy surgery
- Neuromodulation

KEY POINTS

- The prevalence of autism spectrum disorders (ASD) or epilepsy is much higher when these disorders co-exist.
- Chromosomal abnormalities, metabolic disorders, and infections are examples of etiologies that predispose a patient to both ASD and epilepsy—genetic testing in particular can have a high yield in those with ASD and epilepsy.
- The ASD phenotype in epilepsy can look different—ASD may only be diagnosed when seizures are controlled.
- Prompt recognition of seizures in those with ASD or of ASD in those with epilepsy has important treatment implications.
- Epilepsy surgery is an important therapeutic option in patients with ASD and drug-resistant epilepsy.

INTRODUCTION

Autism spectrum disorder (ASD), was first described in 1943 as a disorder consisting of a triad of qualitative impairments of social interaction, communication and restricted repetitive patterns of behavior, interests, and activities.[1] The relationship between ASD and epilepsy is well documented.[2] Patients with ASD have an increased risk of epilepsy, while those with epilepsy have a higher risk of ASD, as compared with the general population.[3] Diagnosing epilepsy in those with ASD can be challenging. For example, stereotyped behaviors could be mistaken as ASD stereotypies, when in

[a] Departments of Neurology, Epidemiology, Neurosurgery, and the Gertrude H. Sergievsky Center, Columbia University Irving Medical Center, 630 W. 168th Street, New York, NY 10032, USA; [b] Division of Epilepsy and Child and Adolescent Neurology, Department of Neurology, Mayo Clinic, 200 First Street Southwest, Rochester MN 55902, USA; [c] Department of Neurology, Icahn school of Medicine at Mount Sinai, One Gustave L. Levy Place, Box 1137, New York, NY 10029, USA
* Corresponding author:
E-mail address: nathalie.jette@mssm.edu

Neurol Clin 40 (2022) 831–847
https://doi.org/10.1016/j.ncl.2022.03.011
0733-8619/22/© 2022 Elsevier Inc. All rights reserved.

fact, they may be due to seizures. Fortunately, in recent years, we have gained a better understanding of the best antiseizure medications (ASMs) to use in this vulnerable population.[4,5] However, more studies are needed to understand how best to screen for ASD in epilepsy, what the various ASD phenotypes are in people with epilepsy, especially those due to de novo genes/mutations,[6] as well as factors influencing the fluctuating nature of ASD symptoms (eg, seizure type, frequency, syndromes, ASMs).[7]

This article begins with an overview of the definitions of epilepsy and ASD. We then discuss commonly shared etiologies and review the epidemiology of these comorbidities. The next section summarizes how ASD is evaluated and treated in people with epilepsy, focusing on both medical and surgical management.

DEFINITIONS

Boxes 1 and **2** provide the latest definitions of epilepsy and ASD. The 2017 ILAE classification also provides etiologic categories for epilepsies including structural, genetic, metabolic, infectious, immune, or unknown causes, as this has substantial treatment implications.[8]

The current DSM-V definition of ASD[9] (see **Box 2**) remains faithful to the original description with added specifications regarding symptoms present in early childhood and that these symptoms collectively limit and impair daily functioning.

DISCUSSION
The epidemiology of autism spectrum disorder and epilepsy

The literature about the bidirectional relationship between epilepsy and ASD is heterogeneous, with variation in ascertainment methods, populations, and definitions of epilepsy or "autism" used. However, studies consistently report a higher estimate of epilepsy in those with ASD and of ASD in those with epilepsy, as compared with population without epilepsy or ASD, respectively. One of the most comprehensive systematic reviews on the topic, incorporating data from 74 studies reporting on more than 283,000 people, found that the median overall period prevalence of epilepsy in ASD was 12.1% while the median overall period prevalence of ASD in epilepsy was 9%.[3] These estimates were slightly lower if those with syndromic epilepsy or developmental delay were excluded. It has also been shown that the prevalence of epilepsy is higher in women with ASD (19%, range 0%–60% compared with 11.4%, range 3.6%–30%; **Fig. 1**A) while the prevalence of ASD is higher in men with epilepsy (**Fig. 1**B).[3] Another systematic review reported a higher prevalence of epilepsy in ASD in clinic-based studies compared with cohort or population-based studies.[11] In this latter review, older age, female sex, intellectual disability and the human development index of countries were all associated with estimates of epilepsy in ASD. These factors, along with "symptomatic etiology of epilepsy" were also found to be associated with a high

---

Box 1
Definitions and classifications of epilepsy

The 2014 ILAE definition of epilepsy states that epilepsy is a disease of the brain with an ongoing predisposition to generate seizures defined by any of the following:[10]

1. At least 2 unprovoked/reflex seizures that occur more than 24 hours apart

2. One unprovoked/reflex seizure and a probability of more seizures similar to the general occurrence risk (≥60%) after 2 unprovoked seizures, occurring over the following 10 years.

3. A diagnosis of an epilepsy syndrome

Box 2
DSM-V definition of ASD spectrum disorder

The definition of ASD consists of the following criteria:

A. Persistent deficits in social communication and social interaction across several contexts that exhibit all 3 deficits in:
   1. Social-emotional reciprocity
   2. Nonverbal communicative behaviors
   3. Developing, maintaining, and understanding relationships

B. Restricted, repetitive patterns of behavior by at least 2 of the following:
   1. Stereotyped/repetitive motor movements, use of objects, or speech
   2. Ritualized patterns of verbal/nonverbal behavior, excessive adherence to routines, and resistant to change
   3. Highly restricted, fixated interests that are abnormal in intensity
   4. Hyper- or hypoactivity to sensory input or unusual interests in sensory aspects of the environment

C. Symptoms must be seen in early childhood

D. Symptoms impair and limit everyday functioning

---

prevalence of ASD in epilepsy, in another systematic review.[12] Finally, the prevalence of ASD in epilepsy was 4.7%, 19.9%, 41.9%, and 47.4%, respectively, in those with generalized epilepsy, infantile spasms, focal seizures, and Dravet syndrome.[12]

Common shared etiologies between epilepsy and autism spectrum disorder

The strong association between epilepsy and ASD is likely due to underlying mechanisms that influence both disease processes. Chromosomal abnormalities, metabolic disorders, and infections are examples of etiologies that predispose to both ASD and epilepsy.

Our understanding of genomic copy number and single-gene causes of ASD and epilepsy help distinguish some of the biological processes that are altered in these disorders.[13–15] Important biological pathways that are vital for neurologic development and that can be affected genetically in both conditions include the regulation of gene transcription, cell growth and proliferation, synapse development, stability and function.[16] The single gene and genomic copy number regions that are frequently linked to ASD and epilepsy are listed in **Box 3**.

Various metabolic disorders, if left untreated, can lead to brain damage. Many children with ASD have underlying metabolic disorders, which in turn are also frequently associated with epilepsy.[17] Metabolic disorders associated with both ASD and epilepsy include amino acid metabolism, biotin, carnitine, cholesterol, creatine, purine, pyridoxine, pyrimidine, and urea cycle disorders.[17] **(Table 1)**

Infectious links are seen in association with intrauterine infection. Congenital rubella has long been associated with an increased risk of ASD, epilepsy and intellectual disability.[18] Brain damage during birth and neonatal jaundice, if inadequately treated, are also associated with ASD and epilepsy.[19,20]

Evaluation of autism spectrum disorder and epilepsy

Which child with epilepsy should be screened, when and how?

The American Academy of Pediatrics (AAP) recommends formal standardized screening for ASD at 18 and 24 months of age in all infants.[21] This recommendation is particularly pertinent to infants with epilepsy given their significantly higher rate of ASD. The recent clinical report from the AAP on Identification, Evaluation, and Management of Children with ASD Spectrum Disorder[21] as well as the AAP Toolkit

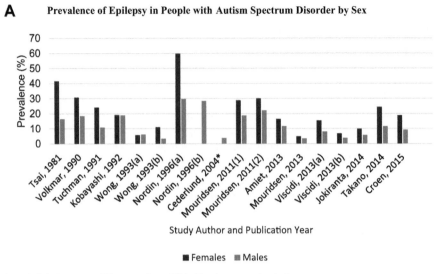

A   Prevalence of Epilepsy in People with Autism Spectrum Disorder by Sex

(1) and (2) indicates two different studies published by the same author in the same year
(a) and (b) indicates multiple estimates reported in the same article
*Only reported on male participants

B   Prevalence of Autism Spectrum Disorder in People with Epilepsy by Sex

Fig. 1. Graph of Trends by Sex and by Year of Publication. (A) Histogram showing the prevalence of epilepsy in people with autism spectrum disorder by sex. (B) Histogram showing the prevalence of autism spectrum disorder in people with epilepsy by sex. (*From* Lukmanji S, Manji SA, Kadhim S, et al. The co-occurrence of epilepsy and autism: A systematic review. Epilepsy Behav. 2019;98:238–248. https://doi.org/10.1016/j.yebeh.2019.07.037; with permission).

(https://toolkits.solutions.aap.org) summarize commonly used screening instruments. The Modified Checklist for ASD in Toddlers—R/F (m-CHAT-R/F) is most often used before 30 months of age and is a two-part screen. The second part, a staff-completed, structured interview is only needed if the first part, a 20-item, parent-completed checklist is positive for indeterminate. This instrument is recommended

---

Box 3
Examples of pathogenic genetic variants that can be seen in persons with epilepsy and autism spectrum disorder

Copy number variants
- 15a11-q13 duplications
- 15q11-q13 deletions
- 16 p11.2 deletion
- 16p13.11 duplication

Trisomy 21

mTORopathies
- TSC1 or 2
- PTEN

Disorders of transcriptional regulation
- FOXG1
- MECP2
- MEF2C

Channelopathies
  Sodium
- SCN1A
- SCN2A
- SCN3A
- SCN8A

  Potassium
- KCNQ3
- KCNMA1

  Calcium
- CACNA1E

  Hyperpolarization-activated cyclic nucleotide-gated
- HCN1

  Glutamate
- GRIN2B

Disorders of synaptic structure
- CASK
- CDKL5
- CNTNAP2
- FMR1
- NRXN1
- SHANK3 (Phelan-McDermid)
- SYNGAP1
- SYN1

Disorders of Neuronal migration
- RELN

---

for all children with epilepsy age 30 months or younger who have not been previously screened.

For children presenting after 30 months of age, who have not undergone prior routine screening, a careful history to evaluate for red flags (lack of response to name by 12 months, lack of pointing at objects to show interest at 14 months, and lack of pretend play at 18 months) should be performed.[21] Other concerning symptoms include avoidance of eye contact, difficulty understanding other people's feelings, delayed speech and language, echolalia, becoming upset about minor changes, obsessive interests, repetitive movements such as hand flapping or rocking and unusual reactions to sensory stimuli.[21] There are no validated screening

Table 1
Metabolic disorders that can be associated with autism spectrum disorder and epilepsy

Disorder	Symptoms	Diagnostic Tests	Treatment
Succinic semialdehyde dehydrogenase deficiency	ID, language delay, hypotonia, ataxia, behavior problems	Urine organic acids – increased 4-hydroxybutyric acid	Symptomatic
Smith–Lemli–Opitz	Growth delay, microcephaly, polydactyly, cleft palate, abnormal genitalia, dysmorphic features, ID	Elevated 7-dehydrocholesterol in blood	Cholesterol supplementation
Cerebral folate deficiency – Primary or Secondary	Regression of motor and cognitive skills, tremor, ataxia, irritability, insomnia, hypotonia	Reduced 5-methyltetrahydrofolate in CSF	Leucovorin
Disorders of creatine transport or metabolism	ID, movement disorders	Urine or serum creatine metabolism screen	Supplemental creatine Dietary manipulation
Adenylsuccinate lyase deficiency	Hypotonia, behavior problems, ID	Succinyl aminoimidazole carboxamide riboside and succinyladenosine in CSF, urine, serum	Symptomatic
Disorders of purine and pyrimidine metabolism -Lesch Nyhan	Self-injurious behavior, ID, dystonia	High uric acid	Symptomatic
Lysosomal storage disorders -Sanfilippo syndrome	ID, regression, movement disorders, mild coarsening of face, hernias, macrocephaly, hepatosplenomegaly, visual and hearing impairment	Urine for mucopolysaccharides	Symptomatic
Mitochondrial disorders	ID, growth deficiency, multiorgan dysfunction, hypotonia, movement disorders, nystagmus	Elevated serum and CSF lactate and alanine Muscle biopsy Genetic testing	Mitochondrial cocktail – Coenzyme Q10, B vitamins, carnitine Avoid valproic acid
Biotinidase deficiency	ID, rash, alopecia	Biotinidase-serum	Biotin supplementation

ID – intellectual disability.

instruments for children more than 30 months of age; however, the Social Communication Questionnaire which is a brief parent-completed checklist can provide helpful data.[22]

The screening instruments do not confirm a diagnosis of ASD but identify children who should be referred for further evaluation to a developmental pediatrician, psychologist, pediatric psychiatrist, or child neurologist with additional expertise in ASD. Tools that are commonly used include lengthier, semi-structured parental questionnaires such as the ASD Diagnostic interview—Revised, as well as structured observation tools such as the ASD Diagnostic Observation Schedule – 2 or the Childhood ASD Rating Scale – 2.

The challenge in diagnosing autism spectrum disorder in children with epilepsy

Autism spectrum disorder can be challenging to identify among children with epilepsy and thus is likely underdiagnosed.[7] A recent commentary identified several factors leading to this challenge:[7]

1. The ASD phenotype in children with epilepsy may be more dynamic and follow an atypical trajectory. In a cohort of 170 children followed through the Developmental Epilepsy Clinic at Great Ormond Street Hospital, only 20% had a trajectory consistent with primary ASD spectrum disorder, whereby symptoms of clear ASD were present before 3 years of age and whereby there was no significant fluctuation in the phenotype. Forty-one percent presented later in the preschool years although they had early onset of seizures in the first 2 years of life and history of atypical social communication development. Of these 58/69 presented with a slowly emerging phenotype with fluctuation in some cases, while 11/69 presented with regression in skills after a period of uncontrolled seizures. Finally, 39% had normal early social communication development and presented with an ASD phenotype after 4 years of age. Of these, 39/67 showed gradual emergence of that phenotype, whereas 28/67 had clear regression in association with uncontrolled seizures or an epileptic encephalopathy. In 5.3% of cases, the ASD phenotype resolved with time.
2. The ASD phenotype may look different. Children with epilepsy may socially approach others; however, still have deficits in understanding verbal and nonverbal cues and socially appropriate behavior. In Dravet syndrome, many children who have been identified with ASD have relatively preserved social skills.[23]
3. Challenging behaviors are often assumed to be either part of epilepsy or a side effect of medication and are not further explored. In some children, behaviors significantly worsened with improved seizure control or seizure cessation, and ASD is only diagnosed at that time.
4. The diagnosis of ASD in the presence of a significant intellectual disability can be challenging as the usual observational tools cannot be used. Intellectual disability, which is often severe, is more frequent in children with epilepsy with comorbid ASD than those with primary ASD.[24] The examiner must identify that social communication skills are more significantly delayed than other developmental skills.
5. Many clinicians are reluctant to give additional diagnoses to a child who already has a very severe seizure disorder often with an associated genetic condition.

Evaluations in persons with comorbid autism spectrum disorder and epilepsy

A careful clinical evaluation, focusing on development, pre and perinatal risk factors, family history, and physical examination (head circumference, dysmorphic features, neurocutaneous lesions, neurologic examination findings) may provide clues to the underlying etiology.

ElectroencephalogramThe main goal of the electroencephalogram (EEG) is to assist in the classification of epilepsy type and etiology, and to evaluate for subtle clinical seizures (such as myoclonic, absence, or focal seizures) that may impact treatment decisions.[25] The rate of epileptiform abnormalities in persons with ASD ranges from 4% to 80%, even without a history of clinical seizures.[26] Discharges can be seen in multiple regions but temporal and central foci are most prevalent.[26] In more than 60%, discharges are seen only during sleep,[27,28] emphasizing the importance of ensuring sleep tracing is obtained.

(Developmental and) Epileptic Encephalopathy with Spike-Wave Activation in Sleep is a relatively rare epilepsy syndrome that presents in childhood and can mimic ASD.[29] Children 2 to 12 years of age (peak age 5–7 years) present with cognitive, behavioral, and/or motor plateauing or regression that occur at the same time or within weeks of the characteristic EEG abnormality. The EEG in wakefulness may be normal or show focal or multifocal discharges, but in sleep, there is marked activation of spike waves, which become nearly continuous, typically occupying more than 50% of slow sleep. Neurocognitive and behavioral improvement is typically seen with a resolution of the continuous spikes and waves during sleep (CSWS) on EEG. This syndrome should be suspected if regression is seen after the first 2 years of life, as regression in ASD is typically seen between 18 and 24 months.[21] Several studies have found that the presence of epileptiform discharges (EDs) in persons with ASD correlates with more severe ASD, lower intellectual function and more severe neuropsychiatric problems.[30,31] Follow-up EEGs should be obtained as clinically indicated. Ictal recordings may be required to confirm the epileptogenic nature of new types of spells, such as staring.

Genetic testing

Genetic testing has a considerable yield in the evaluation of persons with epilepsy and comorbid ASD. The Executive Summary on Identification, Evaluation, and Management of Children With ASD Spectrum Disorder from the AAP recommends that families be offered genetic evaluation, including chromosomal microarray and fragile X testing, with the consideration of other cytogenetic and molecular testing, as indicated.[21] A large number of genes have been implicated and may affect neuronal excitation/inhibition balance, synaptic vesicle release, regulation of ion channels, synaptic physiology, membrane depolarization, control of subcellular signaling pathways and regulation of migration and organization of network connections.[32] A recent systematic review and meta-analysis on use of next-generation sequencing in neurodevelopmental disorders reported a diagnostic yield of 17.1% for ASD, 24% for epilepsy and 28.2% for intellectual disability.[33] Among those with epilepsy, the yield is significantly higher in those with as opposed to without intellectual disability (27.9% vs 9.3%); however, the authors did not report on the yield in those with epilepsy and ASD. The diagnostic yield for whole-exome sequencing was not significantly higher than panel testing. In another study from an outpatient ASD clinic, pathogenic or likely pathogenic variants were found in 17.5% of 137 children with ASD and were significantly more common in the presence of comorbid epilepsy (6/14, 43%).[34]

The results of genetic testing were reviewed in a cohort of 173 children with ASD and an abnormal EEG identified through an ASD clinic.[35] Those with an established diagnosis of epilepsy were more likely to undergo more genetic testing than those without a diagnosis of epilepsy, but had a lower molecular diagnosis rate (9% vs 33%). However, those with epilepsy were more likely to undergo epilepsy gene panels and less likely to receive trio whole-exome sequencing, the latter of which was of higher yield. The authors concluded that exome-based trio testing may be the preferred diagnostic testing for patients with ASD and an abnormal EEG with or without epilepsy.

Neuroimaging
The Executive Summary on Identification, Evaluation, and Management of Children With ASD Spectrum Disorder from the AAP recommends that neuroimaging be considered in persons with ASD based on history and physical examination.[21] The ILAE Subcommittee for Neuroimaging in Children with Epilepsy proposed a list of criteria for structural imaging which include neurologic examination abnormalities and history of developmental delay, arrest or regression.[36] Thus, in the absence of another clear etiology for ASD and seizures, neuroimaging should be strongly considered.

Metabolic studies
The yield of routine metabolic testing for children with ASD alone is low.[21] However, testing should be considered in the appropriate clinical context. **Table 1** contains a list of metabolic disorders that can be associated with both epilepsy and ASD.

Approach to the medical management of seizures with autism spectrum disorder

In general, treatment of epilepsy in persons with ASD should be focused on seizure control, and directed by seizure type(s), epilepsy syndrome (if present), and etiology. Additionally, associated comorbidities should be considered, to minimize the risk of cognitive or behavioral side effects with specific medications. The issue of whether treatment should also focus on the reduction or amelioration of EDs has been debated.[26,37] While EDs may simply be a biomarker of an abnormal brain, there has been concern that they may also have a causal or contributory role in neurocognitive comorbidities such as ASD.

Several studies have evaluated this question in children with neuropsychological dysfunction including ASD with EDs, with conflicting results. This was evaluated in a double-blind, placebo-controlled, crossover study in 61 children with normal IQ but behavioral or cognitive concerns, excluding ASD.[38] Children were treated with lamotrigine versus placebo, and ambulatory EEGs were performed at baseline, and after the end of both the placebo and lamotrigine treatment phases. A significant improvement in behavior was found in those with decreased frequency and duration of EDs. In another study, 70 children with ASD and EDs on EEG but without seizures, were randomized to receive either levetiracetam with educational training or educational training alone.[39] Levetiracetam was associated with a reduction in EDs and with improved behavior and cognition compared with the group treated with educational intervention alone. In a small retrospective study of 14 persons with ASD, some of whom had seizures and/or EDs, 10 were rated as having improved neurocognitive function with valproic acid treatment, and all of these had a history of seizures or EDs on EEG.[40] Conversely, a double-blind, crossover study of 8 children with learning and behavior disorders and EDs, but without seizures, were randomized in another study to either valproic acid or placebo.[41] Children treated with valproic acid had increased distractibility, increased response times, lower memory scores and overall had poorer functioning than those receiving placebo. In summary, in children with neurocognitive dysfunction or regression, a trial of ASMs may be considered, particularly if concerned that the cognitive symptoms may relate to the EDs; however, patients should be carefully evaluated to ensure there is no adverse impact of medication, and medication should only be continued if a clear benefit is seen. The concern for EDs worsening neurocognitive function is most relevant for developmental and epileptic encephalopathies. The term "epileptic encephalopathy" implies that the seizures and/or frequent EDs cause or significantly exacerbate neurocognitive dysfunction such as ASD.

In Infantile Spasms Syndrome, successful treatment is defined by both resolution of infantile spasms and resolution of hypsarrhythmia. However, several investigators have noted that the underlying etiology is even more important than the spasms themselves in predicting ASD.[42-44] In tuberous sclerosis complex (TSC), approximately one-third of cases have both epilepsy and ASD.[45] The risk of ASD is increased by early-onset seizures and intellectual disability, both of which are associated with infantile spasms.[45,46] Furthermore, persistent frontal and temporal EDs seem predictive of the development of ASD in children with TSC-associated infantile spasms.[47,48] The EPISTOP trial investigated whether the initiation of ASMs in infants with TSC at the time EDs were initially found, before the onset of clinical seizures would improve outcomes compared with treatment only after clinical seizures appeared.[49] Eighty infants 4 months and younger, with TSC but without a history of seizures, underwent serial video EEG and developmental testing, which included a Bayley scale of Infant Development and an ASD Diagnostic Observation Schedule. ASD developed in 30% of cases by 24 months and was more commonly seen in infants with epilepsy. However, no significant difference was seen in ASD rates when ASMs were started at the time of ED versus at the time of actual seizure onset.

In (Developmental and) Epilepsy Encephalopathy with Spike-Wave Activation in Sleep, language plateauing or regression is typically seen, and differs from autistic regression in that it typically occurs later, beyond 2 years of age, is more commonly associated with clinical seizures and affects predominantly language with greater preservation of social skills. Early and aggressive treatment targeting the marked activation of EDs in sleep with therapies that include benzodiazepines, steroid, other medications, or surgical options are recommended.[50]

In most cases, ASMs are chosen to target specific seizure type(s), syndromes, or etiologies. There are limited data to guide treatment choice when medications are used solely to attenuate EDs, and such data need to be interpreted in the context of natural fluctuations.[51] In a pediatric study of 213 children who underwent EEG both at baseline and after medication initiation, suppression rates of EDs were 22% for phenobarbital, 33% for carbamazepine and 46% for valproate.[52] Other medications which may also reduce spike counts include lamotrigine,[53] benzodiazepines,[54-57] levetiracetam[58] and steroids.[59] However, ASMs may also exacerbate EDs or seizures.[60]

Approach to the surgical management of epilepsy in patients with autism spectrum disorder

As with all cases of epilepsy, a subset of patients with comorbid epilepsy and ASD develop drug-resistant epilepsy. Epilepsy surgery, when successful, yields greater life expectancy compared with medical treatment in patients with drug-resistant epilepsy, yet it is underutilized.[61] Contrary to the popular belief that epilepsy surgery has limited utility in those with ASD, the feasibility and safety of epilepsy surgery in those with ASD has been reported (see Case 1), emphasizing not only better seizure control but also associated gains in cognition.[62]

The most common open cranial epilepsy surgeries performed in ASD include hemispherotomies, focal/multifocal resections, subpial transections, and disconnections. In the few initial published case series, outcomes have varied. Resective surgery for epilepsy in those with ASD has generally demonstrated improved seizure frequency.[63-65] However, mixed results are seen with behavioral outcomes from drastic improvement[64] to not seeing any overwhelmingly positive gains.[65] Larger more recent case series have also shown decreased seizure burden and the most part either no change or moderate improvement in behavior, again highlighting the importance of extensive neuropsychiatric work-up before surgery.[66-68]

Case 1

This three and a half-year-old boy presented with a history of drug-resistant epilepsy and autism. He was the 1st born child and the pregnancy was complicated by pregnancy-induced hypertension treated with bed rest. Delivery was induced at 36 weeks for maternal hypertension and he was born by spontaneous vaginal delivery with a weight of 5 lb 9 oz and was healthy. He was discharged home at 2 days of age.

At 15 months of age, he presented with a prolonged, focal to bilateral tonic-clonic seizure with fever. The seizure stopped after 25 minutes, following lorazepam, and further workup revealed he had herpes encephalitis. He received 21 days of acyclovir and had no further seizures. He was discharged home off ASMs.

Seizures recurred at 2 years 7 months of age and 2 types were noted:

1. Clusters of epileptic spasms with head flexion, bilateral arm extension, and eye deviation to the left, each lasting 1 to 2 seconds but occurring in clusters lasting 3 to 5 minutes several times per day.
2. Episodes of head drop, arm elevation, and loss of tone lasting 5 to 8 seconds, not occurring in clusters and occurring every 2 to 3 days.

His seizures had persisted despite trials of levetiracetam, oxcarbazepine, topiramate, valproic acid, felbamate, and the ketogenic diet.

His developmental milestones had been normal until 15 months. Following the bout of HSV encephalitis, he was felt to be slightly more clumsy in both fine and gross motor skills, and to have a left exotropia. His language was slowly progressing but since the recurrence of seizures at 2 years 7 months, he had minimal gains in speech and was noted to have poor eye contact.

Neuropsychological testing was performed at three and a half years of age. On the Bayley Scales of Infant and Toddler Development – 3rd edition, his cognitive skills were at the 21 month age equivalent, receptive language at the 6 month age equivalent, and expressive language at the 12 month age equivalent. Parental-reported adaptive functioning showed borderline communication and social skills, with solidly average daily living and motor skills. The BASC-2 showed borderline elevations on the Withdrawal, Attention Problems, Social Skills, and Atypicality scales. The Autism Diagnostic Observation Schedule showed behaviors consistent with autism.

His interictal EEG showed high amplitude generalized slowing, with abundant generalized and multifocal polyspike and wave discharges (**Fig. 2A**). An ictal EEG captured epileptic spasms that were associated with a diffuse generalized spike wave followed by lower amplitude fast activity (**Fig. 2B**).

An MRI showed right temporal encephalomalacia involving the medial temporal region (right uncus and hippocampus) (**Fig. 2C**).

He underwent right temporal lobectomy and achieved seizure freedom. Medications were stopped at 12 months without seizure recurrence.

Repeat neuropsychological testing at 6 years 10 months of age showed low average cognitive abilities (Verbal IQ 88, Performance IQ 96), with mild weakness in attention. However, he was socially appropriate and had no evidence of autism spectrum behaviors. His postoperative EEG showed mild right temporal slowing with the resolution of discharges.

The most studied form of neuromodulation in the treatment of drug-resistant epilepsy in those with ASD is vagus nerve stimulation (VNS). The strongest evidence

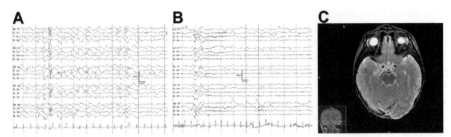

Fig. 2. (*A*) Interictal EEG of case 1 which shows high amplitude generalized slowing, with abundant generalized and multifocal polyspike and wave discharges (see **Fig. 2**A). (*B*) Ictal recording of Case 1, which illustrates epileptic spasms that were associated with a diffuse generalized spike wave followed by lower amplitude fast activity. (*C*) MRI (axial T2) from case 1 demonstrates right temporal encephalomalacia involving the medial temporal region (right uncus and hippocampus).

regarding the efficacy of VNS in patients with ASD comes from 2 retrospective studies that used the same patient registry to track outcomes.[69,70] The first study in 2003 included 59 patients with ASD and reported a median reduction in seizure frequency of 40% at 3 months and 55% at 1 year.[69] More than 50% experienced improvements in achievement, mood, postictal period, seizure clustering 1-year postimplantation. No patients reported significant regression in any aspect of quality of life. This study, however, did not focus on improvement in ASD symptoms.[69] The second study published in 2010 compared outcomes in those with and without ASD. The difference in reduction in seizure frequency between both groups was not statistically significant at 1-year postimplantation. However, a greater proportion of patients with ASD, at 1-year follow-up, had improved mood compared with controls (61.5% vs 47%).[70] While these 2 studies are promising, other work has cast doubt on the efficacy of VNS in this patient population. A prospective study used standardized tools to measure behavioral, cognitive, and seizure frequency in patients with ASD before and 2 years post-VNS implantation (unlike the aforementioned studies).[71] Seizure frequency was unchanged for most of the participants, and neuropsychiatric diagnoses were unchanged from baseline. Only half of the group noticed minor improved social interaction and attention span.

Novel treatments such as responsive neurostimulation (RNS) have added to the neurosurgeon's armamentarium in treating epilepsy.[72] The FDA approved the RNS system following a randomized controlled trial of 191 adults with DRE.[73] After 9 years of follow-up, a 75% median seizure reduction was reported, with over one-quarter of these patients experiencing at least 6 months of seizure freedom,[74] and 44% reporting improvements in their quality of life at 2 years.[75] In the setting of epilepsy and comorbid ASD, the epilepsy is frequently of diffuse onset, multifocal and/or MRI-negative. Although RNS is a relatively new device, there are a few case reports of responsive thalamic stimulation with >50% seizure reduction and improved behavioral outcomes.[76] In such a population whereby surgeries such as palliative disconnections and resections may not be feasible or beneficial, significant gains through better seizure control can be made with the RNS system.[76]

SUMMARY

Autism spectrum disorder and epilepsy are common comorbidities. As the prevalence of each condition is much higher when they co-exist, prompt recognition of ASD in people with epilepsy is important. This is in part because shared etiologies may be identified, in particular genetic etiologists, which can have important treatment implications. Treatment of seizures with medical therapy and, in those with drug-resistant epilepsy, surgery can be associated with important benefits.

CLINICS CARE POINTS

- Autism spectrum disorder is a common comorbidity in children with epilepsy and remains underdiagnosed.
- While it can be associated with a wide variety of epilepsies, children with early-onset, drug-resistant epilepsy are at particularly high risk of ASD.
- Autism spectrum disorder in children with epilepsy often follows an atypical trajectory with later presentation.
- Timely diagnosis is critical to allow appropriate early intervention.
- Etiologies are varied but the genetic evaluation is of particularly high yield.
- Treatment of epilepsy should focus on control of clinical seizures, not the resolution of all EEG abnormalities.
- In epileptic encephalopathies with severely abnormal EEGs, a trial of therapy could be considered to suppress frequent EDs; however, careful clinical correlation is needed to assess the benefit.

DISCLOSURE

Churl-Su Kwon has no relevant disclosures. Nathalie Jette receives grant funding paid to her institution for grants unrelated to this work from NINDS (NIH U24NS107201, NIH IU54NS100064). She is the Bludhorn Professor of International Medicine. She receives an honorarium for her work as an Associate Editor of Epilepsia. Elaine C Wirrell has served as a paid consultant for Encoded Therapeutics and BioMarin. She is the Editor-in-Chief of Epilepsy.com.

REFERENCES

1. Kanner L. Autistic disturbances of affective contact. Nervous Child 1943;2: 217–50.
2. El Achkar CM, Spence SJ. Clinical characteristics of children and young adults with co-occurring autism spectrum disorder and epilepsy. Epilepsy Behav 2015;47:183–90.
3. Lukmanji S, Manji SA, Kadhim S, et al. The co-occurrence of epilepsy and autism: a systematic review. Epilepsy Behav 2019;98:238–48.
4. Alaimo H, Geller E, Mahalingam R, et al. Ictal EEG in patients with autistic spectrum disorder and epilepsy. Epilepsy Res 2020;168:106482.
5. Frye RE, Sreenivasula S, Adams JB. Traditional and non-traditional treatments for autism spectrum disorder with seizures: an on-line survey. BMC Pediatr 2011; 11:37.
6. Bishop SL, Farmer C, Bal V, et al. Identification of developmental and behavioral markers associated with genetic abnormalities in autism spectrum disorder. Am J Psychiatry 2017;174:576–85.
7. Holmes H, Sawer F, Clark M. Autism spectrum disorders and epilepsy in children: a commentary on the occurrence of autism in epilepsy; how it can present

differently and the challenges associated with diagnosis. Epilepsy Behav 2021; 117:107813.

8. Scheffer IE, Berkovic S, Capovilla G, et al. ILAE classification of the epilepsies: position paper of the ILAE commission for classification and terminology. Epilepsia 2017;58:512–21.

9. American psychiatric association: diagnostic and statistical manual of mental disorders. 5th edition. Arlington: American Psychiatric Association; 2013.

10. Fisher RS, Acevedo C, Arzimanoglou A, et al. ILAE official report: a practical clinical definition of epilepsy. Epilepsia 2014;55:475–82.

11. Liu X, Sun X, Sun C, et al. Prevalence of epilepsy in autism spectrum disorders: a systematic review and meta-analysis. Autism 2022;26:33–50.

12. Strasser L, Downes M, Kung J, et al. Prevalence and risk factors for autism spectrum disorder in epilepsy: a systematic review and meta-analysis. Dev Med Child Neurol 2018;60:19–29.

13. Mefford HC, Yendle SC, Hsu C, et al. Rare copy number variants are an important cause of epileptic encephalopathies. Ann Neurol 2011;70:974–85.

14. Olson H, Shen Y, Avallone J, et al. Copy number variation plays an important role in clinical epilepsy. Ann Neurol 2014;75:943–58.

15. Pinto D, Delaby E, Merico D, et al. Convergence of genes and cellular pathways dysregulated in autism spectrum disorders. Am J Hum Genet 2014;94:677–94.

16. Lee BH, Smith T, Paciorkowski AR. Autism spectrum disorder and epilepsy: disorders with a shared biology. Epilepsy Behav 2015;47:191–201.

17. Frye RE. Metabolic and mitochondrial disorders associated with epilepsy in children with autism spectrum disorder. Epilepsy Behav 2015;47:147–57.

18. Chess S. Follow-up report on autism in congenital rubella. J Autism Child Schizophr 1977;7:69–81.

19. Kuban KC, Joseph RM, O'Shea TM, et al. Girls and boys born before 28 weeks gestation: risks of cognitive, behavioral, and neurologic outcomes at age 10 years. J Pediatr 2016;173:69–75 e61.

20. Singh R, Turner RC, Nguyen L, et al. Pediatric traumatic brain injury and autism: elucidating shared mechanisms. Behav Neurol 2016;2016:8781725.

21. Hyman SL, Levy SE, Myers SM. Council on children with disabilities sod, behavioral p. identification, evaluation, and management of children with autism spectrum disorder. Pediatrics 2020;145.

22. Chandler S, Charman T, Baird G, et al. Validation of the social communication questionnaire in a population cohort of children with autism spectrum disorders. J Am Acad Child Adolesc Psychiatry 2007;46:1324–32.

23. Ouss L, Leunen D, Laschet J, et al. Autism spectrum disorder and cognitive profile in children with Dravet syndrome: Delineation of a specific phenotype. Epilepsia Open 2019;4:40–53.

24. Celik H, Acikel SB, Ozdemir MAF, et al. Evaluation of the clinical characteristics of children with autism spectrum disorder and epilepsy and the perception of their parents on quality of life. Epilepsy Res 2021;172:106599.

25. Wirrell EC. Prognostic significance of interictal epileptiform discharges in newly diagnosed seizure disorders. J Clin Neurophysiol 2010;27:239–48.

26. Precenzano F, Parisi L, Lanzara V, et al. Electroencephalographic abnormalities in autism spectrum disorder: characteristics and therapeutic implications. Medicina (Kaunas) 2020;56(9):419.

27. Mulligan CK, Trauner DA. Incidence and behavioral correlates of epileptiform abnormalities in autism spectrum disorders. J Autism Dev Disord 2014;44:452–8.

28. Tuchman RF, Rapin I. Regression in pervasive developmental disorders: seizures and epileptiform electroencephalogram correlates. Pediatrics 1997;99:560–6.
29. Specchio N, Wirrell E, Scheffer I, et al. ILAE classification and definition of epilepsy syndromes with onset in childhood: position paper by the ILAE task force on nosology and definitions. Epilepsia, in press.
30. Ekinci O, Arman AR, Isik U, et al. EEG abnormalities and epilepsy in autistic spectrum disorders: clinical and familial correlates. Epilepsy Behav 2010;17:178–82.
31. Lee H, Kang HC, Kim SW, et al. Characteristics of late-onset epilepsy and EEG findings in children with autism spectrum disorders. Korean J Pediatr 2011;54:22–8.
32. Keller R, Basta R, Salerno L, et al. Autism, epilepsy, and synaptopathies: a not rare association. Neurol Sci 2017;38:1353–61.
33. Stefanski A, Calle-Lopez Y, Leu C, et al. Clinical sequencing yield in epilepsy, autism spectrum disorder, and intellectual disability: a systematic review and meta-analysis. Epilepsia 2021;62:143–51.
34. Lee J, Ha S, Lee ST, et al. Next-Generation sequencing in korean children with autism spectrum disorder and comorbid epilepsy. Front Pharmacol 2020;11:585.
35. Shillington A, Capal JK. Genetic testing in patients with nonsyndromic autism spectrum disorder and EEG abnormalities with or without epilepsy: Is exome trio-based testing the best clinical approach? Epilepsy Behav 2021;114:107564.
36. Gaillard WD, Chiron C, Cross JH, et al. Guidelines for imaging infants and children with recent-onset epilepsy. Epilepsia 2009;50:2147–53.
37. Sanchez Fernandez I, Loddenkemper T, Galanopoulou AS, et al. Should epileptiform discharges be treated? Epilepsia 2015;56:1492–504.
38. Pressler RM, Robinson RO, Wilson GA, et al. Treatment of interictal epileptiform discharges can improve behavior in children with behavioral problems and epilepsy. J Pediatr 2005;146:112–7.
39. Wang M, Jiang L, Tang X. Levetiracetam is associated with decrease in subclinical epileptiform discharges and improved cognitive functions in pediatric patients with autism spectrum disorder. Neuropsychiatr Dis Treat 2017;13:2321–6.
40. Hollander E, Dolgoff-Kaspar R, Cartwright C, et al. An open trial of divalproex sodium in autism spectrum disorders. J Clin Psychiatry 2001;62:530–4.
41. Ronen GM, Richards JE, Cunningham C, et al. Can sodium valproate improve learning in children with epileptiform bursts but without clinical seizures? Dev Med Child Neurol 2000;42:751–5.
42. Saemundsen E, Ludvigsson P, Rafnsson V. Risk of autism spectrum disorders after infantile spasms: a population-based study nested in a cohort with seizures in the first year of life. Epilepsia 2008;49:1865–70.
43. Srivastava S, Sahin M. Autism spectrum disorder and epileptic encephalopathy: common causes, many questions. J Neurodev Disord 2017;9:23.
44. Askalan R, Mackay M, Brian J, et al. Prospective preliminary analysis of the development of autism and epilepsy in children with infantile spasms. J Child Neurol 2003;18:165–70.
45. Specchio N, Pietrafusa N, Trivisano M, et al. Autism and Epilepsy in patients with tuberous sclerosis complex. Front Neurol 2020;11:639.
46. Bolton PF, Park RJ, Higgins JN, et al. Neuro-epileptic determinants of autism spectrum disorders in tuberous sclerosis complex. Brain 2002;125:1247–55.
47. Bitton JY, Demos M, Elkouby K, et al. Does treatment have an impact on incidence and risk factors for autism spectrum disorders in children with infantile spasms? Epilepsia 2015;56:856–63.

48. Riikonen R, Amnell G. Psychiatric disorders in children with earlier infantile spasms. Dev Med Child Neurol 1981;23:747–60.
49. Moavero R, Kotulska K, Lagae L, et al. Is autism driven by epilepsy in infants with Tuberous Sclerosis Complex? Ann Clin Transl Neurol 2020;7:1371–81.
50. van den Munckhof B, van Dee V, Sagi L, et al. Treatment of electrical status epilepticus in sleep: a pooled analysis of 575 cases. Epilepsia 2015;56:1738–46.
51. Libenson MH, Haldar A, Pinto AL. The stability of spike counts in children with interictal epileptiform activity. Seizure 2014;23:454–6.
52. Libenson MH, Caravale B. Do antiepileptic drugs differ in suppressing interictal epileptiform activity in children? Pediatr Neurol 2001;24:214–8.
53. Eriksson AS, Knutsson E, Nergardh A. The effect of lamotrigine on epileptiform discharges in young patients with drug-resistant epilepsy. Epilepsia 2001;42: 230–6.
54. Dahlin M, Knutsson E, Amark P, et al. Reduction of epileptiform activity in response to low-dose clonazepam in children with epilepsy: a randomized double-blind study. Epilepsia 2000;41:308–15.
55. De Negri M, Baglietto MG, Battaglia FM, et al. Treatment of electrical status epilepticus by short diazepam (DZP) cycles after DZP rectal bolus test. Brain Dev 1995;17:330–3.
56. Sanchez Fernandez I, Hadjiloizou S, Eksioglu Y, et al. Short-term response of sleep-potentiated spiking to high-dose diazepam in electric status epilepticus during sleep. Pediatr Neurol 2012;46:312–8.
57. Sanchez Fernandez I, Peters JM, An S, et al. Long-term response to high-dose diazepam treatment in continuous spikes and waves during sleep. Pediatr Neurol 2013;49:163–170 e164.
58. Larsson PG, Bakke KA, Bjornaes H, et al. The effect of levetiracetam on focal nocturnal epileptiform activity during sleep–a placebo-controlled double-blind cross-over study. Epilepsy Behav 2012;24:44–8.
59. Buzatu M, Bulteau C, Altuzarra C, et al. Corticosteroids as treatment of epileptic syndromes with continuous spike-waves during slow-wave sleep. Epilepsia 2009; 50(Suppl 7):68–72.
60. Perucca E, Gram L, Avanzini G, et al. Antiepileptic drugs as a cause of worsening seizures. Epilepsia 1998;39:5–17.
61. Duchowny M. Pediatric epilepsy surgery: past, present, and future. Epilepsia 2020;61:228–9.
62. Kokoszka MA, McGoldrick PE, La Vega-Talbott M, et al. Epilepsy surgery in patients with autism. J Neurosurg Pediatr 2017;19:196–207.
63. Hoon AH Jr, Reiss AL. The mesial-temporal lobe and autism: case report and review. Dev Med Child Neurol 1992;34:252–9.
64. Gillberg C, Uvebrant P, Carlsson G, et al. Autism and epilepsy (and tuberous sclerosis?) in two pre-adolescent boys: neuropsychiatric aspects before and after epilepsy surgery. J Intellect Disabil Res 1996;40(Pt 1):75–81.
65. Szabo CA, Wyllie E, Dolske M, et al. Epilepsy surgery in children with pervasive developmental disorder. Pediatr Neurol 1999;20:349–53.
66. Danielsson S, Viggedal G, Steffenburg S, et al. Psychopathology, psychosocial functioning, and IQ before and after epilepsy surgery in children with drug-resistant epilepsy. Epilepsy Behav 2009;14:330–7.
67. Danielsson S, Rydenhag B, Uvebrant P, et al. Temporal lobe resections in children with epilepsy: neuropsychiatric status in relation to neuropathology and seizure outcome. Epilepsy Behav 2002;3:76–81.

68. McLellan A, Davies S, Heyman I, et al. Psychopathology in children with epilepsy before and after temporal lobe resection. Dev Med Child Neurol 2005;47:666–72.

69. Park YD. The effects of vagus nerve stimulation therapy on patients with intractable seizures and either Landau-Kleffner syndrome or autism. Epilepsy Behav 2003;4:286–90.

70. Levy ML, Levy KM, Hoff D, et al. Vagus nerve stimulation therapy in patients with autism spectrum disorder and intractable epilepsy: results from the vagus nerve stimulation therapy patient outcome registry. J Neurosurg Pediatr 2010;5: 595–602.

71. Danielsson S, Viggedal G, Gillberg C, et al. Lack of effects of vagus nerve stimulation on drug-resistant epilepsy in eight pediatric patients with autism spectrum disorders: a prospective 2-year follow-up study. Epilepsy Behav 2008;12: 298–304.

72. Kwon CS, Jette N, Ghatan S. Perspectives on the current developments with neuromodulation for the treatment of epilepsy. Expert Rev Neurother 2020;20: 189–94.

73. Morrell MJ, Group RNSSiES. Responsive cortical stimulation for the treatment of medically intractable partial epilepsy. Neurology 2011;77:1295–304.

74. Bergey GK, Morrell MJ, Mizrahi EM, et al. Long-term treatment with responsive brain stimulation in adults with refractory partial seizures. Neurology 2015;84: 810–7.

75. Meador KJ, Kapur R, Loring DW, et al. Quality of life and mood in patients with medically intractable epilepsy treated with targeted responsive neurostimulation. Epilepsy Behav 2015;45:242–7.

76. Kwon CS, Schupper AJ, Fields MC, et al. Centromedian thalamic responsive neurostimulation for Lennox-Gastaut epilepsy and autism. Ann Clin Transl Neurol 2020;7:2035–40.

Emerging Technologies for Epilepsy Surgery

Danika L. Paulo, MD*, Tyler J. Ball, MD, Dario J. Englot, MD, PhD

KEYWORDS

- Epilepsy • Epilepsy surgery • Resection • Neuromodulation • Technology

KEY POINTS

- Patients with medically refractory epilepsy should be referred early for consideration of epilepsy surgery.
- Seizure freedom is the best predictor of quality of life.
- Preoperative diagnostic work up optimizes chances for postoperative seizure freedom.
- Many surgical treatment options are available, ranging from resections to noninvasive procedures, and they should be tailored to address patients' individual disease process and preferences.
- Technological advancements in imaging and therapeutic modalities will continue to advance and optimize surgical treatment of epilepsy.

INTRODUCTION

When medical treatments fail to provide patients with seizure freedom, surgical treatment options are a valuable adjunct to therapy, improving patients' quality of life and reducing disease-related morbidity and mortality.[1] Epilepsy is considered drug-resistant if seizures persist despite trials of at least 2 appropriately dosed and tolerated antiseizure medications, which occurs in approximately 30% to 40% of patients.[2,3] These patients should be referred to a comprehensive epilepsy center for multidisciplinary evaluation, diagnostic work-up, and consideration of surgical treatment options.[4,5]

In this review, we aim to highlight recent advances in technology that have enhanced the diagnosis and surgical treatment of epilepsy, leading to novel treatment options for patient-specific and disease-specific therapies. Despite promising developments supported by Class I evidence and consensus guidelines, epilepsy surgery remains underutilized, with some practitioners hesitant to consider invasive surgery for patients due to surgical risk or inefficient referral patterns.[6–8] Here, we review pertinent literature on

Department of Neurological Surgery, Vanderbilt University Medical Center, 1161 21st Avenue So. T4224 Medical Center North, Nashville, TN 37232-2380, USA
* Corresponding author.
E-mail address: danika.l.paulo@vumc.org
Twitter: @danikapaulomd (D.L.P.); @englot (D.J.E.)

Neurol Clin 40 (2022) 849–867
https://doi.org/10.1016/j.ncl.2022.03.012   neurologic.theclinics.com
0733-8619/22/© 2022 Elsevier Inc. All rights reserved.

Abbreviations	
ANT	anterior nucleus of thalamus
ASM	antiseizure medication
ATL	anterior temporal lobectomy
DBS	deep brain stimulaton
DRE	drug resistant epilepsy
EEG	electroencephalography
FDA	Food and Drug Administration
FIAS	focal impaired awareness seizure
fMRI	functional magnetic resonance imaging
FUS	focused ultrasound
IPG	internal pulse generator
LITT	laser interstitial thermal therapy
MRI	magnetic resonance imaging
MTS	mesial temporal sclerosis
RNS	responsive neurostimulation
SAH	selective amygalohippocampectomy
SDE	subdural electrode
SEEG	stereoelectroencephalography
SPECT	single-photon emission computed tomography
SRS	stereotactic radiosurgery
TLE	temporal lobe epilepsy
VNS	vagus nerve stimulation

surgical evaluation, treatment options, and outcomes to highlight the benefits of early surgical consideration, available intervention options and their efficacy.

DIAGNOSTIC TECHNOLOGIES IN THE PREOPERATIVE WORKUP

Diagnostic workup of epilepsy involves a combination of modalities, each of which provides meaningful information about structural lesions, pathologic networks, brain activity, and tissue metabolism that can suggest localization of one or more seizure onset zones.

Imaging Modalities

Evolution of epilepsy treatment into its current form would not have been possible without advancements in neuroimaging. Improved resolution of brain parenchyma afforded by modern magnetic resonance imaging (MRI) has enhanced the ability to localize structural lesions, which is crucial, because identification of an epileptogenic lesion significantly increases chances of postoperative seizure freedom.[9,10] In addition to improved resolution, modern MRI sequences such as T2-weighted short tau inversion recovery, fluid-attenuated inversion recovery, and T2* gradient-recalled echo can help delineate normal from pathologic tissue, and sequences such as 3D volumetric T1-weighted postcontrast can improve safety of surgical procedures, particularly stereotactic procedures, by enabling avoidance of blood vessels.[11,12] Interictal 18F-fluoro-deoxyglucose positron emission tomography can delineate functional deficit zones and ictal single-photon emission computed tomography (SPECT) with subtraction SPECT coregistered to MRI can localize ictal onset zones.[13,14] Functional MRI (fMRI) and Wada testing are useful in lateralization and localization of language functions as well as prediction of postoperative memory or motor deficits.[15] These advanced neuroimaging modalities are paired with neurophysiologic modalities to gather complimentary data for localization.

Neurophysiologic Modalities

Presurgical evaluation begins with noninvasive long-term video scalp electroencephalography (EEG), which has been enhanced with the advent of interictal high-resolution EEG, electrical source imaging, magnetoencephalography, magnetic source imaging, and interictal EEG-fMRI to localize irritative zones.[16] For patients whose localization remains elusive despite noninvasive methods, intracranial EEG in the form of subdural electrodes (SDEs) or depth electrodes may be pursued.

Subdural electrodes

Subdural strips and grids have been used since the 1980s and provide valuable information about the location and extent of an epileptogenic region.[17,18] Subdural strips consist of a single line of 2 to 10 electrodes, 2 to 5 mm in diameter with centers spaced 1 cm apart, whereas subdural grids or arrays consist of multiple rows of electrodes.[19] SDE recordings directly assess cortical activity localizing seizure onset region boundaries with greater precision than scalp electrodes and can also be used for functional mapping.[20] Notable limitations of SDE include inability to target deeper structures, need for craniotomy for placement with its associated complications, and need to perform definitive resection in the same operation as SDE removal.

Stereoelectroencephalography

Minimally invasive stereoelectroencephalography (SEEG), implantation of multiple 8-contact to 16-contact depth electrodes via twist-drill burr holes, arose in the 1950s[21] and has become more prevalent during the past 2 decades.[22] There are several benefits to SEEG, as a craniotomy is not needed, deeper subcortical structures can be targeted, 3D seizure networks can be elucidated, and definitive resection can be performed in a subsequent operation.

Technological advancements including 3D high-resolution MRI, frameless stereotaxy, 3D-printed omnidirectional frames and robot-assisted surgery have increased precision, efficiency, and flexibility of SEEG targeting, driving its increased prevalence.[23] A recent study by Jehi and colleagues[24] comparing 526 SDE and 942 SEEG implants in 2012 patients demonstrated patients who underwent SDE were more likely to both have complications and undergo resection, whereas those who underwent SEEG had greater odds of seizure freedom after resection. Joswig and colleagues[25] retrospectively analyzed 500 SDE and SEEG implants in 450 patients, demonstrating higher albeit nonsignificant rates of favorable seizure outcome after SEEG (80%) compared with SDE (70%) at 2-year follow-up and shorter operative time with SEEG. Other studies have shown higher hemorrhagic complication rates associated with SDE (3%–4%)[26,27] compared to SEEG (1%).[28] SEEG is also more favorable than SDE with regard to infection rates.[26]

THERAPEUTIC TECHNOLOGIES IN SURGICAL TREATMENT

Because resection of epileptic foci offers the best chances of seizure freedom, we will briefly discuss resection and subsequently focus on recently developed surgical treatment options closely intertwined with technology, such as ablation and neuromodulation techniques.

Resection

When seizure onset zones are focal and localizable, resection of the seizure focus can provide excellent seizure freedom rates, drastically improving quality of life. Predictors of favorable surgical outcome include early operative intervention after diagnosis, lack of secondary generalization, concordant MRI/EEG localization, and a visualizable lesion on imaging.[29] In patients with temporal lobe epilepsy (TLE), the most common type of epilepsy, resection via anterior temporal lobectomy (ATL) remains standard of care due to high postoperative seizure freedom rates.[30,31] In previously reported case series, 70% to 80% of TLE patients achieved seizure freedom after ATL.[32,33] Efficacy of ATL was further validated by 3 randomized controlled trials demonstrating significant differences in seizure freedom rates in favor of early resection with continued medical therapy (58%–77%) compared with continued medical therapy alone (0%–8%).[34,35] For patients whose preoperative workup localizes to the hippocampus and/or amygdala, resection of uninvolved temporal structures can be spared via selective amygdalohippocampectomy (SAH; **Fig. 1**). Studies have demonstrated comparable seizure outcomes of SAH to ATL,[36,37] with SAH potentially having reduced chances of visual, memory, and neuropsychological deficits.[38–40] Finally, patients with focal neocortical epilepsy who undergo focus resections have seizure freedom rates of 50% to 66%, albeit less than after ATL or SAH perhaps due to incomplete focus resection or presence of a second unresected focus.[29,41]

Ablation

Ablative procedures for epilepsy offer less invasive, targeted treatment alternatives for patients with focal epilepsy. Multiple minimally invasive or noninvasive ablative therapies have been developed with goals of minimizing surgical risk, hospitalizations, and recovery time while leading to promising surgical outcomes and potential seizure freedom. **Table 1** summarizes subsequently discussed ablation articles.

Laser interstitial thermal therapy

MRI-guided laser interstitial thermal therapy (LITT) is a minimally invasive surgical technique involving stereotactic insertion of a laser probe through a small burr hole into a target to induce time-dependent thermal ablation, visualized in real time with MRI thermography to monitor temperature changes and tissue destruction.[42] Advantages of LITT over traditional radiofrequency thermoablation are related to the ability to monitor the size and borders of the ablation in real time.[43] LITT may be well suited for patients with structurally defined targets such as mesial temporal sclerosis (MTS), hypothalamic hamartomas, focal cortical dysplasias, and cavernous malformations.[44]

LITT was Food and Drug Administration (FDA) approved in the United States for the treatment of brain lesions in 2007 and epilepsy in 2012.[45] Since then, several studies have evaluated the application of LITT for various epileptic causes. It is particularly effective for the treatment of hypothalamic hamartomas, with seizure freedom rates of 66% to 93%.[46,47] Furthermore, the morbidity associated with LITT can be less than approach-related morbidity associated with open surgery. LITT for extratemporal lobe epilepsy has also proven to be effective with a reported 53% meaningful seizure reduction, which is relatively improved with visualizable lesions.[48]

For TLE LITT, studies have reported overall seizure freedom rates of 38% to 78%, with seizure freedom rates of 60% to 89% in patients with evidence of MTS, at 1-year follow-up, noting the advantages of decreased pain, shorter hospital stay, and faster recovery compared with open resection.[49–57] A meta-analysis found TLE LITT seizure freedom rates (57%) to be lower than ATL (69%) or SAH (66%), with the tradeoff of fewer serious complications and improved verbal and neuropsychological outcomes after LITT.[58] Complication rates are low, with a recent systematic review reporting a 16% rate of primarily transient and nondebilitating complications[59] and a recent study supporting superior postoperative verbal memory function with LITT compared with open resection.[60] Analysis of TLE LITT outcomes related to anatomic lesion volumes supported the importance of including the amygdala, hippocampal head, parahippocampal gyrus, and rhinal cortices

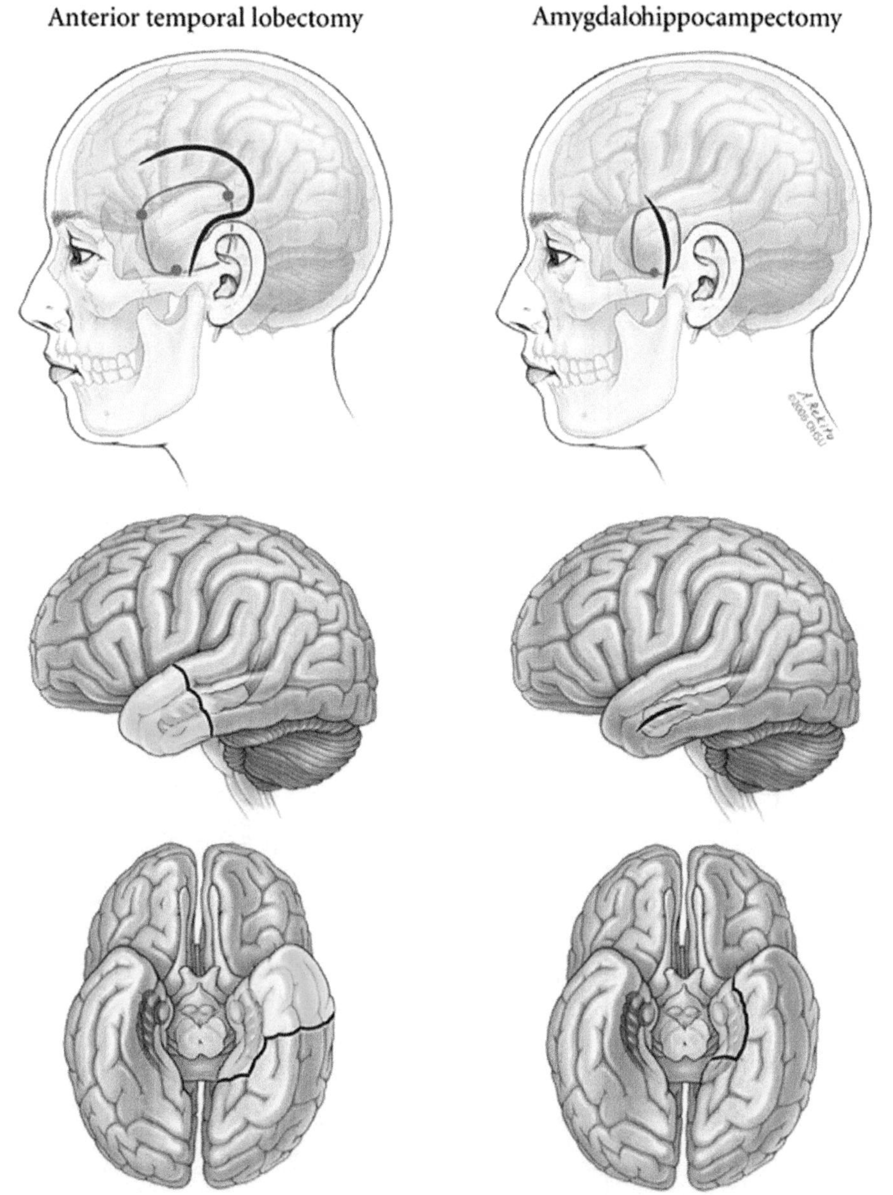

Anterior temporal lobectomy   Amygdalohippocampectomy

Fig. 1. *Common resections for temporal lobe epilepsy.* For anterior temporal lobectomy (left column) and selective amygdalohippocampectomy (right column), this depicts typical incisions and craniotomies (top row) and extents of resection (green) in the lateral (middle row) and inferior (bottom row) view orientation. (*From* David Spencer, Kim Burchiel, "Selective Amygdalohippocampectomy", Epilepsy Research and Treatment, vol. 2012, Article ID 382095, 8 pages, 2012. https://doi.org/10.1155/2012/382095; Copyright © 2012 David Spencer and Kim Burchiel under Creative Commons Attribution License (CC BY 3.0).

in the lesion, with the posterior extent of ablation being less critical.[44] The first prospective, single-arm, multicenter study evaluating safety and efficacy of LITT in 150 TLE patients at 12-month follow-up is underway (Stereotactic Laser Ablation for Temporal Lobe Epilepsy (SLATE) trial, NCT02844465).[61] Refinements to decrease low-temperature cutoffs and

Table 1
Summary of included ablation articles for epilepsy

	Author, year of publication	Type of study	N	Epilepsy Cause	Target(s)	Follow-up duration (mean or median)	Seizure outcomes
LITT	Curry and colleagues,[45] 2012	Retrospective cohort, single center	5	Mixed	Mixed	7 mo	100% seizure free
	Zeller and colleagues,[59] 2021	Retrospective systematic review	303	Mixed	Mixed	15.6 mo	74.1% disabling seizure free
	Curry and colleagues,[46] 2018	Retrospective cohort, single center	71	Hypothalamic hamartoma	Hypothalamic hamartoma	1 y	93% gelastic seizure free
	Xu and colleagues,[47] 2018	Retrospective cohort, single center	18	Hypothalamic hamartoma	Hypothalamic hamartoma	17.4 mo	80% gelastic seizure free, 56% nongelastic seizure free
	Gupta and colleagues,[48] 2020	Retrospective cohort, single center	35	Extratemporal lobe	SOZ	27.3 mo	53% meaningful reduction, 44% seizure free
	Wu and colleagues,[44] 2019	Retrospective cohort, multicenter	234	Temporal lobe epilepsy	Mesial temporal lobe	30 mo	58% disabling seizure free, 77% meaningful seizure reduction
	Kang and colleagues,[49] 2016	Prospective, single center	20	Temporal lobe epilepsy	Mesial temporal lobe	13.4 mo	53% FIAS seizure free at 6 mo, 36.4% at 1 y, 60% at 2 y
	Gross and colleagues,[50] 2018	Retrospective cohort, single center	58	Temporal lobe epilepsy	Mesial temporal lobe	1 y	53% disabling seizure free, 61% with MTS, 33% without MTS
	Donos and colleagues,[51] 2018	Prospective, single center	43	Temporal lobe epilepsy	Mesial temporal lobe	20.3 mo	67% disabling seizure free
	Grewal and colleagues,[52] 2018	Retrospective cohort, multicenter	23	Temporal lobe epilepsy	Mesial temporal lobe	34 mo	65% disabling seizure free
	Jermakowicz and colleagues,[53] 2017	Retrospective cohort, single center	23	Temporal lobe epilepsy	Mesial temporal lobe	22.4 mo	65% disabling seizure free
			30			18 mo	

Study	Study design	N	Epilepsy type	Target	Follow-up	Outcome
Le and colleagues,[54] 2018	Prospective, single center		Temporal lobe epilepsy	Mesial temporal lobe		62% disabling seizure free, 76% > 90% reduction, 97% > 50% reduction
Tao and colleagues,[55] 2018	Prospective, single center	21	Temporal lobe epilepsy	Mesial temporal lobe	24 mo	52% disabling seizure free, 73% with MTS, 30% without MTS
Vakharia and colleagues,[56] 2018	Retrospective cohort, single center	25	Temporal lobe epilepsy	Mesial temporal lobe	24.4 mo	44% disabling seizure free
Willie and colleagues,[57] 2014	Prospective, single center	13	Temporal lobe epilepsy	Mesial temporal lobe	14 mo	54% disabling seizure free, 77% meaningful seizure reduction
Drane and colleagues,[60] 2021	Retrospective systematic review	40	Temporal lobe epilepsy	Mesial temporal lobe	1 y	45% disabling seizure free
SRS Barbaro and colleagues,[65] 2009	Prospective, randomized, multicenter	30	Temporal lobe epilepsy	Mesial temporal lobe	3 y	67% seizure free
Barbaro and colleagues,[66] 2018	Prospective, randomized controlled, single blinded, multicenter	31	Temporal lobe epilepsy	Mesial temporal lobe	4 y	52% seizure remission (seizure free between 25 and 36 mo)

Abbreviation: FIAS, focal impaired awareness seizure; LITT, laser interstitial thermal therapy; MTS, mesial temporal sclerosis; SOZ, seizure onset zone; SRS, stereotactic radiosurgery.

place high-temperature cutoffs further from important structures, paired with improved targeting precision, understanding of tissue thermosensitivity, and experience will continue to optimize this therapy.

Stereotactic radiosurgery

Stereotactic radiosurgery (SRS), first developed in 1949 by Lars Leksell,[62] is a nonsurgical radiation therapy that precisely ablates a planned volume of tissue via convergence of gamma knife or linear accelerator rays while preserving surrounding parenchyma with low radiation exposure.[63,64] This procedure is typically performed in one session, does not require hospitalization and has a short recovery time; however, outcomes may not be evident until months later, which obscures subsequent treatment decisions and may be a driving force behind the recent relative decline of SRS in favor of other noninvasive therapies.

Studies have demonstrated efficacy of SRS targeting mesial temporal structures for TLE. Barbaro and colleagues[65] conducted a multicenter, prospective pilot study evaluating seizure outcomes after SRS for TLE and found 77% of patients who received high-dose treatment and 59% who received low-dose treatment were seizure-free at 1 year. More recently, the randomized, single-blinded, controlled, multicenter Radiosurgery or Open Surgery for Epilepsy (ROSE) trial compared SRS to open surgery in 31 TLE patients followed for 3 years.[66] Seizure remission, defined as absence of disabling seizures between 25 and 36 months postprocedure, was 78% in the temporal lobectomy group and 52% in the SRS group, with no significant differences in verbal memory changes, suggesting SRS is a safe, albeit less effective, therapeutic option in patients unsuitable for or reluctant to undergo open surgery.

Focused ultrasound

Focused ultrasound (FUS) is another noninvasive therapy that has been gaining attention for application in epilepsy treatment. High-intensity FUS applied to a target has precise ablative effects,[67–69] whereas low-intensity FUS has neuromodulatory effects.[70] There are currently 3 ongoing clinical studies of FUS for epilepsy: one evaluating high-intensity FUS anterior nucleus thalamotomy to prevent secondary generalization (NCT03417297), another evaluating high-intensity FUS treatment of subcortical lesional epilepsy (NCT02804230), and another evaluating low-intensity FUS pulsation for TLE. These trials represent the next frontier in noninvasive technology for the treatment of epilepsy.

Neuromodulation

Unlike resection or ablation, neuromodulation remains palliative and may be preferred over resection for patients with seizure foci in or near eloquent areas that would pose risk to speech, motor, or visual functions. Additionally, for generalized or multifocal epilepsy, neuromodulation of central network "hubs" may improve seizure control. For patients opposed to surgical resection, neuromodulation may offer a major improvement in seizure control over medical management alone. Finally, for high-risk surgical patients, neuromodulation may be a better option given its less invasive nature and faster recovery. Although complete seizure freedom is uncommon with neuromodulation, patients may still achieve meaningful seizure reduction and improvement in quality of life and disease-related morbidity. **Table 2** summarizes subsequently discussed neuromodulation articles.

Deep brain stimulation

Deep brain stimulation (DBS) is a surgical open-loop neuromodulation therapy approved by the United States FDA in 2018 for adult patients with focal and

Table 2
Summary of Included neuromodulation articles for epilepsy

	Author, year of publication	Type of study	N	Type of epilepsy	Target(s)	Follow-up duration (mean or median)	Seizure outcomes
DBS	Fisher and colleagues,[73] 2010	Prospective, randomized, double-blind, multicenter	110	Generalized	ANT	2 y	56% median seizure frequency reduction, 54% with ≥50% reduction, 14% seizure free for >6 mo
	Salanova and colleagues,[74] 2015	Prospective, long-term follow-up, multicenter	83	Generalized	ANT	5 y	69% median seizure frequency reduction, 68% with ≥50% reduction, 16% seizure free for >6 mo
	Salanova and colleagues,[75] 2021	Prospective, long-term follow-up, multicenter	62	Generalized	ANT	10 y	75% median seizure frequency reduction, 74% with ≥50% reduction, 18% seizure free for >6 mo
	Son and colleagues,[77] 2016	Retrospective, nonblinded, single center	14	Generalized	CM	18.2 mo	68% mean seizure frequency reduction, 79% with ≥50% reduction
RNS	Bergey and colleagues,[83] 2015	Prospective, long-term, open label, multicenter	230	Focal	SOZ	5.4 y	66% median seizure reduction, 59% with ≥50% reduction
	Nair and colleagues,[82] 2020	Prospective, long-term, open label, multicenter	162	Focal	SOZ	9 y	75% median seizure reduction, 73% with ≥50% reduction, 35% with ≥90% reduction, 18% with ≥ 1 y seizure free
	Burdette and colleagues,[84] 2020	Retrospective, nonblinded, single center	7	Regional neocortical	CM, SOZ	17 mo	88% median seizure reduction of disabling seizures, 73% median reduction of all seizures, 100% with ≥50% reduction
	Burdette and colleagues,[85] 2021	Retrospective, nonblinded, single center	3	Regional neocortical	Pulvinar, SOZ	12.5 mo	100% with ≥50% reduction, 67% with ≥90% reduction

(continued on next page)

Table 2
(continued)

	Author, year of publication	Type of study	N	Type of epilepsy	Target(s)	Follow-up duration (mean or median)	Seizure outcomes
VNS	Ben-Menachem and colleagues,[88] 1994	Prospective, randomized, parallel, double-blinded, multicenter	114	Partial	L vagus nerve	3 mo	31% with ≥50% reduction
	Handforth and colleagues,[89] 1998	Prospective, randomized controlled, double-blinded, multicenter	196	Partial	L vagus nerve	3 mo	23% with ≥50% reduction
	Amar et al,[87] 1998	Prospective, randomized controlled, double-blinded, single center	17	Partial	L vagus nerve	3 mo	57% with ≥50% reduction
	Klikenberg and colleagues,[90] 2012	Prospective, randomized controlled, double-blinded, single center	41	Mixed	L vagus nerve	3 mo	26% with ≥50% reduction
	Tzadok and colleagues,[93] 2019	Retrospective cohort, nonblinded, single center	46	Mixed	L vagus nerve	13 mo	61% with ≥50% reduction, 11% with complete seizure freedom, 67% with shorter seizure duration

Abbreviations: ANT, anterior nucleus of thalamus; CM, centromedian nucleus of thalamus; DBS, deep brain stimulation; L, left; RNS, responsive neurostimulation; SOZ, seizure onset zone; VNS, vagus nerve stimulation.

secondarily generalized drug resistant epilepsy (DRE). DBS typically uses 4-contact electrodes implanted into a surgical target connected to a subclavicular internal pulse generator (IPG) that supplies continuous low-voltage, high-frequency electrical pulses, altering network dynamics, and decreasing frequency of seizures (**Fig. 2**A). The most common and well-studied DBS target for epilepsy is the anterior nucleus of the thalamus (ANT), an anatomic hub in the limbic network (**Fig. 2**B, C).

Since the initial study by Kerrigan and colleagues[71] demonstrating the efficacy of ANT DBS for epilepsy in 2004, several studies have evaluated this DBS target, reporting responder rates of 44% to 100%.[72] The primary study prompting FDA approval was a prospective, randomized, double-blinded trial by the Stimulation of the Anterior Nucleus of the Thalamus for Epilepsy (SANTE) Study Group.[73] In month 3 of the blinded phase, active stimulation patients had 29% greater reduction in seizures compared with controls, and at 2-year follow-up, there was a 56% median reduction in seizure frequency with 54% having 50% or greater reduction in seizures and 14% being seizure-free for more than 6 months. Complication rates were low, with no patients experiencing acute perioperative symptomatic hemorrhage or infection and 1.8% experiencing acute, transient stimulation-associated seizures. Five and 7-year follow-up studies demonstrated continued and improved efficacy, with 75% median seizure frequency reduction, 74% having 50% or greater seizure reduction and 18% seizure-free for more than 6 months.[74,75]

Recent studies have evaluated efficacy and safety of targeting the centromedian (CM) nucleus of the thalamus, due to its diffuse cortical connections.[76] Son and colleagues[77] evaluated CM DBS in 14 DRE patients, with mean seizure reduction from baseline to mean follow-up of 18.2 months of 68 ± 22% and 79% achieving greater than 50% reduction. This and other DBS targets are being evaluated for efficacy with promising results, yet optimal targeting remains to be further refined.

A

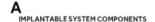

IMPLANTABLE SYSTEM COMPONENTS

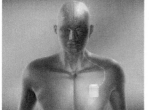

Three Components*

1. Implantable Neurostimulator (INS): Power
2. Extension: connects the INS to the lead
3. Lead: Implanted in the brain, electrodes in contact with target tissue

B

ANT: EFFECTIVELY-PLACED LEADS (DORSAL VIEW)

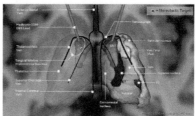

C

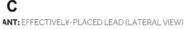

ANT: EFFECTIVELY-PLACED LEAD (LATERAL VIEW)

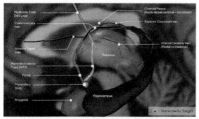

Fig. 2. *Deep brain stimulation for epilepsy.* Complete DBS system (*A*) with 2 electrodes connected to a subclavicular internal pulse generator with dorsal (*B*) and lateral (*C*) views of an effectively placed anterior nucleus of thalamus lead with key surrounding anatomic structures. (*Courtesy of* Medtronic, Minneapolis, MN; with permission).

Responsive neurostimulation

Another implantable surgical treatment option is responsive neurostimulation (RNS), which was FDA approved in 2013 and is suitable for patients with 1 or 2 seizure foci that may not be favorable for resection without risking deficits.[78] RNS consists of a neurostimulator lying flush with the skull in a craniectomy defect connected to two 4-contact electrodes, depth electrodes or cortical strips, implanted in or overlying seizure onset zones (**Fig. 3**). The novelty of this system is its closed-loop capability of detecting abnormal electrocorticographic (ECoG) patterns preceding a seizure and applying bursts of stimulation to prevent or terminate seizures.[79] Furthermore, chronic EcoG recordings stored in the neurostimulator can be transferred wirelessly to an online platform so that patient-specific biomarkers can be analyzed to guide programming and optimize therapy. This adaptive capability makes RNS efficient and well-tolerated, especially as total stimulation time is typically less than 5 minutes per day.[80,81]

Two long-term prospective clinical trials demonstrated safety and efficacy of RNS in patients with focal DRE.[82,83] Bergey and colleagues[83] studied 230 RNS patients with median 5.4-year follow-up, reporting 66% median seizure reduction. Nair and colleagues[82] studied 162 patients with 9-year follow-up, achieving 75% median seizure reduction, with 35% achieving 90% or greater reduction and 18% achieving 1 year or greater of seizure freedom. Importantly, overall quality of life and cognitive function were significantly improved. Alternative targets for RNS therapy specific to certain disease subtypes are being evaluated with encouraging results, such as the CM nucleus for regional neocortical epilepsy.[84] Burdette and colleagues[84] evaluated 7 patients with RNS using a hybrid approach targeting a cortical seizure onset zone and a central network hub (CM). They found 88% reduction in disabling seizures and 73% median reduction in all seizures, with more than 50% overall reduction in seizure severity.[84] The same group reported encouraging results in 3 patients with posterior quadrant epilepsy using an analogous paradigm of a neocortical electrode paired with a pulvinar

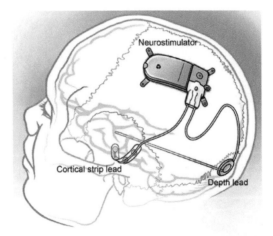

Fig. 3. *Responsive neurostimulation system* depicting the neurostimulator sitting within a tray flush with the skull in a craniectomy defect connected to one depth lead placed into a deep surgical target and one cortical strip lead overlaying cortex of seizure onset zone. (*From* Loring DW, Kapur R, Meador KJ, Morrell MJ. Differential neuropsychological outcomes following targeted responsive neurostimulation for partial-onset epilepsy. Epilepsia. 2015;56(11):1836–1844. https://doi.org/10.1111/epi.13191; with permission).

depth electrode, with greater than 50% seizure reduction in all patients and greater than 90% reduction in 2 patients.[85] Recently, RNS was authorized for emergency use by the FDA in 2021 for the RNS® System Responsive Thalamic Stimulation for Primary Generalized Seizures (NAUTILUS) study (NCT05147571) evaluating its use for the treatment of idiopathic generalized epilepsy. This therapy will likely continue to improve in efficacy as appropriate individualized targets and stimulation parameters are better understood and optimized.

Vagal nerve stimulation

An extracranial neuromodulation option for epilepsy is the vagal nerve stimulator (VNS) system, which consists of an electrode wrapped around the left vagus nerve connected to a subclavicular IPG. Continuous stimulation is delivered using various configurations and additional stimulation can be applied via an external magnet over the pulse generator when seizure onset is anticipated. Its proposed mechanism of action is alteration of epinephrine release by solitary tract projections to the locus coeruleus and increased gamma aminobutyric acid levels in the brainstem, thereby decreasing ictal events and desynchronizing cortical activity.[86] Similar to DBS and RNS, the primary goal of VNS is seizure reduction and improved quality of life.[5]

VNS was FDA approved in 1997 for adjunctive therapy in patients aged 12 years or greater with medically refractory focal onset seizures. Subsequently, 4 blinded, randomized controlled trials were conducted yielding Class I evidence of efficacy, with mean seizure reduction from baseline to 3-month follow-up ranging from 6% to 71% and a responder rate of greater than 50% seizure reduction ranging from 23% to 57%.[87–90] Larger reviews demonstrate that efficacy of VNS increases with long-term follow-up.[91] Predictors of good response to VNS include epilepsy onset at age greater than 12 years, nonlesional epilepsy, generalized seizures, and posttraumatic epilepsy.[29,92]

Recent technological advancements have paired closed-loop VNS with heart rate detection, as heart rates typically increase before and during the seizure activity. VNS with heart rate detection was FDA approved in 2015 (**Fig. 4**) and uses a customizable cardiac algorithm to detect heart rate increases predicting ictal onset and apply autostimulation to prevent or abort seizures. Studies have reported a 59% to 62% responder rate of 50% or greater reduction in seizures with closed-loop therapy compared with 44% to 56% responder rate with open-loop therapy.[93] In 2017, a

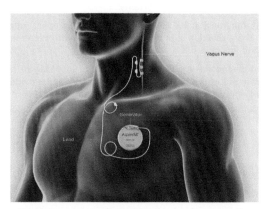

Fig. 4. *Vagal nerve stimulator system* depicting the lead wrapped around the left vagus nerve connected to a subclavicular internal pulse generator. (*Courtesy of* LivaNova, Houston, TX; with permission).

newer VNS device was FDA approved, which offers similar autostimulation therapy with the benefits of smaller size, data-gathering capabilities allowing clinicians to tailor stimulation parameters, and a tablet-based interface.

DISCUSSION

Medically refractory epilepsy patients should be referred for early surgical evaluation at a comprehensive epilepsy center because surgical intervention leads to excellent outcomes and remains underutilized despite compelling evidence and consensus guideline recommendations. Technological advancements in diagnostic tools have resulted in improved detection and localization of epileptogenic foci for surgical targeting. Although resection of epileptogenic foci continues to yield highest chances of seizure freedom, multiple minimally invasive and noninvasive therapies have transformed the field of epilepsy surgery in recent years and may be viable alternatives for select patients. The field of surgical epilepsy is closely intertwined with neuroimaging, EEG, and therapeutic technology and will continue to coevolve to provide the best results for patients.

SUMMARY

Technological advancements in epilepsy surgery have led to increases in surgical treatment options, thereby capturing a larger number of patients and improving their quality of life to a greater extent. In light of this rapid expansion of the surgical epilepsy field, it is imperative that clinicians develop a broader understanding of these technologies and the importance of early referral to a comprehensive epilepsy center capable of extensive preoperative workup and a variety of surgical treatment options.

CLINICS CARE POINTS

- Consider referral for surgical evaluation after 2 antiseizure medication (ASMs) have been tried and failed.

- Imaging modalities paired with noninvasive electrocorticography can often localize seizure onset zones, and intracranial monitoring such as subdural electrode and stereoelectroencephalography can be used in cases with unclear localization.

- Identification and resection of the epileptogenic zones can lead to seizure freedom and reduce epilepsy-related morbidity and mortality.

- There are multiple minimally invasive and noninvasive therapies with promising results, albeit less efficacy than resection, and typically associated with decreased surgical risk, shorter recovery, and less pain.

- Future advances in diagnostic workup and treatment of medically refractory epilepsy will increase the accuracy of localization of epileptogenic zones and provide alternative effective treatment options to improve outcomes and patient quality of life.

DISCLOSURE

The authors have nothing to disclose.

REFERENCES

1. Choi H, Sell RL, Lenert L, et al. Epilepsy surgery for pharmacoresistant temporal lobe epilepsy: a decision analysis. JAMA 2008;300(21):2497–505.

2. Kwan P, Brodie MJ. Early identification of refractory epilepsy. N Engl J Med 2000; 342(5):314–9.
3. Kwan P, Sperling MR. Refractory seizures: try additional antiepileptic drugs (after two have failed) or go directly to early surgery evaluation? Epilepsia 2009; 50(Suppl 8):57–62.
4. Engel J Jr, Wiebe S, French J, et al. Practice parameter: temporal lobe and localized neocortical resections for epilepsy: report of the Quality Standards Subcommittee of the American Academy of Neurology, in association with the American Epilepsy Society and the American Association of Neurological Surgeons. Neurology 2003;60(4):538–47.
5. Englot DJ. A modern epilepsy surgery treatment algorithm: Incorporating traditional and emerging technologies. Epilepsy Behav 2018;80:68–74.
6. Kwon CS, Blank L, Mu L, et al. Trends in lobectomy/amygdalohippocampectomy over time and the impact of hospital surgical volume on hospitalization outcomes: A population-based study. Epilepsia 2020;61(10):2173–82.
7. Engel J Jr. What can we do for people with drug-resistant epilepsy? The 2016 Wartenberg Lecture. Neurology 2016;87(23):2483–9.
8. Englot DJ, Ouyang D, Garcia PA, et al. Epilepsy surgery trends in the United States, 1990-2008. Neurology 2012;78(16):1200–6.
9. de Tisi J, Bell GS, Peacock JL, et al. The long-term outcome of adult epilepsy surgery, patterns of seizure remission, and relapse: a cohort study. Lancet 2011; 378(9800):1388–95.
10. Tellez-Zenteno JF, Hernandez Ronquillo L, Moien-Afshari F, et al. Surgical outcomes in lesional and non-lesional epilepsy: a systematic review and meta-analysis. Epilepsy Res 2010;89(2–3):310–8.
11. Duncan JS, Winston GP, Koepp MJ, et al. Brain imaging in the assessment for epilepsy surgery. Lancet Neurol 2016;15(4):420–33.
12. Wellmer J, Quesada CM, Rothe L, et al. Proposal for a magnetic resonance imaging protocol for the detection of epileptogenic lesions at early outpatient stages. Epilepsia 2013;54(11):1977–87.
13. O'Brien TJ, So EL, Mullan BP, et al. Subtraction ictal SPECT co-registered to MRI improves clinical usefulness of SPECT in localizing the surgical seizure focus. Neurology 1998;50(2):445–54.
14. Capraz IY, Kurt G, Akdemir O, et al. Surgical outcome in patients with MRI-negative, PET-positive temporal lobe epilepsy. Seizure 2015;29:63–8.
15. Baumgartner C, Koren JP, Britto-Arias M, et al. Presurgical epilepsy evaluation and epilepsy surgery. F1000Res 2019;8:1–13.
16. Baroumand AG, van Mierlo P, Strobbe G, et al. Automated EEG source imaging: a retrospective, blinded clinical validation study. Clin Neurophysiol 2018;129(11): 2403–10.
17. Levy WJ, Hahn JH, Lueders H, et al. Chronic cortical electrode array for seizure investigation. Childs Brain 1982;9(1):48–52.
18. Wyler AR, Ojemann GA, Lettich E, et al. Subdural strip electrodes for localizing epileptogenic foci. J Neurosurg 1984;60(6):1195–200.
19. Lesser RP, Crone NE, Webber WRS. Subdural electrodes. Clin Neurophysiol 2010;121(9):1376–92.
20. Ikeda A, Taki W, Kunieda T, et al. Focal ictal direct current shifts in human epilepsy as studied by subdural and scalp recording. Brain 1999;122(Pt 5):827–38.
21. Bancaud J, Dell MB. [Technics and method of stereotaxic functional exploration of the brain structures in man (cortex, subcortex, central gray nuclei)]. Rev Neurol (Paris) 1959;101:213–27.

22. Rolston JD, Ouyang D, Englot DJ, et al. National trends and complication rates for invasive extraoperative electrocorticography in the USA. J Clin Neurosci 2015; 22(5):823–7.

23. Englot DJ. Surface or depth: a paradigm shift in invasive epilepsy monitoring. Epilepsy Curr 2020;20(6):348–50.

24. Jehi L, Morita-Sherman M, Love TE, et al. Comparative effectiveness of stereotactic electroencephalography versus subdural grids in epilepsy surgery. Ann Neurol 2021;90(6):927–39.

25. Joswig H, Lau JC, Abdallat M, et al. Stereoelectroencephalography versus subdural strip electrode implantations: feasibility, complications, and outcomes in 500 intracranial monitoring cases for drug-resistant epilepsy. Neurosurgery 2020;87(1):E23–30.

26. Arya R, Mangano FT, Horn PS, et al. Adverse events related to extraoperative invasive EEG monitoring with subdural grid electrodes: a systematic review and meta-analysis. Epilepsia 2013;54(5):828–39.

27. Tebo CC, Evins AI, Christos PJ, et al. Evolution of cranial epilepsy surgery complication rates: a 32-year systematic review and meta-analysis. J Neurosurg 2014; 120(6):1415–27.

28. Mullin JP, Shriver M, Alomar S, et al. Is SEEG safe? A systematic review and meta-analysis of stereo-electroencephalography-related complications. Epilepsia 2016;57(3):386–401.

29. Englot DJ, Chang EF. Rates and predictors of seizure freedom in resective epilepsy surgery: an update. Neurosurg Rev 2014;37(3):389–404 [discussion: 404-385].

30. Engel J Jr. Surgery for seizures. N Engl J Med 1996;334(10):647–52.

31. Spencer S, Huh L. Outcomes of epilepsy surgery in adults and children. Lancet Neurol 2008;7(6):525–37.

32. Englot DJ, Lee AT, Tsai C, et al. Seizure types and frequency in patients who "fail" temporal lobectomy for intractable epilepsy. Neurosurgery 2013;73(5):838–44, quiz 844.

33. Englot DJ, Rutkowski MJ, Ivan ME, et al. Effects of temporal lobectomy on consciousness-impairing and consciousness-sparing seizures in children. Childs Nerv Syst 2013;29(10):1915–22.

34. Engel J Jr, McDermott MP, Wiebe S, et al. Early surgical therapy for drug-resistant temporal lobe epilepsy: a randomized trial. JAMA 2012;307(9):922–30.

35. Wiebe S, Blume WT, Girvin JP, et al. Effectiveness, Efficiency of surgery for temporal lobe epilepsy study G. A randomized, controlled trial of surgery for temporal-lobe epilepsy. N Engl J Med 2001;345(5):311–8.

36. Schramm J. Temporal lobe epilepsy surgery and the quest for optimal extent of resection: a review. Epilepsia 2008;49(8):1296–307.

37. Yasargil MG, Krayenbuhl N, Roth P, et al. The selective amygdalohippocampectomy for intractable temporal limbic seizures. J Neurosurg 2010;112(1):168–85.

38. Clusmann H, Kral T, Gleissner U, et al. Analysis of different types of resection for pediatric patients with temporal lobe epilepsy. Neurosurgery 2004;54(4):847–59 [discussion: 859-860].

39. Mengesha T, Abu-Ata M, Haas KF, et al. Visual field defects after selective amygdalohippocampectomy and standard temporal lobectomy. J Neuroophthalmol 2009;29(3):208–13.

40. Morino M, Uda T, Naito K, et al. Comparison of neuropsychological outcomes after selective amygdalohippocampectomy versus anterior temporal lobectomy. Epilepsy Behav 2006;9(1):95–100.

41. Englot DJ, Raygor KP, Molinaro AM, et al. Factors associated with failed focal neocortical epilepsy surgery. Neurosurgery 2014;75(6):648-645 [discussion: 655]; quiz 656.
42. Hoppe C, Witt JA, Helmstaedter C, et al. Laser interstitial thermotherapy (LiTT) in epilepsy surgery. Seizure 2017;48:45–52.
43. Sun XR, Patel NV, Danish SF. Tissue ablation dynamics during magnetic resonance-guided, laser-induced thermal therapy. Neurosurgery 2015;77(1): 51–8 [discussion: 58].
44. Wu C, Jermakowicz WJ, Chakravorti S, et al. Effects of surgical targeting in laser interstitial thermal therapy for mesial temporal lobe epilepsy: a multicenter study of 234 patients. Epilepsia 2019;60(6):1171–83.
45. Curry DJ, Gowda A, McNichols RJ, et al. MR-guided stereotactic laser ablation of epileptogenic foci in children. Epilepsy Behav 2012;24(4):408–14.
46. Curry DJ, Raskin J, Ali I, et al. MR-guided laser ablation for the treatment of hypothalamic hamartomas. Epilepsy Res 2018;142:131–4.
47. Xu DS, Chen T, Hlubek RJ, et al. Magnetic resonance imaging-guided laser interstitial thermal therapy for the treatment of hypothalamic hamartomas: a retrospective review. Neurosurgery 2018;83(6):1183–92.
48. Gupta K, Cabaniss B, Kheder A, et al. Stereotactic MRI-guided laser interstitial thermal therapy for extratemporal lobe epilepsy. Epilepsia 2020;61(8):1723–34.
49. Kang JY, Wu C, Tracy J, et al. Laser interstitial thermal therapy for medically intractable mesial temporal lobe epilepsy. Epilepsia 2016;57(2):325–34.
50. Gross RE, Stern MA, Willie JT, et al. Stereotactic laser amygdalohippocampotomy for mesial temporal lobe epilepsy. Ann Neurol 2018;83(3):575–87.
51. Donos C, Breier J, Friedman E, et al. Laser ablation for mesial temporal lobe epilepsy: Surgical and cognitive outcomes with and without mesial temporal sclerosis. Epilepsia 2018;59(7):1421–32.
52. Grewal SS, Zimmerman RS, Worrell G, et al. Laser ablation for mesial temporal epilepsy: a multi-site, single institutional series. J Neurosurg 2018;130(6): 2055–62.
53. Jermakowicz WJ, Kanner AM, Sur S, et al. Laser thermal ablation for mesiotemporal epilepsy: Analysis of ablation volumes and trajectories. Epilepsia 2017; 58(5):801–10.
54. Le S, Ho AL, Fisher RS, et al. Laser interstitial thermal therapy (LITT): seizure outcomes for refractory mesial temporal lobe epilepsy. Epilepsy Behav 2018;89: 37–41.
55. Tao JX, Wu S, Lacy M, et al. Stereotactic EEG-guided laser interstitial thermal therapy for mesial temporal lobe epilepsy. J Neurol Neurosurg Psychiatry 2018; 89(5):542–8.
56. Vakharia VN, Sparks R, Li K, et al. Automated trajectory planning for laser interstitial thermal therapy in mesial temporal lobe epilepsy. Epilepsia 2018;59(4): 814–24.
57. Willie JT, Laxpati NG, Drane DL, et al. Real-time magnetic resonance-guided stereotactic laser amygdalohippocampotomy for mesial temporal lobe epilepsy. Neurosurgery 2014;74(6):569–84 [discussion: 584-565].
58. Kohlhase K, Zollner JP, Tandon N, et al. Comparison of minimally invasive and traditional surgical approaches for refractory mesial temporal lobe epilepsy: a systematic review and meta-analysis of outcomes. Epilepsia 2021;62(4):831–45.
59. Zeller S, Kaye J, Jumah F, et al. Current applications and safety profile of laser interstitial thermal therapy in the pediatric population: a systematic review of the literature. J Neurosurg Pediatr 2021;28(3):360–7.

60. Drane DL, Willie JT, Pedersen NP, et al. Superior verbal memory outcome after stereotactic laser amygdalohippocampotomy. Front Neurol 2021;12:779495.
61. Sperling MR, Gross RE, Alvarez GE, et al. Stereotactic laser ablation for mesial temporal lobe epilepsy: a prospective, multicenter, single-arm study. Epilepsia 2020;61(6):1183–9.
62. Leksell L. The stereotaxic method and radiosurgery of the brain. Acta Chir Scand 1951;102(4):316–9.
63. Regis J, Bartolomei F, Hayashi M, et al. The role of gamma knife surgery in the treatment of severe epilepsies. Epileptic Disord 2000;2(2):113–22.
64. Regis J, Bartolomei F, Rey M, et al. Gamma knife surgery for mesial temporal lobe epilepsy. J Neurosurg 2000;93(Suppl 3):141–6.
65. Barbaro NM, Quigg M, Broshek DK, et al. A multicenter, prospective pilot study of gamma knife radiosurgery for mesial temporal lobe epilepsy: seizure response, adverse events, and verbal memory. Ann Neurol 2009;65(2):167–75.
66. Barbaro NM, Quigg M, Ward MM, et al. Radiosurgery versus open surgery for mesial temporal lobe epilepsy: The randomized, controlled ROSE trial. Epilepsia 2018;59(6):1198–207.
67. Abe K, Yamaguchi T, Hori H, et al. Magnetic resonance-guided focused ultrasound for mesial temporal lobe epilepsy: a case report. BMC Neurol 2020; 20(1):160.
68. Parker WE, Weidman EK, Chazen JL, et al. Magnetic resonance-guided focused ultrasound for ablation of mesial temporal epilepsy circuits: modeling and theoretical feasibility of a novel noninvasive approach. J Neurosurg 2019;133(1): 63–70.
69. Yamaguchi T, Hori T, Hori H, et al. Magnetic resonance-guided focused ultrasound ablation of hypothalamic hamartoma as a disconnection surgery: a case report. Acta Neurochir (Wien) 2020;162(10):2513–7.
70. Brinker ST, Preiswerk F, White PJ, et al. Focused Ultrasound Platform for Investigating Therapeutic Neuromodulation Across the Human Hippocampus. Ultrasound Med Biol 2020;46(5):1270–4.
71. Kerrigan JF, Litt B, Fisher RS, et al. Electrical stimulation of the anterior nucleus of the thalamus for the treatment of intractable epilepsy. Epilepsia 2004;45(4): 346–54.
72. Zhou JJ, Chen T, Farber SH, et al. Open-loop deep brain stimulation for the treatment of epilepsy: a systematic review of clinical outcomes over the past decade (2008-present). Neurosurg Focus 2018;45(2):E5.
73. Fisher R, Salanova V, Witt T, et al. Electrical stimulation of the anterior nucleus of thalamus for treatment of refractory epilepsy. Epilepsia 2010;51(5):899–908.
74. Salanova V, Witt T, Worth R, et al. Long-term efficacy and safety of thalamic stimulation for drug-resistant partial epilepsy. Neurology 2015;84(10):1017–25.
75. Salanova V, Sperling MR, Gross RE, et al. The SANTE study at 10 years of follow-up: Effectiveness, safety, and sudden unexpected death in epilepsy. Epilepsia 2021;62(6):1306–17.
76. Velasco F, Velasco AL, Velasco M, et al. Deep brain stimulation for treatment of the epilepsies: the centromedian thalamic target. Acta Neurochir Suppl 2007; 97(Pt 2):337–42.
77. Son BC, Shon YM, Choi JG, et al. Clinical outcome of patients with deep brain stimulation of the centromedian thalamic nucleus for refractory epilepsy and location of the active contacts. Stereotact Funct Neurosurg 2016;94(3):187–97.
78. Ma BB, Rao VR. Responsive neurostimulation: Candidates and considerations. Epilepsy Behav 2018;88:388–95.

79. Sisterson ND, Wozny TA, Kokkinos V, et al. Closed-loop brain stimulation for drug-resistant epilepsy: towards an evidence-based approach to personalized medicine. Neurotherapeutics 2019;16(1):119–27.

80. Morrell MJ, Halpern C. Responsive direct brain stimulation for epilepsy. Neurosurg Clin N Am 2016;27(1):111–21.

81. Sun FT, Morrell MJ. Closed-loop neurostimulation: the clinical experience. Neurotherapeutics 2014;11(3):553–63.

82. Nair DR, Laxer KD, Weber PB, et al. Nine-year prospective efficacy and safety of brain-responsive neurostimulation for focal epilepsy. Neurology 2020;95(9): e1244–56.

83. Bergey GK, Morrell MJ, Mizrahi EM, et al. Long-term treatment with responsive brain stimulation in adults with refractory partial seizures. Neurology 2015; 84(8):810–7.

84. Burdette DE, Haykal MA, Jarosiewicz B, et al. Brain-responsive corticothalamic stimulation in the centromedian nucleus for the treatment of regional neocortical epilepsy. Epilepsy Behav 2020;112:107354.

85. Burdette D, Mirro EA, Lawrence M, et al. Brain-responsive corticothalamic stimulation in the pulvinar nucleus for the treatment of regional neocortical epilepsy: a case series. Epilepsia Open 2021;6(3):611–7.

86. Vonck K, Van Laere K, Dedeurwaerdere S, et al. The mechanism of action of vagus nerve stimulation for refractory epilepsy: the current status. J Clin Neurophysiol 2001;18(5):394–401.

87. Amar AP, Heck CN, Levy ML, et al. An institutional experience with cervical vagus nerve trunk stimulation for medically refractory epilepsy: rationale, technique, and outcome. Neurosurgery 1998;43(6):1265–76 [discussion: 1276-1280].

88. Ben-Menachem E, Manon-Espaillat R, Ristanovic R, et al. Vagus nerve stimulation for treatment of partial seizures: 1. A controlled study of effect on seizures. First International Vagus Nerve Stimulation Study Group. Epilepsia 1994;35(3):616–26.

89. Handforth A, DeGiorgio CM, Schachter SC, et al. Vagus nerve stimulation therapy for partial-onset seizures: a randomized active-control trial. Neurology 1998; 51(1):48–55.

90. Klinkenberg S, Aalbers MW, Vles JS, et al. Vagus nerve stimulation in children with intractable epilepsy: a randomized controlled trial. Dev Med Child Neurol 2012;54(9):855–61.

91. Gonzalez HFJ, Yengo-Kahn A, Englot DJ. Vagus Nerve Stimulation for the Treatment of Epilepsy. Neurosurg Clin N Am 2019;30(2):219–30.

92. Englot DJ, Rolston JD, Wang DD, et al. Efficacy of vagus nerve stimulation in posttraumatic versus nontraumatic epilepsy. J Neurosurg 2012;117(5):970–7.

93. Tzadok M, Harush A, Nissenkorn A, et al. Clinical outcomes of closed-loop vagal nerve stimulation in patients with refractory epilepsy. Seizure 2019;71:140–4.

Prevalence and Diagnosis of Sexual Dysfunction in People with Epilepsy

Chaturbhuj Rathore, MD, DM[a],
Kurupath Radhakrishnan, MD, DM, FAMS, FAAN, FANA[b],*

KEYWORDS

- Antiseizure medicines • Diagnosis • Epilepsy • Epilepsy surgery • Prevalence
- Sexual dysfunction • Treatment

KEY POINTS

- Sexual dysfunctions occur 2 to 4 times more frequently in people with epilepsy (PWE) as compared with normal controls, and are similarly prevalent in men and women.
- While men with epilepsy generally have arousal disorders such as erectile dysfunction and premature ejaculation, women usually have dysfunction in the domains of desire.
- Epilepsy-related and medication-related factors, and psychiatric and psychosocial co-morbidities contribute to sexual dysfunction in PWE.
- Sexual dysfunctions are more common with drug-resistant epilepsy and in those receiving enzyme-inducing antiseizure medicines (ASMs); sexual function often improves in seizure-free patients following epilepsy surgery.
- Because the physicians are reluctant to inquire and the patients are hesitant to complain about it during routine clinic visits, sexual dysfunctions largely remain unrecognized.

INTRODUCTION

One of the principal characteristics that define all living beings is their ability to reproduce which in turn is intimately related to sexual functions. Sexual functioning is one of the basic human drives apart from eating and sleeping. Normal sexual functioning is essential for the optimal quality of life in all human beings. Sexual dysfunction is associated with impaired quality of life in adults and has become an issue of immense public health importance over the last few decades.[1] The fact that epilepsy is associated with impaired sexual functions is known for more than 70 years.[2] Despite this, sexual dysfunctions in people with epilepsy (PWE) are

a Department of Neurology, Smt. B. K. Shah Medical Institute and Research Center, Sumandeep Vidyapeeth, Vadodara, Gujarat 391760, India; b Department of Neurosciences, Avitis Institute of Medical Sciences, Palakkad, Kerala 678508, India
* Corresponding author.
E-mail addresses: kurupath.radhakrishnan@gmail.com; drradhakrishnan.k@avitishospital.com

Neurol Clin 40 (2022) 869–889
https://doi.org/10.1016/j.ncl.2022.03.013
neurologic.theclinics.com

grossly under-recognized, under-reported, and under-treated.[3,4] One of the main reasons for this is the hesitation from the physicians and patients to talk about sexual functions. Most of the patients feel inhibited in disclosing their sexual inadequacy and may consider it a part of their disease. Additionally, there is a poor understanding of sexual dysfunction, its causes, and appropriate treatment strategies among physicians. For optimizing the sexual health in PWE, neurologist should regularly inquire about sexual functions during outpatient consultations and should have a proper understanding of its causes and management strategies. In this review, we deliberate on the present understanding of sexual dysfunction in PWE with an emphasis on its prevalence and diagnosis.

DEFINITION AND CLASSIFICATION OF SEXUAL DYSFUNCTIONS

Precise definition and classification of sexual dysfunctions are essential for proper diagnosis, for planning optimal management strategies, and for designing clinical studies on this scantily researched area of epilepsy care. Sexual dysfunction is defined by the World Health Organization (WHO) as "the various ways in which an individual is unable to participate in a sexual relationship as he or she would wish."[4] Normal sexual functioning is highly subjective and is dependent on multiple social, cultural, psychological, intrapersonal, and interpersonal factors. Henceforth, it is almost impossible to define sexual dysfunction in a quantitative way without introducing a good deal of subjectivity. Nonetheless, it is recognized that any difficulty experienced by an individual during any stage of normal sexual activity which causes distress and strained interpersonal relationship can be defined as sexual dysfunction.

Several attempts have been made to classify sexual dysfunctions.[5,6] The International Classification of Diseases-10 (ICD-10) by WHO, Diagnostic and Statistical Manual of Mental Disorders (DSM)-V classification proposed by the American Psychiatric Association, and the classification offered by the International Consultation on Sexual Medicine are the 3 most widely used and elaborate classification systems.[5,7–9] Regardless of the variable terminologies put forward by the different classification systems, the sexual disorders are customarily categorized into one of the 4 broad domains: disorders of desire, disorders of arousal, orgasmic disorders, and sexual pain disorders (**Box 1**). Nevertheless, this type of categorization may be arbitrary and an individual might have a mixture of different sexual disorders. The ICD-10 classification further subdivides sexual disorders into organic and nonorganic disorders. However, in a given patient there may be a combination of psychological and organic factors accountable for sexual dysfunction. The DSM-V classification also supplements the presence or absence of marked distress or interpersonal difficulty with each type of sexual dysfunction.

For the precise diagnosis, sexual dysfunction is concluded when it is present for at least 6 months and is present 75% to 100% of the sexual intercourses.[7] Hyposexuality is defined as diminished sexual drive and is further quantified as sexual activity less than once per month.[7] Furthermore, sexual dysfunction may be generalized when it occurs during all situations and with all the partners, while it may be situational when it occurs in specific situations. This type of distinction helps us in understanding the social and psychological aspects of sexual dysfunction. To gauge the severity of the sexual dysfunction, a simple yes/no scale may be too restrictive and can lead to the overestimation of its severity. Massachusetts Male Aging Study (MMAS), which ranks erectile dysfunction on a four-grade scale (no/mild/moderate/complete), is widely used to grade the severity of other sexual dysfunctions as well.[10]

Box 1
Classification of sexual dysfunctions

1. Disorders of desire (both men and women)
   i. Hypoactive sexual desire disorder
   ii. Sexual aversion disorder
   iii. Excessive sexual drive

2. Disorders of arousal (vaginal dryness/erectile dysfunction)
   i. Female sexual arousal disorder
   ii. Male erectile disorder

3. Orgasmic disorders (absence/delay/premature)
   i. Male orgasmic disorder
   ii. Female orgasmic disorder
   iii. Premature ejaculation

4. Sexual pain disorders
   i. Dyspareunia
   ii. Vaginismus
   iii. Other sexual pain disorders

5. Sexual dysfunctions not otherwise specified

Modified from Rathore C, Henning OJ, Luef G, Radhakrishnan K. Sexual dysfunction in people with epilepsy. Epilepsy Behav. 2019;100(Pt A):106495. https://doi.org/10.1016/j.yebeh.2019.106495; with permission.

SCREENING FOR SEXUAL DYSFUNCTION

More than 50 scales, either self-reported or interview-based, have been developed to ascertain the presence and pattern of sexual dysfunctions, and to assess their severity in the general population and in many chronic diseases.[6,11] These scales measure different domains of sexual functioning, estimate their severity, and also provide a composite score to judge the overall sexual functioning in an individual. However, none of these scales have been validated in PWE and different studies in PWE have used diverse scales to measure sexual dysfunction. Dawson and colleagues[12] reported that the International Index of Erectile Function (IIEF) tool can be used to assess the sexual functions in men with epilepsy. However, they only reported the face and content validity of the tool and did not attempt to validate it against the more standard clinical tools or clinical interviews. An ideal scale should be brief, simple, easy to administer, unobtrusive, should measure all domains of sexual functioning, should be applicable to people of all genders and sexual orientations, and should have good reliability. None of the available scales fulfill all these requirements. Nonetheless, certain scales are used commonly in PWE, especially in the clinical and research settings (**Table 1**).[13–19]

Of all the available scales, Arizona Sexual Experience Scale (ASEX) is a good initial screening tool for sexual dysfunction in PWE.[19] It is simple, brief, least intrusive, and takes about 5 minutes to administer. It was validated in 107 normal subjects and 58 psychiatric patients.[19] It demonstrated good internal consistency, reliability, and construct validity. It is a 5-item rating scale with scores varying from 5 to 30 and higher scores indicate greater dysfunction. It can be used in busy outpatient clinics to screen all PWE. Those patients found to have sexual dysfunction can be further evaluated with one of the more elaborate measures. The Derogatis Interview for Sexual Functioning is a 25-item semi-structured interview to assess various domains of sexual functioning.[18] It takes 12 to 15 minutes to administer this scale and it also has a

Table 1
Screening scales for sexual dysfunction in people with epilepsy

Name of Scale	Target Population	Items	Domains	Time to Administer	Comments
Brief Sexual Symptom Checklist for Men and women (BSSC-M; BSSC-W)[13]	All	4 questions	Desire, arousal, orgasm, pain	5 min	Brief screening questionnaire
Sexual Complaints Screener for Men and women (SCS)[13]	All	10 questions for men; 11questions for women; each graded on a scale of 5	Desire, arousal, orgasm, pain	10 min	Brief screening questionnaire
Female Sexual Function Index (FSFI)[14]	Women	19 & 6 (abbreviated version)	Desire, arousal, orgasm, pain	10–15 min	Widely used; considered gold standard for the evaluation of SD in women
Sexual Function Questionnaire (SFQ)[15]	Women	28	Desire, arousal, orgasm, pain	15–20 min	Good for the evaluation of SD in women
International Index of Erectile Function (IIEF)[16]	Men	15 & 5 (Brief)	Erection, orgasm, desire, satisfaction, and overall satisfaction	10–15 min	Widely used; can be used to quantify treatment response
Premature Ejaculation Profile (PEP)[17]	Men	4	Ejaculation	5 min	To assess severity of premature ejaculation
Derogatis Interview for Sexual Function (DISF)[18]	All	25	Desire, arousal, orgasm, pain	15–20 min	Good tool for individual components and overall sexual functions
Arizona Sexual Experiences Scale (ASEX)[19]	All	5	Desire, arousal, orgasm, overall satisfaction	5 min	Good initial screening tool

Abbreviation: SD, sexual dysfunction

Adapted from Rathore C, Henning OJ, Luef G, Radhakrishnan K. Sexual dysfunction in people with epilepsy. Epilepsy Behav. 2019;100(Pt A):106495. https://doi.org/10.1016/j.yebeh.2019.106495; with permission.

self-reported version. It provides measures of sexual functioning in individual domains and a composite score for measuring the overall sexual functioning in an individual. It is applicable to both genders and has good sensitivity and discriminative validity.

PREVALENCE OF SEXUAL DYSFUNCTION IN PEOPLE WITH EPILEPSY

The fact that PWE are more likely to have sexual dysfunction as compared with the general population is known for the last 7 decades.[2] Reports published in the 1950s and 1960s surmised that 50%–70% of the patients with temporal lobe epilepsy have hyposexuality.[2,20] Subsequently multiple other studies have reported the prevalence of sexual dysfunctions in PWE. We have summarized their salient features in **Table 2**.[3,12,21–42] Despite large amount of information gathered over the last 70 years, the prevalence and pattern of sexual dysfunction in PWE are indeterminate. This is largely related to the marked heterogeneity in the studies with regard to the population studied and the methods used to define and ascertain sexual dysfunction. The study subjects varied with regard to gender distribution, age group, type of epilepsy, seizure control, and number and type of antiseizure medicines (ASMs) used. Likewise, the studies have used different tools to identify sexual dysfunction including screening scales, semi-structured interviews, and clinical interviews. Generally, the studies which have used quantitative screening scales with definite cut-off values to define sexual dysfunction have reported higher prevalence of sexual dysfunction in PWE as compared with the studies using semi-structured interviews. Even though this difference may suggest superior sensitivity of quantitative screening scales in identifying sexual dysfunction, these scales may overestimate the prevalence by falsely classifying many patients with sexual difficulties as having sexual dysfunctions. Finally, variable prevalence of sexual dysfunction in PWE reported from different geographic regions may be related to diverse social and cultural influences.

A recent meta-analysis that included 9 studies with 1556 normal subjects and 599 PWE has reported that the prevalence of sexual dysfunction in PWE is 58.1% as compared with 16.5% in the control group.[43] Compared with controls, while women with epilepsy had a 2.7 (95% confidence interval, 1.5–4.9) times higher risk of having sexual dysfunction, men with epilepsy had a 4.9 (95% confidence interval, 2.0–11.7) times higher risk of sexual dysfunction. However, most of the studies included in this meta-analysis did not have details of epilepsy-related factors and henceforth it is difficult to determine the differential rates of sexual dysfunction in patients with different epilepsy types, in relation to seizure control and various ASMs used. A recent study that compared sexual dysfunctions among 299 PWE (mostly with poor seizure control) and 1671 normal adult Norwegians in the general population revealed that problems with orgasm, dyspareunia, erectile dysfunction, and feelings of sexual deviance were more prevalent in PWE as compared with the general population.[44]

Sexual Dysfunctions in Women with Epilepsy

Even though many studies have estimated the prevalence and type of sexual dysfunction in women with epilepsy, because of the limitations detailed above it is difficult to draw reliable conclusions. The reported prevalence of sexual dysfunction in women with epilepsy has varied from 18% to 70%.[21,27,29] In an older study from Egypt, comprising 700 women with epilepsy and 100 controls, sexual dysfunction was perceived by only 18% of the women with epilepsy.[21] In this study, patients were evaluated through a clinical interview and the majority were on enzyme-inducing ASMs. On the other hand, a recent study that evaluated sexual functions in 196 married

Table 2
Major studies reporting the prevalence of sexual dysfunction in men and women with epilepsy

Reference (First Author/year)	Subjects	Type of Epilepsy	Assessment Tool	Prevalence of SD	Type of SD	Factors Associated with SD	Comments
Demerdash et al.,[21] 1991	700 women; 100 controls	Mixed	Clinical interview	127 (18%)	Sexual dysfunction:83% All domains equally affected; Paraphilias (16%)	Longer duration of epilepsy; Focal epilepsy	Majority on enzyme-inducing ASMs; Seizure control was not reported
Bergen et al.,[22] 1992	50 women; Age matched controls	Mixed (64% focal epilepsy)	Self-reported questionnaire	17 (34%)	Hyposexuality; 20% with no desire at all.	None	Seizure control not reported; 44% on >1ASM; 94% on enzyme-inducing ASM
Morrell &Guldner,[23] 1996	116 women	Predominantly focal epilepsy (85%)	Sexual Arousability Inventory-Expanded; Sexual Behavior Inventory; Sexual Functioning Inventory	30%	Desire (16%); (Arousal 42%); Pain (25%); Orgasm (18%)	None	Seizure not controlled in 62%; 27% on polytherapy; Used published norms as control
Morrell et al.,[24] 2005	57 women; 17 controls	Mixed; On monotherapy	Sexual Arousability Inventory-Expanded; Sexual Behavior Inventory; Sexual Anxiety Interview;	20% vs 9% in controls	Arousal and anxiety	Focal epilepsy; Phenytoin therapy; depression; Low estradiol levels	Seizure control not reported; 43% on non-enzyme-inducing drugs

Study	Sample	Type	Scale	Prevalence	Domains	Risk factors	Seizure control
Duncan et al.,[25] 1997	195 women; 48 controls	Mixed; 36 not on AED	Sexuality Experience Scales; Hormonal levels	No difference between patients and controls	Not provided	None	75% on monotherapy; Seizure control and frequency not mentioned
Zelena et al.,[26] 2011	78 women	Mixed	Female Sexual Function Index	23%	All domains mainly desire and arousal	Depression	Majority had uncontrolled epilepsy and were on polytherapy
Atarodi-Kashani et al.,[27] 2017	196 married women	Mixed	Female Sexual Function Index	74.5%	All 4 components; Maximum dysfunction in orgasm and sexual satisfaction	Age >40 y; Low education and income; higher seizure frequency; Polypharmacy; Enzyme-inducing drugs	56% had uncontrolled epilepsy; 45% on more than one ASM
Ogunjimi et al.,[28] 2018	70 women and 70 controls	Mixed	Arizona Sexual Experience Scale	50% in patients and 38% in controls	All domains; Patients had a high score in all domains	Lesional epilepsy; older age; Motor weakness	50% had uncontrolled epilepsy;
Tao et al.,[29] 2018	112 women and 120 controls	Mixed	Female Sexual Function Index	70% in patients and 24% in controls	Desire (85.7%); All other domains: 40%-60%	Poor economic status; presence of anxiety; nonadherence to medicines	50% had uncontrolled epilepsy; 45% on more than one ASM
Hamed et al.,[30] 2020	120 women and 80 matched controls	Focal epilepsy (63% temporal lobe epilepsy) receiving either CBZ or OXCBZ	Female Sexual Function Index	~80% with CBZ; ~60% with OXCBZ	All domains	Higher seizure frequency and mood disorders	Mostly (82%) had good seizure control

(continued on next page)

Table 2
(*continued*)

Reference (First Author/year)	Subjects	Type of Epilepsy	Assessment Tool	Prevalence of SD	Type of SD	Factors Associated with SD	Comments
Mazdeh et al.,[31] 2020	80 married women	Mixed; Predominantly generalized seizures	Female Sexual Function Index	78%	Satisfaction in 70%; Rest of the domains in 40%–50%	Older age, longer epilepsy duration, polypharmacy	Not well-characterized cohort
Santos et al.,[32] 2021	55 women with epilepsy and 55 controls	Mixed	Female Sexual Function Index; Female Genital Self Image Scale	19.3% in patients vs 21% in controls	All domains	Enzyme-inducing ASMs; Depression	Small cohort
Jensen et al.,[33] 1990	86 (38 men; 48 women); Historical controls	Mixed; 73% on single or no drug	Self-reported questionnaire; Hormonal assessment	8% in men; 29% in women; Normal hormones in both	Desire (22%); Orgasmic (19%); ED (3%); Some had combination	None	Majority had good seizure control
Souza et al.,[34] 2000	60 patients of both genders and 60 controls	Mixed with majority (58) on monotherapy	Sexual Behavior Interview	50% patients and 25% controls	Not reported	Depression	50% had uncontrolled epilepsy
Herzog et al.,[35] 2003	36 patients; 9 untreated; 12 controls	Uncontrolled TLE	Arizona Sexual Experience Scale; Hormonal analysis	39%	Not reported	Right TLE; Low bioactive testosterone	Uncontrolled TLE
Henning et al.,[36] 2016	171 patients; 594 controls	Mixed	Self-reported questionnaire	75% vs 12% in women; 63% vs 10% in men	All domains mainly reduced desire in women (50%) and ED in men (34%)	None of the epilepsy-related factors predicted dysfunction	Majority of patients had uncontrolled epilepsy
Ejigu et al.,[37] 2019	576 patients	Mixed	Changes in Sexual Functioning Questionnaires (CSFQ-14)	63.9%; 67.4% in men & 55.6% in women	Arousal dysfunction in 98%	Age>51 y; depression; being jobless; Khat (local stimulant) use	40% had uncontrolled epilepsy & 74% were on monotherapy

Study	Sample	Epilepsy type	Assessment tool	Prevalence/Finding	Domains	Risk factors	Population notes
Kumar et al,[38] 2020	108 patients	Mixed	Sexual Functioning Questionnaire	60.2%	Not specified	Presence of anxiety and depression; Drugs other than valproate	Mixed epilepsy population from clinic
Pellinen et al,[3] 2021	89 patients	Mostly focal epilepsy admitted to epilepsy monitoring units	Self-reported questionnaire	22.5%	Not specified	Being obese; Enzyme-inducing ASMs	Most drug-resistant epilepsy
Nikoobakht et al,[39] 2007	80 married men	Mixed	International Index of Erectile Function-15	43% had ED; 11% had premature ejaculation	Desire and arousal	Higher seizure frequency; generalized seizures	70% had controlled epilepsy (seizure free for 6 mo)
Duncan et al,[40] 2009	69 men and 50 controls	Mixed on single AED	Sexual Desire Inventory; Sexual Self-Efficacy Scale Erectile Function; Sexual response inventory	Patients had higher scores than controls	Desire and arousal	Anxiety and depression	Two-third of the patients had uncontrolled epilepsy
Calabro et al,[41] 2013	30 men and 30 controls	Mixed	Semi-structured questionnaire and Sex-relation Evaluation Schedule Assessment Monitoring	28% in patients and 18% in controls	All domains; ED in 5%	High seizure frequency	Majority had well-controlled epilepsy. 70% were seizure free for more than 5 y

(continued on next page)

Table 2
(continued)

Reference (First Author/year)	Subjects	Type of Epilepsy	Assessment Tool	Prevalence of SD	Type of SD	Factors Associated with SD	Comments
Dawson et al.,[12] 2020	164 men	Mixed	International Index of Erectile Function	18%	All domains	NA	Majority on polytherapy
Sureka et al.,[42] 2021	100 men	Idiopathic generalized epilepsy	Arizona Sexual Experience Scale	60%	ED (36%); Premature ejaculation (26%); Decreased libido (4%)	Longer epilepsy duration; Polypharmacy	Seizure freedom for 1 year; psychiatric comorbidities excluded

Abbreviations: ASM, antiseizure medicine; CBZ, carbamazepine; ED, erectile dysfunction; NA, not available; OXCBZ, oxcarbazepine; SD, sexual dysfunction; TLE, temporal lobe epilepsy.

From Rathore C, Henning OJ, Luef G, Radhakrishnan K. Sexual dysfunction in people with epilepsy. Epilepsy Behav. 2019;100(Pt A):106495. https://doi.org/10.1016/j.yebeh.2019.106495; with permission.

Iranian women with epilepsy (56% with uncontrolled epilepsy) using the Female Sexual Function Index reported sexual dysfunction in 74.5% of the women.[27] In another recent study from Addis Ababa, Ethiopia, 576 PWE were assessed by interviewer-administered Changes in Sexual Functioning Questionnaire (CSFQ-14).[37] Compared with 67.4% (95%CI = 62.8–72.1) of men, 55.6% (95%CI = 49.1–62.6) women participants reported sexual dysfunction.[37] Whether the striking difference in the prevalence of sexual dysfunction in women with epilepsy observed between these studies from developing countries is an artifact of ascertainment or additionally influenced by region-specific socio-cultural factors is uncertain. In the Norwegian study, women with drug-resistant epilepsy sought consultation for their sexual problems significantly more compared with well-controlled epilepsy and women without epilepsy.[44] Unexpectedly, this study did not find an association between the frequency of sexual dysfunction and the level of seizure control, use of enzyme-inducing AEDs or their adverse effects. The small sample size in most of the studies may be responsible for the inconsistent influence of the type of epilepsy and ASM profile on the prevalence of sexual dysfunction. This also indicates that sexual functions are controlled by multiple personal and cultural factors which are difficult to measure in clinical studies.

In general, it can be surmised that sexual dysfunctions are present in nearly half of the unselected women with epilepsy. Women with drug-resistant epilepsy, longer duration of epilepsy, receiving polytherapy and enzyme-inducing medicines, higher seizure frequency, and those with focal epilepsy are more likely to have sexual dysfunction (**Box 2**). On the other hand, those women with well-controlled epilepsy and receiving single ASM are more likely to have normal sexual functions. Although all types of sexual dysfunctions can occur in women with epilepsy, disorders of sexual desire and arousal are more frequent as compared with disorders of orgasm. Nonetheless, more studies with a larger number of patients having different epilepsy syndromes, different epilepsy severity, and residing in different geographic regions should be undertaken before drawing any firm conclusions.

Sexual Dysfunctions in Men with Epilepsy

Men with epilepsy are 3 to 4 times more likely to have sexual dysfunction as compared with the controls.[43] The prevalence of sexual dysfunction in men with epilepsy varies from 18% to 60% in different studies.[12,42] A study from Taiwan using health insurance database involving 6427 men with erectile dysfunction and 32,135 controls reported that epilepsy was 1.8 times more common in patients

---

Box 2
Factors commonly associated with sexual dysfunction in people with epilepsy

- High seizure frequency
- Uncontrolled epilepsy
- Focal epilepsy
- Use of polypharmacy
- Use of enzyme-inducing antiseizure medicines
- Presence of anxiety and depression
- Older age
- Longer epilepsy duration
- Low education and economic status

with erectile dysfunction as compared with the controls.[45] Overall, the number of studies evaluating sexual functions exclusively in men with epilepsy is less as compared with the studies in women (see **Table 2**). Most of the studies have included a mixed population of both men and women and have studied a small number of patients. These studies have shown that men are more likely to have disorders of arousal and orgasm in the form of erectile dysfunction and premature ejaculation. One of the earliest Veterans Administration Cooperative Study reported the effects of various ASMs on sexual functions in men and reported decreased libido in 11%-22% of them.[46] In a study of 80 married men with epilepsy evaluated using the International Index of Erectile Function-15, erectile dysfunction was reported in 43% of the patients.[39] In an earlier Norwegian study comprising 171 patients with drug-resistant epilepsy, women had a higher prevalence of sexual dysfunction compared with men (75.3% vs 63.3%).[36] Overall, it can be concluded that sexual dysfunctions occur in nearly half of unselected men with epilepsy. Patients with poor seizure control and higher seizure frequency are more likely to have sexual dysfunctions as compared with men with well-controlled epilepsy.

Sexual Dysfunction and Epilepsy Surgery

Patients undergoing epilepsy surgery have uncontrolled seizures and often receive multiple ASMs. Institutively, seizure freedom and reduction in ASM following epilepsy surgery should improve sexual functions in these patients. However, evidence in this regard is largely sparse and has mainly come from few cross-sectional studies in the postoperative period.

In 1967, Blume and Walker reported that 7 of the 11 patients with marked hyposexuality in the preoperative period improved following temporal lobectomy.[20] In a larger study involving 100 patients, Taylor reported improved sexual function in 22% of the patients following temporal lobectomy.[47] In a cross-sectional study of 58 patients evaluated in the postoperative period, Baird and colleagues[48] reported improved sexual functions in 40% of patients and decreased sexual function in 24% of patients while others did not report any change in sexual functions following surgery. The present authors used a self-reported quantitative questionnaire to assess the sexual behavior of 50 married male patients who had undergone temporal lobectomy and compared it with 50 controls.[49] Although the sexual desire and satisfaction levels improved in the postoperative period, they did not match with the levels of control subjects. In this study, postoperative seizure freedom, use of single or no ASMs, and the absence of interictal discharges on postoperative EEG were associated with better sexual functions.[49] Longitudinal studies with a large number of patients are required to better define the effects of epilepsy surgery on sexual functions.

There are few old reports of hypersexuality following temporal lobectomy.[50] This has been assumed to occur as a part of partial Klüver–Bucy syndrome due to bilateral temporal dysfunctions, which is unlikely to occur in patients selected for surgery based on modern presurgical evaluation strategies.

To our knowledge, there are no studies that have assessed the effects of vagus nerve stimulation (VNS) and deep brain stimulation (DBS) on sexual functions in PWE. The VNS by reducing ASM burden and by improving depression may have a positive effect on sexual functions in PWE. The experimental data suggest that vagus nerve indeed exerts control over the sexual functions in normal people.[51] Although few studies have assessed the effect of subthalamic nucleus stimulation on sexual dysfunctions in patients with Parkinson's disease with variable results,[52] there has been no study of sexual function in patients undergoing DBS for epilepsy.

FACTORS AFFECTING SEXUAL FUNCTIONS IN PEOPLE WITH EPILEPSY

Even though the emphasis of this review is on the prevalence and diagnosis, it is important to understand the mechanism and underlying factors causing sexual dysfunction in PWE to plan diagnostic evaluation and management strategies. A complex interaction between epilepsy-related and medication-related factors, and psychiatric and psycho-social comorbidities contribute to sexual dysfunction in PWE (**Fig. 1**). From the management perspective, it is often difficult to delineate the cause(s) of sexual in an individual patient, and expectedly, studies that have inquired about the causal dimensions of sexual dysfunction have come up with inconsistent results.

Epilepsy-Related Factors

Epilepsy may cause sexual dysfunctions through both central and peripheral mechanisms. Centrally, repeated seizures and interictal epileptiform discharges propagating through amygdalo-hypothalamic pathways can affect the pituitary–hypothalamic axis leading to reduced secretion of luteinizing hormone (LH) and hypogonadotropic hypogonadism.[53] The experimental evidence suggests that reproductive pathways are more lateralized to the right hypothalamus which may explain the higher prevalence of sexual dysfunction in patients with right temporal lobe epilepsy.[54] The evidence for this has come from the studies reporting lower levels of LH in patients with right temporal lobe epilepsy and sexual dysfunctions.[53] In these studies, the sexual dysfunction occurred independently of the ASM usage or the presence of psychiatric disorders.

Peripherally, a few studies have reported low testosterone levels in PWE having sexual dysfunctions. Bauer and colleagues[55] compared serum levels of gonadotropic hormones and free testosterone in 200 men with epilepsy and 105 controls. All the patients were receiving either single or no ASM. Most of the PWE had focal epilepsy and more than half of them had temporal lobe epilepsy. Patients had lower free testosterone levels and low testosterone/LH ratio as compared with the controls. Patients

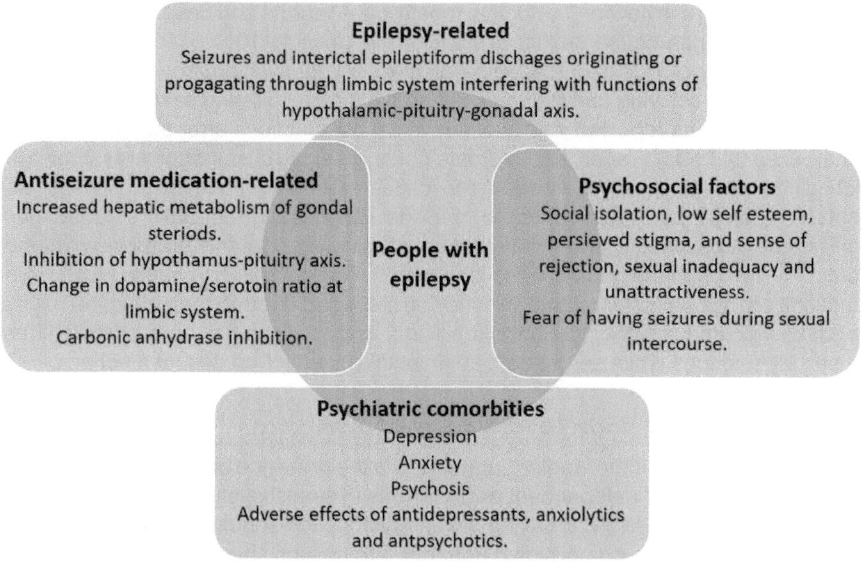

Epilepsy-related
Seizures and interictal epileptiform dischages originating or progagating through limbic system interfering with functions of hypothalamic-pituitry-gonadal axis.

Antiseizure medication-related
Increased hepatic metabolism of gondal steriods.
Inhibition of hypothamus-pituitry axis.
Change in dopamine/serotoin ratio at limbic system.
Carbonic anhydrase inhibition.

People with epilepsy

Psychosocial factors
Social isolation, low self esteem, persieved stigma, and sense of rejection, sexual inadequacy and unattractiveness.
Fear of having seizures during sexual intercourse.

Psychiatric comorbities
Depression
Anxiety
Psychosis
Adverse effects of antidepressants, anxiolytics and antpsychotics.

Fig. 1. Causal dimensions of sexual dysfunctions in people with epilepsy.

with temporal lobe epilepsy and those receiving carbamazepine had the lowest levels of testosterone. However, the authors did not assess sexual dysfunction in this study. In contrast, another study involving 60 men with epilepsy and 60 controls found no difference in the levels of free and bioactive testosterone between patients and the controls.[56] Nonetheless, a significant correlation was found between the presence of anxiety and depression and sexual dysfunctions. A recent study involving 112 married women and 120 controls from China showed that low levels of testosterone and the presence of estrogen receptor gene polymorphisms were associated with sexual dysfunction.[57] These variable results indicate that there is a complex interaction between disease- and treatment-related factors, genetic predisposition, hormonal levels, and psychosocial comorbidities in instigating sexual dysfunction in PWE.

Antiseizure Medicines and Sexual Dysfunction

Enzyme-inducing ASMs increase the hepatic clearance of gonadal and adrenal steroids.[58–60] These drugs also increase the levels of sex hormone-binding globulin (SHBG) leading to low levels of free testosterone.[58–60] ASMs also inhibit the pituitary–hypothalamic axis leading to low levels of LH and subsequent hypogonadotropic hypogonadism.[53] Additionally, experimental evidence suggests that ASMs influence sexual functions by their effect on monoaminergic and serotoninergic pathways.[58,61]

Both carbamazepine and phenytoin have been shown to increase the levels of SHBG and lower the levels of bioactive testosterone in multiple studies.[59,60] This is further substantiated by the studies showing improvement in levels of free testosterone and sexual functions after withdrawal of carbamazepine.[62] A study of 141 subjects who were either initiated or switched to lamotrigine showed improvement in sexual functions.[63] This improvement might have been related to better seizure control or improved mood after lamotrigine use. Other studies have also shown better sexual functions in patients receiving valproate, lamotrigine, and levetiracetam as compared with those receiving carbamazepine or phenytoin.[38,64]

Data regarding the effects of other newer ASMs on sexual functions are rather limited. A systemic review of 17 studies, mostly case reports and case series, revealed that topiramate can cause sexual dysfunction in close to 10% of PWE.[61] Although there are rare reports of oxcarbazepine causing sexual dysfunction, in a large study of 228 subjects receiving carbamazepine and having pre-existing sexual dysfunction, 80% of the patients reported improvement in sexual functions after switching over to oxcarbazepine.[65] Data regarding valproate causing sexual dysfunction are rather conflicting, but overall it has been shown to cause erectile dysfunction in 10% of patients.[66] There are isolated case reports implying pregabalin, gabapentin, zonisamide, lacosamide, and levetiracetam causing erectile and orgasmic dysfunctions.[67–71] Although the mechanisms by which the new ASMs can cause sexual dysfunctions are not well understood, this may be mediated through their effect on central dopaminergic and serotoninergic transmission, as dopamine has an excitatory effect on sexual functions while serotonin has an inhibitory effect on sexual functions.[70,71]

Psychiatric and Psycho-Social Issues and Sexual Dysfunction

The evidence from multiple studies suggests that the presence of depression and anxiety is one of the major independent determinants of sexual dysfunction in PWE.[24,56] It is imperative that all the PWE having sexual dysfunction should be screened for the presence of psychiatric comorbidity. Patients with epilepsy have a 2- to 3-fold higher risk of developing depression and 10-fold higher risk of developing psychosis as compared with normal controls.[72,73] Sexual dysfunctions can be further aggravated by the use of antidepressant and antipsychotic medicines.[74]

Additionally, various psycho-social issues affecting the lives of PWE can contribute to sexual dysfunction. In a survey of 89 patients admitted to an epilepsy monitoring unit, feeling of being overweight or obese was independently associated with sexual dysfunction.[3] PWE often have low self-esteem, perceived stigma, and lower socio-economic development. All these factors may contribute to sexual dysfunction. In a recent study, positive personality traits such as extraversion and agreeableness were associated with better sexual functions in women with epilepsy.[75]

EVALUATION AND DIAGNOSIS OF SEXUAL DYSFUNCTIONS

The objectives of the evaluation of sexual functioning in PWE are to ascertain the presence or absence of sexual dysfunction, characterize the type of sexual dysfunction, assess the severity of sexual dysfunction, and assess the possible etiologic factors. The clinical interview is the gold standard tool for diagnosing the nature of sexual dysfunction, ascertaining the likely etiology, and to plan the management of sexual dysfunction in PWE. While evaluation and management of psychological factors are in the domain of psychologists and psychiatrists, the treating neurologists should be able to find out the presence of sexual dysfunction in a person with epilepsy and should be able to judge the likely contribution of epilepsy- or treatment-related factors contributing to the sexual dysfunction. As multiple factors contribute to sexual dysfunctions, a multidisciplinary approach should be undertaken for the evaluation of patients with sexual dysfunctions. In **Fig. 2**, we have provided an algorithmic approach to the diagnosis and treatment of sexual dysfunction in PWE.

Initial Assessment and the Clinical Interview

The first and foremost step in the evaluation of sexual dysfunctions is to discuss it with the patients. Most of the patients do not come forward to discuss sexual dysfunctions and the treating physicians usually do not inquire about it. The best way is to screen all the patients for the presence of sexual dysfunctions using a brief and nonintrusive screening questionnaire such as the Arizona Sexual Experiences (ASEX) Scale. The second step is to conduct a detailed clinical interview of the patients and their partners by a trained psychologist. Those patients with associated anxiety, depression, and psychosis should be counseled appropriately and should be initiated on pharmacologic treatment, if indicated.

Patients, especially male patients with erectile dysfunction, should also be evaluated for the presence of systemic illnesses such as cardiac disease, diabetes, and hypertension, which all can contribute to sexual dysfunction. Likewise, a drug history is important as certain drugs such as beta-blockers, antidepressants, and diuretics are associated with sexual dysfunction. In indicated cases, a urogenital evaluation should be undertaken by a urologist or a gynecologist.

Optimizing Epilepsy Treatment

As patients with well-controlled epilepsy are less likely to have sexual dysfunction, every attempt should be made to optimize seizure control with a single non–enzyme-inducing ASM, as far as possible. Those patients receiving enzyme-inducing ASMs such as phenytoin and carbamazepine can be switched over to non–enzyme-inducing ASMs such as levetiracetam, lamotrigine, lacosamide, oxcarbazepine, or valproate. However, a balance should always be maintained between optimal seizure control and optimal sexual function. Patients with drug-resistant

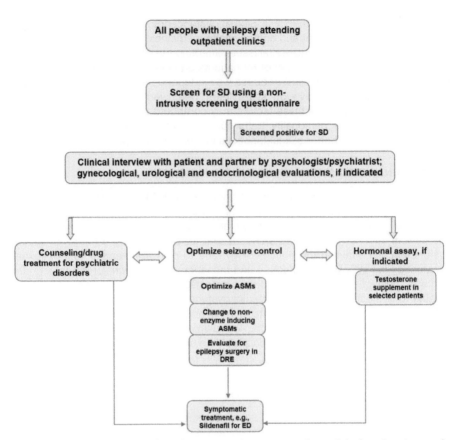

Fig. 2. An algorithmic approach to diagnosis and treatment of sexual dysfunctions in people with epilepsy (ASM, antiseizure medicine; DRE, drug-resistant epilepsy; ED, erectile dysfunction; SD, sexual dysfunction).

epilepsy should undergo presurgical evaluation and selected patients should be offered epilepsy surgery to improve seizure control and prospect of reduction in ASM.

Hormonal Assessment

As many patients with sexual dysfunction have associated hormonal disturbances, a complete hormonal assay is desirable. However, in a developing country set-up, whereby more than three-fourths of the global PWE reside, because of the lack of availability and affordability, hormonal assessment may have to be limited to those with no apparent drug-related or psychiatric and psychosocial comorbidities. Levels of thyroid hormones, total and free testosterone, SHBG, prolactin, follicle-stimulating hormone (FSH), and LH should, if possible, be measured in consultation with an endocrinologist. Those patients with low testosterone levels can benefit from testosterone supplements.[76]

Symptomatic Treatment

Male patients with erectile dysfunction can benefit from symptomatic treatment with phosphodiesterase type-5 inhibitor drugs such as sildenafil and vardenafil. Caution should be exercised in their usage, as there are isolated reports of them precipitating seizures in nonepilepsy patients.[77] Patients with premature ejaculation can improve with selective serotonin reuptake inhibitor drug paroxetine.[78] These patients and female patients with sexual pain disorders should be managed in close collaboration with the urologists and gynecologists.

SUMMARY

Sexual dysfunctions in PWE are grossly under-reported and under-recognized. Overall, nearly half of the unselected PWE have sexual dysfunction. Patients with uncontrolled epilepsy and those receiving enzyme-inducing ASMs have a higher prevalence of sexual dysfunctions. A complex interaction between disease-related, and medicine-related factors, and psychiatric and psychosocial comorbidities contribute to sexual dysfunction in PWE. A multidisciplinary and comprehensive diagnostic evaluation is required to individualize treatment strategies to improve the sexual health of PWE.

CLINICS CARE POINTS

- Routine screening of all the PWE for sexual dysfunctions during outpatient clinic visits using a brief, nonintrusive scale is recommended.
- All patients with sexual dysfunction should be evaluated for underlying anxiety and depression, and for psychosocial problems.
- Switching from enzyme-inducing ASMs to non–enzyme-inducing medicine and early epilepsy surgery in those who are drug-resistant may improve sexual function.
- Although hormonal evaluation is desirable in all patients with sexual dysfunction, in developing countries this may have to be restricted to those without obvious causes.
- Seizure freedom by medical or surgical treatment improves sexual function; symptomatic treatment may improve sexual function even in patients who are not seizure-free.

DISCLOSURE

The authors have nothing to disclose.

REFERENCES

1. Flynn KE, Lin Li, Bruner DW, et al. Sexual satisfaction and the importance of sexual health to quality of life throughout the life course of U.S. adults. J Sex Med 2016;13:1642–50.
2. Gastaut H, Collomb H. Sexual behavior in psychomotor epileptics. Ann Med Psychol (Paris) 1954;112:657–96.
3. Pellinen J, Chong DJ, Elder C, et al. The impact of medications and medical comorbidities on sexual function in people with epilepsy. Epilepsy Res 2021;172: 106596.
4. Reed GM, Drescher J, Krueger RB, et al. Disorders related to sexuality and gender identity in the ICD-11: revising the ICD-10 classification based on current scientific evidence, best clinical practices, and human rights considerations. World Psychiatry 2016;5:205–21.
5. Hatzimouratidis K, Hatzichristou D. Sexual dysfunctions: classifications and definitions. J Sex Med 2007;4:241–50.

6. Bhugra D, Colombini G. Sexual dysfunction: classification and assessment. Adv Psychiatr Treat 2013;19:48–55.

7. American Psychiatric Association. Diagnostic and statistical manual of mental disorders. 5th edition. Washington, DC: Author; 2013.

8. Lue TF, Giuliano F, Montorsi F, et al. Summary of the recommendations on sexual dysfunctions in men. J Sex Med 2004;1:6–23.

9. Basson R, Althof S, Davis S, et al. Summary of the recommendations onsexual dysfunctions in women. J Sex Med 2004;1:24–34.

10. Feldman HA, Goldstein I, Hatzichristou DG, et al. Impotence and its medical and psychosocial correlates: results of the Massachusetts Male Aging Study. J Urol 1994;151:54–61.

11. Hatzichristou D, Kirana PS, Banner L, et al. Diagnosing sexual dysfunction in men and women: sexual history taking and the role of symptom scales and question-naires. J Sex Med 2016;13:1166–82.

12. Dawson E, Stutzman SE, Olson DM, et al. Performance of the International Index of Erectile Function tool in men with epilepsy. Epilepsy Behav 2019;94:78–81.

13. Hatzichristou D, Rosen RC, Derogatis LR, et al. Recommendations for the clinical evaluation of men and women with sexual dysfunction. J Sex Med 2010;7:337–48.

14. Rosen R, Brown C, Heiman J, et al. The Female Sexual Function Index (FSFI): a multidimensional self-report instrument for the assessment of female sexual func-tion. J Sex Marital Ther 2000;26:191–208.

15. Quirk FH, Heiman J, Rosen RC, et al. Development of a sexual function question-naire for clinical trials of female sexual function. J Womens Health Gend Based Med 2002;11:277–85.

16. Rosen RC, Riley A, Wagner G, et al. The International Index of Erectile Function (IIEF): a multi-dimensional scale for assessment of sexual dysfunction. Urology 1997;49:822–30.

17. Patrick D, Giuliano F, Ho K, et al. The Premature Ejaculation Profile: validation of self-reported outcome measures for research and practice. BJU Int 2009;103:358–64.

18. Derogatis LR. The Derogatis Interview for Sexual Functioning (DISF/DISF-SR): an introductory report. J Sex Marital Ther 1997;23:291–304.

19. McGahuey C, Gelenberg A, Laukes CA, et al. The Arizona Sexual Experience Scale (ASEX) reliability and validity. J Sex Marital Ther 2000;26:25–40.

20. Blumer D, Walker AE. Sexual behaviour in temporal lobe epilepsy: a study of the effects of temporal lobectomy on sexual behavior. Arch Neurol 1967;16:37–43.

21. Demerdash A, Shaalon M, Midori A, et al. Sexual behavior of a sample of females with epilepsy. Epikpsia 1991;32:82–5.

22. Bergen D, Daugherty S, Eckenfels E. Reduction of sexual activities in females taking antiepileptic drugs. Psychopathology 1992;25:1—4.

23. Morrell MJ, Guldner GT. Self-reported sexual function and sexual arousability in women with epilepsy. Epilepsia 1996;37:1204—10.

24. Morrell MJ, Flynn KL, Done S, et al. Sexual dysfunction, sex steroid hormone ab-normalities, and depression in women with epilepsy treated with antiepileptic drugs. Epilepsy Behav 2005;6:360–5.

25. Duncan S, Blacklaw J, Beastall GH, et al. Sexual function in women with epilepsy. Epilepsia 1997;38:1074—81.

26. Zelená V, Kuba R, Soška V, et al. Depression as a prominent cause of sexual dysfunction in women with epilepsy. Epilepsy Behav 2011;20:539–44.

27. Atarodi-Kashani Z, Kariman N, Ebadi A, et al. Sexual function and related factors in Iranian woman with epilepsy. Seizure 2017;52:147–53.
28. Ogunjimi L, Yaria J, Makanjuola A, et al. Sexual dysfunction among Nigerian women with epilepsy. Epilepsy Behav 2018;83:108–12.
29. Tao L, Zhang X, Duan Z, et al. Sexual dysfunction and associated factors in Chinese Han women with epilepsy. Epilepsy Behav 2018;85:150–6.
30. Hamed SA, Attiah FA, Gabra RH, et al. Sexual functions in women with focal epilepsy: Relationship to demographic, clinical, hormonal and psychological variables. Clin Neurol Neurosurg 2020;191:105697.
31. Mazdeh M, Taheri M, Ghafouri-Fard S. Investigation of sexual satisfaction in women with epilepsy and its clinical correlates. J Mol Neurosci 2021;71:1193–6.
32. Santos AMC, Castro Lima Filho H, Siquara GM, et al. Sexual function in women of fertile age with epilepsy. Epilepsy Behav 2021;125:108399.
33. Jensen P, Jensen SB, Sorensen PS, et al. Sexual dysfunction in male and female patients with epilepsy: a study of 86 outpatients. Arch Sex Behav 1990;19:1–14.
34. Souza EA, Keiralla DM, Silveira DC, et al. Sexual dysfunction in epilepsy identifying the psychological variables. Arq Neuropsiquiatr 2000;58:214–20.
35. Herzog AG, Coleman AE, Jacobs AR, et al. Relationship of sexual dysfunction to epilepsy laterality and reproductive hormone levels in women. Epilepsy Behav 2003;4:407–13.
36. Henning OJ, Nakken KO, Traeen B, et al. Sexual problems in people with refractory epilepsy. Epilepsy Behav 2016;61:174–9.
37. Ejigu AK, Zewlde KH, Muluneh NY, et al. Sexual dysfunction and associated factors among patients with epilepsy at Amanuel Mental Specialty Hospital, Addis Ababa – Ethiopia. BMC Neurol 2019;19:255.
38. Kumar DP, Wadwekar V, Nair PP, et al. Study of sexual dysfunction in people living with epilepsy at a tertiary care center of South India. Neurol India 2020;68:861–6.
39. Nikoobakht M, Motamedi M, Orandi A, et al. Sexual dysfunction in epileptic men. Urol J 2007;4:111–7.
40. Duncan S, Talbot A, Sheldrick R, et al. Erectile function, sexual desire, and psychological well-being in men with epilepsy. Epilepsy Behav 2009;15:351–7.
41. Calabro RS, Grisolaghi J, Quattrini F, et al. Prevalence and clinical features of sexual dysfunction in male with epilepsy: the first southern Italy hospital-based study. Int J Neurosci 2013;123:732–7.
42. Sureka RK, Gaur V, Purohit G, et al. Sexual dysfunction in male patients with idiopathic generalized tonic clonic seizures. Annl Ind Aca Neurol 2021;24:726–31.
43. Zhao S, Tang Z, Xie Q, et al. Association between epilepsy and risk of sexual dysfunction: a meta-analysis. Seizure 2019;65:80–8.
44. Henning O, Johannessen Landmark C, Traeen B, et al. Sexual function in people with epilepsy: Similarities and differences with the general population. Epilepsia 2019;60:1984–92.
45. Keller J, Chen YK, Lin HC. Association between epilepsy and erectile dysfunction: evidence from a population-based study. J Sex Med 2012;9:2248–55.
46. Mattson RH, Cramer JA, Collins JF, et al. Comparison of carbamazepine, phenobarbital, phenytoin, and primidone in partial and secondarily generalized tonic-clonic seizures. N Engl J Med 1985;313:145–51.
47. Taylor DC. Sexual behavior and temporal lobe epilepsy. Arch Neurol 1969;21:510–6.
48. Baird AD, Wilson SJ, Baldin PF, et al. Sexual outcome after epilepsy surgery. Epilepsy Behav 2003;4:268–78.

49. Ramesha KN, Radhakrishnan A, Jiayaspathi A, et al. Sexual desire and satisfaction after resective surgery in patients with mesial temporal lobeepilepsy with hippocampal sclerosis. Epilepsy Behav 2012;25:374–80.

50. Baird AD, Wilson SJ, Bladin PF, et al. Hypersexuality after temporal resection. Epilepsy Behav 2002;3:173–81.

51. Stanton AM, Pulverman CS, Meston CM. Vagal activity during physiological sexual arousal in women with and without sexual dysfunction. J Sex Marital Ther 2017;43:78–89.

52. Pedro T, Sousa M, Rito M, et al. The impact of deep brain stimulation on the sexual function of patients with Parkinson's disease. Neurologist 2020;25:55–61.

53. Herzog AG, Seibel MM, Schomer DL, et al. Reproductive endocrine disorders in women with partial seizures of temporal lobe origin. Arch Neurol 1986;43:341–6.

54. Gerendai I, Halasz B. Neuroendocrine asymmetry. Front Neuroendocrinol 1997; 18:354–81.

55. Bauer J, Blumenthal S, Reuber M, et al. Epilepsy syndrome, focus location, and treatment choice affect testicular function in men with epilepsy. Neurology 2004; 62:243–6.

56. Talbot JA, Sheldrick R, Caswell H, et al. Sexual function in men with epilepsy: how important is testosterone? Neurology 2008;70:1346–52.

57. Tao L, Duan Z, Liu Y, et al. Correlation of sexual dysfunction with sex hormone and estrogen receptor gene polymorphism in Chinese Han women with epilepsy. Epilepsy Res 2021;169:106527.

58. Rathore C, Henning OJ, Luef G, et al. Sexual dysfunction in people with epilepsy. Epilepsy Behav 2019;100:106495.

59. Connell JM, Rapeport WG, Beastall GH, et al. Changes in circulating androgens during short term carbamazepine therapy. Br J Clin Pharmacol 1984;17:347–51.

60. Herzog AG, Drislane FW, Schomer DL, et al. Differential effects of antiepileptic drugs on sexual function and hormones in men with epilepsy.Neurology 2005;65:1016-1020.

61. Chen LW, Chen MY, Chen KY, et al. Topiramate-associated sexual dysfunction: a systematic review. Epilepsy Behav 2017;73:10–7.

62. Lossius MI, Taubøll E, Mowinckel P, et al. Reversible effects of antiepileptic drugs on reproductive endocrine function in men and women with epilepsy–a prospective randomized double-blind withdrawal study. Epilepsia 2007;48:1875–82.

63. Gil-Nagel A, Lopez-Munoz F, Serratosa JM, et al. Effect of lamotrigine on sexual function in patients with epilepsy. Seizure 2006;15:142–9.

64. Svalheim S, Tauboll E, Luef G, et al. Differential effects of levetiracetam, carbamazepine, and lamotrigine on reproductive endocrine function in adults. Epilepsy Behav 2009;16:281–7.

65. Luef G, Kramer G, Stefan H. Oxcarbazepine treatment in male epilepsy patients improves pre-existing sexual dysfunction. Acta Neurol Scand 2009;119:94–9.

66. Mattson RH, Cramer JA, Collins JF. A comparison of valproate with carbamazepine for the treatment of complex partial seizures and secondarily generalized tonic clonic seizures in adults. The Department of Veterans Affairs Epilepsy Cooperative Study No. 264 Group. N Engl J Med 1992;327:765–71.

67. Grant AC, Oh H. Gabapentin-induced anorgasmia in women. Am J Psychiatry 2002;159:1247.

68. Hamed SA. Sexual Dysfunctions Induced by Pregabalin. Clin Neuropharmacol 2018;41:116–22.

69. Maschio M, Saveriano F, Dinapoli L, et al. Reversible erectile dysfunction in a patient with brain tumor-related epilepsy in therapy with zonisamide in add-on. J Sex Med 2011;8:3515–7.

70. Calabrò RS, Magaudda A, Nibali VC, et al. Sexual dysfunction induced by lacosamide: an underreported side effect? Epilepsy Behav 2015;46:252–3.

71. Calabrò RS, Italiano D, Militi D, et al. Levetiracetam-associated loss of libido and anhedonia. Epilepsy Behav 2012;24:283–4.

72. Fiest KM, Dykeman J, Patten SB, et al. Depression in epilepsy: a systematic review and meta-analysis. Neurology 2013;80:590–9.

73. Qin P, Xu H, Laursen TM, et al. Risk for schizophrenia and schizophrenia-like psychosis among patients with epilepsy: population based cohort study. BMJ 2005; 331:23.

74. Atlantis E, Sullivan T. Bidirectional association between depression and sexual dysfunction: a systematic review and meta-analysis. J Sex Med 2012;9: 1497–507.

75. Sheikhalishahi A, Jahdi F, Haghani H. The relationship between sexual health and personality type in women with epilepsy. J Educ Health Promot 2021;10:257.

76. Herzog AG, Farina EL, Drislane FW, et al. A comparison of anastrozole and testosterone versus placebo and testosterone for treatment of sexual dysfunction in men with epilepsy and hypogonadism. Epilepsy Behav 2010;17:264–71.

77. Gilad R, Lampl Y, Eshel Y, et al. Tonic-clonic seizures in patients taking sildenafil. Br Med J 2002;325:869.

78. Zhang D, Cheng Y, Wu K, et al. Paroxetine in the treatment of premature ejaculation: a systematic review and meta-analysis. BMC Urol 2019;19:2.

Epilepsy in Older Persons

Sofia Toniolo, MD, FEBN[a,1], Michele Romoli, MD, PhD, FEBN[b,1],
Arjune Sen, MD, PhD, FRCPE[c,]*

KEYWORDS

- Comorbidity • Dementia • Elderly • Psychosocial impact • Seizure

KEY POINTS

- Epilepsy in older people is increasingly common across the world and consists of late-onset epilepsy as well as people with early-onset epilepsy living into later life.
- Older people with epilepsy often have multiple comorbidities, which may obscure the diagnosis of seizures and limit treatment options.
- The complex relationship between epilepsy, dementia, vascular disease, and psychosocial impact in older people with seizures mandates a comprehensive and holistic approach to clinical management.
- Older people with epilepsy must be included in clinical trials of new medications and devices to help optimize treatment in this demographic.

INTRODUCTION

Perhaps one reason that the World Health Organization declared epilepsy a public health imperative in 2019[1] is that the condition is much more common in older people. Populations are aging across the world with the rate of increase in older demographics three times higher in low to middle-income countries (LMICs) compared with more developed economies. Given that 80% to 85% of people with epilepsy live in LMICs,[1,2] the combined pressures of increasing prevalence and inequity may result in widening diagnostic and treatment gaps in a neurological illness for which multiple management strategies exist to improve morbidity and decrease mortality.

In the current review, we aim to provide a holistic insight into epilepsy as it affects older people. We explore epidemiology, presentation, clinical management and focus on links with comorbidity. While cognitive, psychological, and psychosocial factors

[a] Cognitive Neurology Group, Nuffield Department of Clinical Neurosciences, University of Oxford, John Radcliffe Hospital, 3rd Floor, West Wing, Oxford OX3 9DU, UK; [b] Neurology and Stroke Unit, Department of Neuroscience, Bufalini Hospital, viale Ghirotti 286, Cesena 47521, Italy; [c] Oxford Epilepsy Research Group, NIHR Biomedical Research Centre, Nuffield Department of Clinical Neurosciences, University of Oxford, Oxford OX3 9DU, UK
[1] joint first authors
* Corresponding author. Department of Neurology, John Radcliffe Hospital, 3rd Floor, West Wing, Oxford OX3 9DU. UK.
E-mail address: arjune.sen@ndcn.ox.ac.uk

Neurol Clin 40 (2022) 891–905
https://doi.org/10.1016/j.ncl.2022.03.014
0733-8619/22/© 2022 Elsevier Inc. All rights reserved.

impinge on people with epilepsy of all ages, there are specific difficulties in older people. We also discuss how the increasing links between vascular disease, dementia and late-onset epilepsy may offer therapeutic opportunities in older populations.

Epidemiology

Older people with epilepsy consist of two rather distinct groups–those who develop epilepsy once they are older and individuals with epilepsy, including complex epilepsy syndromes, who are now increasingly living into older age. The incidence of epilepsy demonstrates a bimodal distribution with case numbers being highest in those under 5 years of age and in later life.[3,4] Data also suggest that the incidence of adult-onset epilepsy may be increasing in later life across both sexes.[5] The exact age at which a person may be defined as having "late-onset epilepsy" (LOE) remains poorly specified, although there is a likely inflection point at around the age of 50 years with a progressive increase in incidence thereafter.[3,6] The Cardiovascular Health Study estimated an incidence rate of around 2.5 cases per 1000 person years in older adults.[7] Similarly, once standardized for age, the prevalence of "idiopathic epilepsy" as captured by the Global Burden of Disease report shows a bimodal pattern across high and low-income countries with an overall prevalence of epilepsy of 5.4 per 100 older people.[6]

These figures cannot, though, be considered homogenously. Epilepsy is most common in the very elderly, nursing home residents and can also be separated by race, being more frequent in African Americans and less common in Asian and Native American people compared with white populations.[8–10] Underpinning all of this, the actual incidence and prevalence of epilepsy in older people are likely under-estimated. Older people may be more likely to live alone, meaning events are not witnessed; are prone to present with nonconvulsive seizures which may be harder to recognize than convulsive epilepsy; and may have comorbid conditions, particularly dementia, that further cloud the diagnosis of a seizure disorder.

Causes of Late-Onset Epilepsy

Identification of a specific etiology is critical to defining the best medical approach and understanding long-term prognosis in LOE. Stroke represents the main cause of new-onset epilepsy in older people with up to 50% of LOE cases related to either ischemic or hemorrhagic stroke.[11] Early seizures present within the first 7 days after a stroke and are strictly related to local cytotoxic damage. Treatment of such events is limited to symptomatic medications. By contrast, a single seizure more than 7 days from the index stroke carries a >60% risk of recurrence within 10 years,[12,13] is thought to represent the result of brain remodeling after stroke and qualifies as poststroke epilepsy (PSE).[11] PSE occurs in 2% to 14% of stroke survivors,[14,15] has a detrimental impact on quality of life,[16] and requires treatment with antiseizure medications (ASMs), the choice of which has to be carefully considered owing to potential interactions with secondary prevention medications, including anticoagulants.[15] The SELECT score has been validated to provide a possible prediction of the risk of PSE, assimilating certain key risk factors: stroke severity, large-vessel atherosclerosis, cortical involvement, anterior circulation stroke, and early seizure occurrence.[17]

Several risk factors for stroke have also been found as independent risk factors for LOE[18,19] (Fig. 1). The Atherosclerosis Risk in Communities (ARIC) Study, which followed a broad biracial cohort for more than 25 years, highlighted that there are several midlife vascular and lifestyle risk factors associated with LOE. Most of these factors are modifiable, including hypertension, diabetes, smoking, lack of physical activity, and alcohol use, while only APOE ε4 allele number and being of black ethnicity emerged as nonmodifiable items.[18] As these factors were associated with LOE

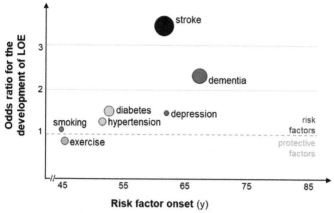

Fig. 1. Middle-age modifiable risk factors for developing late-onset epilepsy.
Stroke represents the strongest risk factors for developing LOE. Among middle-age modifiable risk factors, cardiovascular risk factors (including hypertension, smoking, and diabetes mellitus) represent potentially preventable contributors to LOE. We created this figure using data from a large prospective study[18] and from a recent meta-analysis.[19] Circle diameter displays the relative risk of LOE carried by each factor, and appears in correspondence to the mean age of incidence in mid-adulthood (eg, stroke carries a 3.5 higher risk of developing LOE,[18] and has a progressive increase in incidence in mid-adulthood up to 64 years).

independently from the development of either stroke or dementia, it seems reasonable to derive person-centered implications for primary prevention measures. Policies promoting lifestyle changes and preventing vascular risk factors might, therefore, cost-effectively reduce the burden of dementia, stroke, and epilepsy.[18,20]

Among other causes of LOE, primary brain cancer or metastasis (15%) and metabolic/toxic causes (10%) are the most common.[21,22] Also, there is increasing evidence of a close relationship between neurodegenerative disorders and LOE[22–24](see comorbidity in older people with epilepsy section). Of the rarer causes of LOE, autoimmune encephalitis is important to recognize as early treatment may prevent cognitive decline.[25]

Presentation of Seizures in Older People

Older people are more likely to have seizures with focal onset, with or without impaired awareness or secondary generalization, reflecting the increased incidence of a structural etiology to epilepsy in this cohort.[26]

The clinical diagnosis of seizures can be particularly challenging in older adults who may present with events of atypical semiology.[27] Seizures in older people may be of short duration[28] increasing the rate of late or misdiagnosis.[29] The clinical features of seizures in LOE can also be less overt, or even masked by cognitive impairment.[28,30] Staring spells, repeated movements of hands/orofacial automatisms together with lapses in memory and transient alteration in mental status tend to be more frequent in older people with epilepsy.[28,30] Symptoms of seizures arising from the temporal lobes might be limited to confusional or wandering episodes, poorly distinguishable from "sundowning" or fluctuations in cognitive status in people with dementia. Isolated and brief spells of amnesia due to transient epileptic amnesia can also be mistaken for the more common transient global amnesia[31] resulting in delayed diagnosis and treatment.[32]

The number and range of differential diagnoses also increase in LOE. The main chameleons of seizures become more frequent with aging, and seizure mimics can represent up to 50% of cases.[33] Episodes of confusion/delirium can have alternative causes, including toxins, electrolyte disturbances, and medication side effects. Similarly, limb or facial jerking may have several differentials, ranging from other neurologic conditions to psychiatric disorders (**Table 1**).[28] By corollary, acute episodes of confusion in older people may, not infrequently, associated with electroencephalographic changes.[34]

Determining whether a transient loss of consciousness is cardiological or neurological in etiology is often difficult. Syncope can cause convulsive movements secondary to anoxia from low cardiac output.[35] Similarly, seizures can be complicated by asystole, and the conditions can coexist in isolated cases.[36] A study using implantable electrocardiographic monitoring demonstrated that 1 in 10 people with transient loss of consciousness in adulthood is misdiagnosed as having epilepsy, receiving inappropriate treatment with ASMs.[37] In older populations, in whom both cardiac and neurologic cardiovascular and neurological dysfunction may be more likely, being able to identify the underlying cause of a collapse becomes both more challenging and more important.

Postictal states tend to be prominent and can be particularly prolonged in the elderly.[38,39] Postictal aphasia may occur in up to 15% of people with LOE, while

Table 1	
Main differential diagnosis in cases of atypical seizure semiology in LOE	
Clinical Presentation	**Main Differential Diagnosis**
Fainting, falling, and transient loss of consciousness	• *Cerebrovascular disease:* transient ischemic attack, posterior circulation stroke (although loss of consciousness not common with TIA or stroke) • *Cardiovascular disease:* arrhythmias, sick sinus syndrome, vasovagal syncope, postural hypotension, pulmonary embolism • *Metabolic causes:* hypo/hyperglycemia, acute thyroid disturbances, acute kidney failure
Confusional state, delirium	• *Other neurological/psychiatric disorders:* cognitive disturbances, dementia, sundowning, mania/bipolar disorder, psychosis • *Metabolic:* hypo/hyperglycemia, acute thyroid disturbances, acute kidney failure, electrolyte disturbances • *Toxins:* cocaine, 3,4-Methylenedioxymethamphetamine (MDMA), nitric oxide inhalation, heavy metal poisoning (less commonly seen in older populations but detailed alcohol and recreational substance misuse history should still be sought) • *Medications:* antidepressants, antipsychotic, beta-blockers
Repetitive movements, abnormal behaviors	• *Other neurological/psychiatric disorders:* parkinsonism, tics, neuropathic tremor, limb-shaking transient ischaemic attacks, psychogenic nonepileptic seizures • *Metabolic:* tremor due to thyroid disturbances, uremia • *Toxins:* cocaine, MDMA, heavy metal poisoning • *Medications:* antidepressants, antipsychotics (tardive dyskinesia), acetyl-cholinesterase inhibitors

confusion (45% of cases) and Todd's paralysis (19%), which can last for hours in this population, represent other frequent types of postictal state in older individuals.[38,40] Acute perfusion computerized tomography (CT) or arterial spin labeling (ASL) magnetic resonance imaging (MRI) might help differentiate post-ictal phenomenon from stroke, ruling out areas of hypoperfusion and showing potential hyper-perfused regions corresponding to an epileptic focus, although the accuracy of this approach is currently limited.[41] Further complicating the differential diagnosis, post-event phenomena can also occur after vasovagal syncope.[42]

Status epilepticus is a common presentation of LOE.[28] Convulsive status epilepticus is easier to recognise and more usually diagnosed and treated within an appropriate timeframe. Nonconvulsive status epilepticus (NCSE), though, can pass unnoticed or misdiagnosed.[28,43,44] In a 10-year study, 64% of people with NCSE were misdiagnosed at first evaluation, with age and no previous history of seizures being the main independent predictors of misdiagnosis.[44] A low threshold for suspecting NCSE should, therefore, be adopted in older people presenting with acute confusional states, and an electroencephalogram (EEG) performed promptly.[44]

How to Evaluate Seizures in Older People?

The diagnostic work-up in LOE should mirror the specific epidemiological profile of its causes. As always in epilepsy, but even more so in older people, accurate history from the affected individual and witnesses is crucial. Neurological examination may reveal subtle asymmetric deficits suggestive of underlying structural pathology, while bedside cognitive testing for early signs of impairment also aids diagnostic formulation. Evaluation of vascular risk factors in terms of history, bedside examination (for example pulse and blood pressure), and investigations are crucial in LOE.

First-line investigations in LOE should include blood tests, an electrocardiogram (ECG), EEG, and brain imaging[22] (**Table 2**). In those presenting with explosive onset seizures and cognitive decline, or other risk factors for autoimmune encephalitis, antibody testing should be sent promptly. CT brain imaging, with or without angiography (CTA), might be a sufficient, time- and cost-effective option in the Emergency Department. CT perfusion can help in excluding stroke and identifying hyper-perfused areas corresponding to regions involved by epileptic activity thereby helping recognize NCSE and postictal status in the hyperacute setting.[41] Brain MRI should be considered in people with LOE, especially when CT fails to detect a salient epileptogenic lesion. EEG remains important in LOE as it can help identify an epileptogenic focus and, occasionally, may uncover genetic generalized epilepsy.[45]

Second-line diagnostics should be equitably available for older people with suboptimal seizure control, including EEG-telemetry, nuclear medicine investigations in cases of focal onset and drug-resistant epilepsy, prolonged cardiac-monitoring, and more extensive laboratory investigations (see **Table 2**). Cerebrospinal fluid (CSF) examination may be considered whenever, even subtle, cognitive deficits are present, to exclude autoimmune etiology and better identify neurodegenerative disorders potentially manifesting with seizures.[23]

Treatment of Seizures in Older People Including Surgical Management

The choice of ASMs in older individuals poses many challenges owing to the multiple underlying seizure etiologies; comorbidities; polypharmacy; and pharmacokinetic considerations, with an overall narrower therapeutic window between seizure control and risk of adverse events (AE) compared to younger people with epilepsy.[22] A "start low, go slow" approach, with "end low" addendum, might be beneficial, as older people often require lower doses of ASMs to achieve seizure control.[46] Monotherapy

Table 2
First-level and second-level diagnostics in late-onset epilepsy

	Diagnostics	Acute vs Elective	Specific Points
First-level diagnostics	Blood tests	Acute setting	Including complete blood count, C-reactive protein, electrolytes, renal and liver function. Antibody testing should be performed if underlying autoimmune encephalitis is possible (consider toxicology screening in specific cases)
	ECG	Acute setting	Exclude arrhythmia and atrioventricular block
	EEG	Acute setting and elective	In acute setting: exclude nonconvulsive status epilepticus, subclinical seizures (video plus EEG advised) In elective setting, identify adult-onset generalized genetic epilepsy; localize seizure focus.
	Brain imaging	CT in the acute setting	Exclude ischemic/hemorrhagic stroke and mass lesions
		MRI (whenever needed in the acute setting, and in elective setting in other cases)	Identify changes suggestive of rarer causes (eg, T2-weighted hyperintense changes in autoimmune encephalitis, superficial siderosis in cases of cerebral amyloid angiopathy) Localize subtle abnormalities (small gliomas, focal cortical dysplasia)
Second-level diagnostics	Cerebrospinal fluid examination	Acute setting whenever infectious or autoimmune disease suspected; Consider in elective setting in cases of cognitive decline. Assess biomarkers of neurodegeneration.	Exclude infection and identify specific pathogens. Search for autoimmune antibodies (blood and CSF examination).
	Cardiovascular testing	Elective	ECG monitoring, tilt-test, cardiac ultrasound as diagnostic work-up in unclear cases/cardiac disease within differential diagnosis.
		Elective (PET or SPECT)	

(continued on next page)

Table 2 (continued)		
Diagnostics	**Acute vs Elective**	**Specific Points**
Nuclear medicine investigations		^{18}F-FDG-PET and Amyloid-β PET to identify areas of brain hypometabolism and brain amyloid deposition. SPECT can be used as a further ascertainment in people with LOE with focal onset, especially if drug-resistant epilepsy with potential for epilepsy surgery.
Neuropsychological testing	Elective	Diagnose and identify subtle cognitive deficits in the context of LOE.

should also be encouraged whenever possible.[47] In some cases it may be appropriate to consider treatment in older people after a single seizure, even if a clear underlying substrate is not identified, given the high rate of missing focal seizures in this demographic[48] and the potential disruptive impact of a traumatic convulsive seizure (eg, hip fracture, subdural hematoma). Older people who live alone may be particularly keen to avoid any further events. The decision to start an ASM should, as in all people with epilepsy, be person-centered and approached holistically.

In older people with epilepsy, the likely medications of choice are lamotrigine (LTG) or levetiracetam (LEV) and then lacosamide (LCM)[49,50](Fig. 2). Older ASMs, perhaps carbamazepine (CBZ) in particular, have been associated with poorer tolerability.[49,50] More recent studies that have evaluated LCM, eslicarbazepine acetate (ESL), perampanel (PER), and brivaracetam (BRV) in older populations, show promise. LCM has good efficacy and tolerability, and both PER and BRV seem reasonably tolerated in older people. ESL has comparable efficacy and AEs to that seen in younger people and associates with less vascular risk than oxcarbazepine.[48] In particular, certain medications may not suit older individuals owing to cognitive or psychiatric AE. Data on drug-naïve older people with epilepsy suggest, for example, that up to 58% have evidence of cognitive impairment before treatment is initiated, perhaps indicating less cognitive reserve to help cope with ASM AEs.[51,52] Topiramate (TPM), zonisamide (ZNS), and valproate (VPA)- which may associate with hyperammonemia encephalopathy-are likely less preferred in this cohort.

Age-related pharmacokinetic considerations in the choice of ASMs include reduced renal clearance (eg, LEV; reduce dose accordingly), hepatic impairment (eg, CBZ) and hypoalbuminemia (eg, phenytoin (PHT)).[51] Long-term use of older ASMs, and particularly enzyme-inducing drugs such as CBZ, PHT, phenobarbital (PHB), and primidone (PMD), has been shown to increase cardiovascular risk factors such as vascular inflammatory markers, homocysteine levels, cholesterol levels, and carotid intima-media thickness.[53] Enzyme-inhibiting medications such as VPA can cause a metabolic syndrome-including abdominal obesity, glucose intolerance, elevated triglycerides, low high density lipoprotein C, and hypertension-especially in women.[54] Older people are particularly susceptible to adverse impacts on bone health. Vitamin D

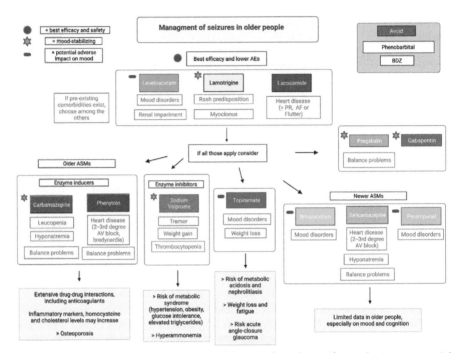

Fig. 2. Medical management of seizures in older people with specific emphasis on potential adverse effects. Antiseizure medications are listed in hierarchical order alongside principal side effects. Levetiracetam, Lamotrigine, and Lacosamide represent the drugs of choice in older people as achieve the best efficacy and tolerability. If all 3 are contraindicated, consider other ASMs according to pre-existing comorbidities. AE, adverse event; AF, atrial fibrillation; ASMs, anti-seizure medications; BDZ, benzodiazepines.

levels should be monitored and replenished, especially in those taking enzyme-inducing ASMs and pregabalin (PGB).[22] Hyponatremia, which is common in the elderly and can adversely impact cognition, is frequently observed with CBZ, OXC and ESL; moderately with PHT; sometimes with LEV and VPA, and less frequently with LTG and gabapentin (GBP).[55]

Current surgical options for people with drug-resistant epilepsy include resective surgery, magnetic resonance-guided laser interstitial thermal therapy, vagal nerve stimulation (VNS), responsive neurostimulation (RNS), and deep brain stimulation (DBS).[56–59] In older people, there has been a historical reticence to explore epilepsy surgery owing to perceptions that outcomes are poorer and complications increased in this age group.[22,56] Approximately 90% of individuals aged over 60 years, however, achieve good seizure control with resective surgery with comparable efficacy compared with younger people.[56] Rates of postoperative cognitive impairment need to be factored in to the decision process, with newer and less invasive procedures showing some promise.[57–59]

Comorbidity in Older People with Epilepsy

Cognitive, psychiatric, and systemic comorbidities have a huge impact on the diagnosis, management, and prognosis of older people with epilepsy (**Fig. 3**). Aging and epilepsy are independently associated with increased prevalence of cognitive impairment,[60] but have also been shown to exert a synergistic detrimental impact on

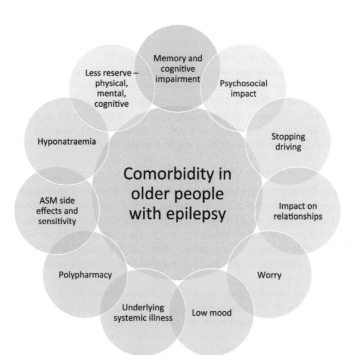

Fig. 3. The complex cycle of interdependent comorbidities in older people with epilepsy. Multiple factors contribute to comorbidity in older populations with epilepsy and these tend to interact closely. Having to stop driving, reduces independence for people who may be less able to utilize public transport thereby adversely impacting on psychosocial factors and relationships–for example, being less able to visit grandchildren. Similarly, low serum sodium levels, which can be exacerbated by a multitude of antiseizure medications and other drugs, may have much greater cognitive impact on those with less reserve.

pathophysiological cascades involved in amyloid deposition and neurodegeneration. Early network hyperexcitability can be followed by tau-induced hypoexcitability, potentially leading to the development of Alzheimer's disease (AD).[46,61] People with LOE are more likely to have a multi-domain cognitive impairment, to have increased pathologic amyloid deposition, and higher rates of conversion to AD compared with older people who do not have epilepsy. Recent studies suggest that there may be traits that long predate seizure onset that contribute to cognitive difficulties, while seizures are also more prevalent in individuals with AD compared with age-matched controls.[23,62] Cerebrovascular disease adds to a complex multimodal interaction, whereby white matter changes are more frequently observed in older people and people with epilepsy. Such changes can worsen the prognosis of individuals with AD.[63,64] People with late-onset Aβ-related epilepsy (LAβE) and cognitive decline should be monitored closely for evidence of conversion to AD, especially as people with AD and epilepsy decline more rapidly than people who have AD without experiencing seizures.[23,65]

Psychiatric comorbidities are highly prevalent in older individuals with epilepsy. Depression and anxiety are more frequently observed when compared with age-matched controls and younger people with epilepsy. Those with poor ASM adherence and uncontrolled seizures may be particularly prone to mood disorders.[66–68] Pre-existing psychiatric comorbidities should also help guide the choice of ASMs in older people, as some ASMs may have a beneficial/stabilizing impact on mood (for example VPA, CBZ, LTG, PGB, GBP), while others should be used with caution in those with relevant psychiatric history (eg, LEV, PER, TPM, ZNS).[69]

Older ASMs, especially enzyme-inducing ASMs, have frequent drug–drug interactions and should be used with caution in older people, especially those taking complex poly-pharmacological regimens that often include statins, diuretics, anticoagulants, and antiarrhythmics.[22] Newer ASMs should also be scrutinized for possible contraindications in the elderly, as, for example, coadministration of LCM with drugs that alter cardiac AV conduction such as digoxin might be harmful.[48]

Broader Impact of Epilepsy in Older Age

Epilepsy in later life aggravates key determinants of frailty including isolation, cognitive impairment, low mood, and reduced independence.[70] Loss of independence secondary to driving restrictions is often listed as the major stressor related to an epilepsy diagnosis in older people. Other stressors include lack of control over ASM management, being a burden rather than a positive contributor to family life, the expense and side effects associated with ASM usage, personal safety, social embarrassment, and cognitive decline.[71]

Stigma associated with epilepsy has a 2-fold impact on the life of older persons with epilepsy. First, the rates of people seeking medical attention are reduced, perhaps partly contributed to by concern over not being allowed to drive, which may lead to an increase in underdiagnosed, untreated seizures. Second, epilepsy may cause a breakdown of normal social interactions, as people feel ashamed of disclosing their condition. Stigma seems more pronounced in people that have received a diagnosis earlier in life and then transition to older age as well as in those from backgrounds where traditional beliefs can lead to reduced disclosure of epilepsy.[70]

Possible strategies to minimize the psychosocial impact of epilepsy on older people include greater education of the public about epilepsy to reduce stigma; empowering older people in self-management; and treating pharmacologically modifiable targets, such as uncontrolled seizures and depression, as these are important predictors of lower quality of life.[72]

Prognosis

New-onset seizures in older people can, relatively speaking, be easier to control than in younger people.[73] Also, recent data show that even complex epilepsies can associate with seizure freedom in later life.[74] This should not, though, be taken to mean that epilepsy in older individuals is benign. As well as the complexities surrounding the choice of medication, comorbidities and psychosocial impact, epilepsy in older people is also associated with an increased risk of mortality.[75] Lower mortality can associate with female sex, Asian race, and Hispanic ethnicity while comorbid disease, especially a neurologic condition being present before the onset of seizures, associates with higher mortality.[75] Also, the rates of status epilepticus are substantially higher in older people and the mortality associated with prolonged seizures also rises with age.[76,77] Perhaps owing to the presence of other comorbidities, sudden unexpected death in epilepsy (SUDEP) tends to be underestimated in older people,[78] potentially meaning that preventative interventions are not discussed in this vulnerable group.

CONCLUSIONS AND FUTURE DIRECTIONS

Although relatively overlooked for decades, epilepsy in older people is now recognized as a major and complex health burden. Not only is LOE common and increasing in frequency globally, but the inter-relationship between seizures and comorbidities in later life also creates multi-layered challenges. In particular, the intersections between dementia, mental health difficulties, vascular disease, and psychosocial factors as pertains to older people with epilepsy require disentangling. Clinicians can be hampered by a lack of data on how to optimally manage this patient group with, for example, trials of novel ASMs not being performed in older people, and a historical nervousness about surgical or other novel interventions in this cohort. As demographics shift across the world, there will need to be increasing distinction made between biological and chronological age as well as an imperative to ensure that people with early-onset complex epilepsies are enabled to achieve their full potential in older life.

CLINICS CARE POINTS

- Seizures in older people can present with atypical semiologies, requiring clinicians to be very alert to epilepsy as a possible diagnosis, particularly in people presenting with recurrent stereotyped attacks
- Confusional states in older people may be a manifestation of nonconvulsive status epilepticus
- The choice of anti-seizure medication can be more limited in older people with epilepsy owing to pre-existing comorbidities. Lamotrigine, levetiracetam and lacosamide are preferred
- In older people with epilepsy, enzyme inducing medications should generally be avoided owing to multiple interactions, including with novel anticoagulants, and adverse impacts on, for example, bone health
- The psychosocial impact of epilepsy on older people can be profound, so it is essential to enquire about and address adverse consequences such as driving restrictions, impacts on relationships, mental health difficulties, and stigmatization

DISCLOSURE

The authors have nothing to disclose.

ACKNOWLEDGEMENTS

This work is supported by the Oxford NIHR Biomedical Research Centre.

REFERENCES

1. World Health Organization. WHO | epilepsy: A Public Health Imperative.; 2019.
2. World Health Organization. Atlas: epilepsy care in the world.; 2005.
3. Cloyd J, Hauser W, Towne A, et al. Epidemiological and medical aspects of epilepsy in the elderly. Epilepsy Res 2006;68 Suppl 1:S39–48.
4. Hauser WA, Annegers JF, Kurland LT. Incidence of epilepsy and unprovoked seizures in Rochester, Minnesota: 1935–1984. Epilepsia 1993;34(3):453–8.
5. Sipilä JOT, Kälviäinen R. Adult onset epilepsy incidence in Finland over 34 years: a nationwide registry study. Eur J Neurol 2021;(October):1–4.
6. Feigin VL, Abajobir AA, Abate KH, et al. Global, regional, and national burden of neurological disorders during 1990–2015: a systematic analysis for the Global Burden of Disease Study 2015. Lancet Neurol 2017;16(11):877–97.

7. Choi H, Pack A, Elkind MSV, et al. Predictors of incident epilepsy in older adults: The Cardiovascular Health Study. Neurology 2017;88(9):870–7.

8. Fiest KM, Sauro KM, Wiebe S, et al. Prevalence and incidence of epilepsy: A systematic review and meta-analysis of international studies. Neurology 2017;88(3): 296–303.

9. Birnbaum AK, Leppik IE, Svendsen KH, et al., Prevalence of epilepsy/seizures as a comorbidity of neurologic disorders in nursing homes. Neurology 2017; 88(8):750–757.

10. Hussain SA, Haut SR, Lipton RB, et al. Incidence of epilepsy in a racially diverse, community-dwelling, elderly cohort: Results from the Einstein aging study. Epilepsy Res 2006;71(2–3):195–205.

11. Zelano J. Poststroke epilepsy: Update and future directions. Ther Adv Neurol Disord 2016;9(5):424–35.

12. Fisher RS, Acevedo C, Arzimanoglou A, et al. ILAE official report: a practical clinical definition of epilepsy. Epilepsia 2014;55(4):475–82.

13. Holtkamp M, Beghi E, Benninger F, et al. European stroke organisation guidelines for the management of post-stroke seizures and epilepsy. Eur Stroke J 2017;2(2): 103–15.

14. Weng SW, Chen TL, Yeh CC, et al. The effects of bu yang huan wu tang on post-stroke epilepsy: a nationwide matched study. Clin Epidemiol 2018;10:1839–50.

15. Costa C, Nardi Cesarini E, Eusebi P, et al. Incidence and antiseizure medications of post-stroke epilepsy in umbria: a population-based study using healthcare administrative databases. Front Neurol 2022;12(January):1–7.

16. Arntz RM, Rutten-Jacobs LCA, Maaijwee NAM, et al. Poststroke epilepsy is associated with a high mortality after a stroke at young age: follow-up of transient ischemic attack and stroke patients and unelucidated risk factor evaluation Study. Stroke 2015;46(8):2309–11.

17. Galovic M, Döhler N, Erdélyi-Canavese B, et al. Prediction of late seizures after ischaemic stroke with a novel prognostic model (the SeLECT score): a multivariable prediction model development and validation study. Lancet Neurol 2018; 17(2):117.

18. Johnson EL, Krauss GL, Lee AK, et al. Association between midlife risk factors and late-onset epilepsy: results from the atherosclerosis risk in communities study. JAMA Neurol 2018;75(11):1375–82.

19. Yuan S, Tomson T, Larsson SC. Modifiable risk factors for epilepsy: a two-sample Mendelian randomization study. Brain Behav 2021;11(5):1–7.

20. Lane CA, Barnes J, Nicholas JM, et al. Associations between vascular risk across adulthood and brain pathology in late life. JAMA Neurol 2020;77(2):175.

21. Huberfeld G, Vecht CJ. Seizures and gliomas — towards a single therapeutic approach. Nat Rev Neurol 2016;12(4):204–16. Published online 2016.

22. Sen A, Jette N, Husain M, et al. Epilepsy in older people. Lancet 2020; 395(10225):735–48.

23. Romoli M, Sen A, Parnetti L, et al. Amyloid-β: a potential link between epilepsy and cognitive decline. Nat Rev Neurol 2021;17(8):469–85.

24. Keret O, Hoang TD, Xia F, et al. Association of late-onset unprovoked seizures of unknown etiology with the risk of developing dementia in older veterans. JAMA Neurol 2020;77(6):710–5.

25. Gastaldi M, Mariotto S, Giannoccaro M, et al. Subgroup comparison according to clinical phenotype and serostatus in autoimmune encephalitis: a multicenter retrospective study. Eur J Neurol 2019;8:ene.14139. Published online December.

26. Lawn N, Kelly A, Dunne J, et al. First seizure in the older patient: clinical features and prognosis. Epilepsy Res 2013;107(1–2):109–14.

27. Godfrey JBW. Misleading presentation of epilepsy in elderly people. Age Ageing 1989;18(1):17–20.

28. Vu LC, Piccenna L, Kwan P, et al. New-onset epilepsy in the elderly. Br J Clin Pharmacol 2018;84(10):2208–17.

29. Neligan A, Heaney D, Rajakulendran S. Is a separate clinical pathway for first seizures justified? Appraisal of the first seizure pathway at a tertiary neuroscience centre. Seizure 2021;84(September 2020):108–11.

30. Ramsay RE, Rowan AJ, Pryor FM. Special considerations in treating the elderly patient with epilepsy. Neurology 2004;62(Issue 5):S24–9.

31. Romoli M, Tuna MA, McGurgan I, et al. Long-term risk of stroke after transient global amnesia in two prospective cohorts. Stroke 2019;50(9):2555–7.

32. Savage SA, Butler CR, Hodges JR, et al. Transient epileptic amnesia over twenty years: Long-term follow-up of a case series with three detailed reports. Seizure 2016;43:48–55.

33. Green SF, Loefflad N, Heaney DC, et al. New-onset seizures in older people: clinical features, course and outcomes. J Neurol Sci 2021;429(May):118065.

34. Sambin S, Gaspard N, Legros B, et al. Role of epileptic activity in older adults with delirium, a prospective continuous EEG study. Front Neurol 2019;10.

35. Ozkara C, Metin B, Kucukoglu S. Convulsive syncope: a condition to be differentiated from epilepsy. Epileptic Disord 2009;11(4):315–9.

36. Pasini E, Michelucci R. Fit and faint or faint and fit? Clin Neurophysiol 2021; 132(1):178–9.

37. Petkar S, Hamid T, Iddon P, et al. Prolonged implantable electrocardiographic monitoring indicates a high rate of misdiagnosis of epilepsy-REVISE study. Europace 2012;14(11):1653–60.

38. Theodore WH. The postictal state: Effects of age and underlying brain dysfunction. Epilepsy Behav 2010;19(2):118–20.

39. Villanueva V, Serratosa JM. Temporal lobe epilepsy: clinical semiology and age at onset. Epileptic Disord 2005;7(2):83–90.

40. Stefan H, May TW, Pfäfflin M, et al. Epilepsy in the elderly: comparing clinical characteristics with younger patients. Acta Neurol Scand 2014;129(5):283–93.

41. Gugger JJ, Llinas RH, Kaplan PW. The role of CT perfusion in the evaluation of seizures, the post-ictal state, and status epilepticus. Epilepsy Res 2020; 159(November 2019):106256.

42. Moloney D, Pérez-Denia LP, Kenny RA. Todd's paresis following vasovagal syncope provoked by tilt-table testing. BMJ Case Rep 2020;13(6):1–3.

43. Rossetti AO, Waterhouse E. Missed diagnosis of prehospital status epilepticus. Neurology 2017;89(4):314–5.

44. Semmlack S, Yeginsoy D, Spiegel R, et al. Emergency response to out-of-hospital status epilepticus. Neurology 2017;89(4):376–84.

45. Pimentel J, Varanda S, Guimarães P, et al. Idiopathic generalised epilepsies of adult onset: a reappraisal and literature review. Epileptic Disord 2018;20(3): 169–77.

46. Sen A, Capelli V, Husain M. Cognition and dementia in older patients with epilepsy. Brain 2018;141(6):1592–608.

47. Faught E. Monotherapy in adults and elderly persons. Neurology 2007;69(24 suppl 3):S3–9.

48. Rohracher A, Kalss G, Kuchukhidze G, et al. New anti-seizure medication for elderly epilepsy patients - a critical narrative review. Expert Opin Pharmacother 2021;22(5):621–34.

49. Lattanzi S, Trinka E, Del Giovane C, et al. Antiepileptic drug monotherapy for epilepsy in the elderly: a systematic review and network meta-analysis. Epilepsia 2019;60(11):2245–54.

50. Lezaic N, Gore G, Josephson CB, et al. The medical treatment of epilepsy in the elderly: a systematic review and meta-analysis. Epilepsia 2019;60(7):1325–40.

51. Witt JA, Werhahn KJ, Krämer G, et al. Cognitive-behavioral screening in elderly patients with new-onset epilepsy before treatment. Acta Neurol Scand 2014; 130(3):172–7.

52. Foster E, Malpas CB, Ye K, et al. Antiepileptic drugs are not independently associated with cognitive dysfunction. Neurology 2020;94(10):e1051–61.

53. Chuang YC, Chuang HY, Lin TK, et al. Effects of long-term antiepileptic drug monotherapy on vascular risk factors and atherosclerosis. Epilepsia 2012; 53(1):120–8.

54. Kim JY, Lee HW. Metabolic and hormonal disturbances in women with epilepsy on antiepileptic drug monotherapy. Epilepsia 2007;48:1366–70.

55. Falhammar H, Lindh JD, Calissendorff J, et al. Differences in associations of antiepileptic drugs and hospitalization due to hyponatremia: a population–based case–control study. Seizure 2018;59:28–33.

56. Bialek F, Rydenhag B, Flink R, et al. Outcomes after resective epilepsy surgery in patients over 50 years of age in Sweden 1990-2009–a prospective longitudinal study. Seizure 2014;23(8):641–5.

57. Waseem H, Osborn KE, Schoenberg MR, et al. Laser ablation therapy: an alternative treatment for medically resistant mesial temporal lobe epilepsy after age 50. Epilepsy Behav 2015;51:152–7.

58. Petito GT, Wharen RE, Feyissa AM, et al. The impact of stereotactic laser ablation at a typical epilepsy center. Epilepsy Behav 2018;78:37–44.

59. Nair DR, Laxer KD, Weber PB, et al. Nine-year prospective efficacy and safety of brain-responsive neurostimulation for focal epilepsy. Neurology 2020;95(9): e1244–56.

60. Subota A, Jetté N, Josephson CB, et al. Risk factors for dementia development, frailty, and mortality in older adults with epilepsy – a population-based analysis. Epilepsy Behav 2021;120:108006.

61. Toniolo S, Sen A, Husain M. Modulation of Brain Hyperexcitability: Potential New Therapeutic Approaches in Alzheimer's Disease. Int J Mol Sci 2020;21(23):1–37.

62. Costa C, Romoli M, Liguori C, et al. Alzheimer's disease and late onset epilepsy of unknown origin: two faces of beta amyloid pathology. Neurobiol Aging 2018;73. A5-A7.

63. Hatton SN, Huynh KH, Bonilha L, et al. White matter abnormalities across different epilepsy syndromes in adults: anENIGMA-Epilepsy study. Brain 2020;143(8): 2454.

64. Attems J, Jellinger KA. The overlap between vascular disease and Alzheimer's disease - lessons from pathology. BMC Med 2014;12(1):1–12.

65. Baker J, Libretto T, Henley W, et al. A Longitudinal study of epileptic seizures in Alzheimer's disease. Front Neurol 2019;10:1266.

66. Haut SR, Katz M, Masur J, et al. Seizures in the elderly: impact on mental status, mood, and sleep. Epilepsy Behav 2009;14(3):540–4.

67. Hernández-Ronquillo L, Adams S, Ballendine S, et al. Epilepsy in an elderly population: Classification, etiology and drug resistance. Epilepsy Res 2018;140:90–4.

68. Jones RM, Butler JA, Thomas VA, et al. Adherence to treatment in patients with epilepsy: Associations with seizure control and illness beliefs. Seizure 2006; 15(7):504–8.
69. Ettinger AB. Psychotropic effects of antiepileptic drugs. Neurology 2006;67(11): 1916–25.
70. Wojewodka G, McKinlay A, Ridsdale L. Best care for older people with epilepsy: a scoping review. Seizure 2021;85(December 2020):70–89.
71. Martin R, Vogtle L, Gilliam F, et al. What are the concerns of older adults living with epilepsy? Epilepsy Behav 2005;7(2):297–300.
72. Canuet L, Ishii R, Iwase M, et al. Factors associated with impaired quality of life in younger and older adults with epilepsy. Epilepsy Res 2009;83(1):58–65.
73. Besocke AG, Rosso B, Cristiano E, et al. Outcome of newly-diagnosed epilepsy in older patients. Epilepsy Behav 2013;27(1):29–35.
74. Rajakulendran S, Belluzzo M, Novy J, et al. Late-life terminal seizure freedom in drug-resistant epilepsy: "Burned-out epilepsy. J Neurol Sci 2021;431(April): 120043.
75. Blank LJ, Acton EK, Willis AW. Predictors of mortality in older adults with epilepsy. Neurology 2021;96(1):e93–101.
76. DeLorenzo RJ, Hauser WA, Towne AR, et al. A prospective, population-based epidemiologic study of status epilepticus in Richmond, Virginia. Neurology 1996;46(4):1029–35.
77. Greenlund SF, Croft JB, Kobau R. Epilepsy by the Numbers: Epilepsy deaths by age, race/ethnicity, and gender in the United States significantly increased from 2005 to 2014. Epilepsy Behav 2017;69:28–30.
78. Sveinsson O, Andersson T, Carlsson S, et al. The incidence of SUDEP: A nationwide population-based cohort study. Neurology 2017;89(2):170–7.

Electrographic Seizures in the Critically Ill

Smitha K. Holla, MD[a],*, Parimala Velpula Krishnamurthy, MD[a],
Thanujaa Subramaniam, MD[b], Monica B. Dhakar, MD, MS[c], Aaron F. Struck, MD[a,d]

KEYWORDS

- Electrographic seizures • IIC pattern • Critical illness • Continuous EEG
- 2HELPS2B score

KEY POINTS

- There is growing evidence indicating that electrographic seizures cause neuronal damage, leading to secondary brain injury so early identification of patients at risk is necessary.
- Electrographic seizures and patterns on the ictal-interictal continuum are now better defined, and their associated risks, supported by ancillary tests, are under investigation.
- Choice of medications and duration of treatment need to be tailored to the individual patient.

Video content accompanies this article at http://www.neurologic.theclinics.com.

INTRODUCTION

Electroencephalography (EEG)[1] has become an integral component of neurologic care since it was first used by Hans Berger to record surface human brain activity in 1924. In the 1990s, the advent of digitalized EEG revolutionized inpatient continuous EEG (cEEG) monitoring. The scale and scope of cEEG has expanded exponentially over the last several decades.[2] The expansion of cEEG is driven in part by the recognition that non-convulsive electrographic seizures are relatively common in hospitalized patients.[3]

In critically ill patients, seizure incidence has been reported to be between 3.3% and 34%,[4] with more recent large studies suggesting an incidence closer to 12.0%.[5] Most

[a] Department of Neurology, UW Medical Foundation Centennial building, 1685 Highland Avenue, Madison, WI 53705, USA; [b] Division of Neurocritical Care and Emergency Neurology, Department of Neurology, Yale School of Medicine, 15 York Street, Building LLCI, 10th Floor, Suite 1003 New Haven, CT 06520, USA; [c] Department of Neurology, The Warren Alpert Medical School of Brown University, 593 Eddy St, APC 5, Providence, RI 02903, USA; [d] William S Middleton Veterans Hospital, Madison WI, USA
* Corresponding author.
E-mail address: holla@neurology.wisc.edu

Neurol Clin 40 (2022) 907–925
https://doi.org/10.1016/j.ncl.2022.03.015
0733-8619/22/© 2022 Elsevier Inc. All rights reserved.
neurologic.theclinics.com

of these seizures (75%) are nonconvulsive.[3,6,7] It requires a high index of suspicion from the clinician to warrant EEG for days. Alternatively, using prophylactic antiseizure medications (ASMs) without EEG tends to fall short in preventing and stopping seizures in those patients at risk and can cause unnecessary side effects and even poor outcomes in those at low risk of seizure.[8–10]

American Clinical Neurophysiology Society (ACNS) Standardized Critical Care EEG terminology-2021[11] introduced standardized terminology to define electrographic seizures, ictal-interictal continuum (IIC), and terms such as brief potentially ictal rhythmic discharges (BIRDs). These terms and seizure risk stratification tools such as 2HELPS2B[12] offer more clarity in identifying potentially ictal patterns and those that may warrant longer cEEG monitoring and aggressive treatment. The presence of electrographic seizures and associated patterns has been tied to local metabolic failure[7,13,14] and poor clinical outcomes.[15,16]

A personalized approach to treatment of seizures and IIC patterns is essential, and cEEG, clinical examination, along with ancillary testing with neuroimaging, multimodal monitoring, or serum biomarkers maybe necessary, but more study is required. There is still no strong evidence guiding the selection and aggressiveness of treatment of a given EEG pattern.

Abbreviations	New Terms	Definitions—ACNS Standardized Critical Care EEG Terminology 2021
ESz	Electrographic seizures	a. Epileptiform discharges averaging >2.5 Hz for $\geq$10 s (>25 discharges in 10 s), OR b. Any pattern with definite evolution marked by at least two unequivical changes in frequency (by at least 0.5 Hz), morphology or location and lasting 10 s
ESE	Electrographic status epilepticus	An ESz for $\geq$10 continuous minutes or for a total duration of $\geq$20% of any 60-min period of recording
ECSz	Electroclinical seizures	Any EEG pattern with either: a. Definite clinical correlate time-locked to the pattern (of any duration), OR b. EEG AND clinical improvement with a parenteral (typically IV) antiseizure medication
ECSE	Electroclinical status Epilepticus	An ECSz seizure for $\geq$10 continuous minutes or for a total duration of $\geq$20% of any 60-min period of recording. An ongoing seizure with bilateral tonic-clonic (BTC) motor activity only needs to be present for $\geq$5 continuous minutes to qualify as ECSE. This is also referred to as "convulsive SE," a subset of "SE with prominent motor activity."
BIRDs	Brief potentially ictal Rhythmic discharges	Focal (including lateralized [L], bilateral independent [BI], unilateral independent [UI] or multifocal [Mf]) or generalized rhythmic activity >4 Hz (at least 6 waves at a regular rate) lasting $\geq$0.5 to <10 s, not consistent with a known normal pattern or benign variant, not part of burst-suppression or burst-attenuation, without definite clinical correlate, and that has at least one of the following features: a. Evolution ("evolving BIRDs," a form of definite BIRDs)

(continued on next page)

(continued)		
Abbreviations	New Terms	Definitions—ACNS Standardized Critical Care EEG Terminology 2021
		b. Similar morphology and location as interictal epileptiform discharges or seizures in the same patient (definite BIRDs)
		c. Sharply contoured but without (a) or (b) (possible BIRDs)
IIC	Ictal-interictal continuum	Synonymous with "possible Esz" or "possible electrographic SE," is a purely electrographic term and not a diagnosis and can have the following patterns:
		a. Any PD or SW pattern that averages >1.0 and ≤2.5 Hz over 10 s (>10 and ≤25 discharges in 10 s); or
		b. Any PD or SW pattern that averages ≥0.5 Hz and ≤1.0 Hz over 10 s (≥5 and ≤10 discharges in 10 s) and has a plus modifier or fluctuation; or
		c. Any lateralized RDA averaging >1 Hz for at least 10 s (at least 10 waves in 10 s) with a plus modifier or fluctuation. This includes any LRDA, BIRDs, UIRDA, and MfRDA, but not GRDA. AND
		d. Does not qualify as ESz or ESE

Abbreviations: GRDA, generalized rhythmic delta activity; IV, intravenous.

PATIENTS AT RISK/SEIZURE PROGNOSTICATION

Around 12% to 25% of critically ill patients placed on continuous EEG monitoring will have at least one electrographic seizure detected.[3,14,17–26] The underlying conditions that can be associated with seizures are varied and include systemic medical illnesses such as sepsis, liver and kidney failure as well as primary neurologic injuries such as stroke, intracranial hemorrhage, brain tumor, or traumatic brain injury.[3,14,17,19,21,22,24,27–33] Clinical risk factors that have been associated with an increased chance of seizure include a history of epilepsy, age less than 18 years, coma, and suspected acute symptomatic seizure.[3]

In comparison to clinical factors, EEG factors are more accurate predictors.[34] For example, coma is associated with an increased seizure risk but once EEG features are accounted for, the added predictive power of coma is lessened. Similarly, the type of brain injury can influence the risk of seizure,[35] but this variance is less powerful when EEG factors are taken into account.[34]

Relevant EEG findings for seizure prediction include sporadic epileptiform discharges, lateralized periodic discharges (LPDs), generalized periodic discharges (GPDs), bilateral independent discharges (BIPDs), BIRDs, and lateralized rhythmic delta activity (LRDAs).

LPDs are seen most commonly in acute structural brain injuries[36–39] such as central nervous system infection, stroke, and brain tumors and, carry an increased risk of seizures.[36–40] LPDs with higher frequency (>2 Hz) and/or with rhythmic or fast activity— so called "plus" features—pose a higher risk[40,41] of seizures. LRDA is found in similar patient populations as LPDs and presents a similar risk for seizures.[13,37] GPDs occur more frequently in toxic-metabolic encephalopathy and anoxic brain injury.[42,43] And similar to LPD, higher frequency (>1.5 Hz)[5] and associated plus features portend increased risk of seizures, but their presence in of themselves does not have the same risk as the lateralized findings (LPD, BIPDs, LRDA). Generalized rhythmic delta activities, even with higher frequency and plus modifiers, do not seem to increase risk for seizures.[5] BIRDs[44] are brief seizurelike patterns lasting less than 10 seconds and highly associated with seizures and may be conceptualized as an incompletely formed seizure.[11]

2HELPS2B[12,45] is a scoring system that combines several of these EEG markers and a single clinical factor (history of clinical seizure) into a risk stratification scheme to guide seizure monitoring and decision to use prophylactic antiseizure medications.[10] The variables in 2HELPS2B are (1) frequency greater than 2 Hz, (2) sporadic Epileptiform discharges, (3) LPD/BIPD/LRDA, (4) Plus features, (5) prior Seizure, and (6) BIRDs(2). BIRDs are assigned 2 points, whereas the rest of the variables get 1 point each, and the total score ranges from 0 to 7. A score of 0 confers a seizure risk less than 5% and a score of 7 a risk of greater than 95%, with the scores in the range predicting a risk in between. 2HELPS2B score has been validated in an independent cohort study,[12] and its proposed clinical algorithm can be used to assess seizure risk based on 1 hour of EEG. For a score greater than or equal to 2, cEEG of 24 hours is recommended; for score = 1, 12 hours of cEEG; and for score = 0, no cEEG is recommended.[12] Further areas of study include developing updated real-time seizure risk assessment aided by automated or semiautomated EEG interpretation.

ICTAL-INTERICTAL CONTINUUM AND ELECTROGRAPHIC SEIZURES

There is growing evidence indicating that electrographic seizures cause neuronal damage leading to secondary brain injury.[46,47] MRI of patients with status epilepticus have been found to have restricted diffusion on diffusion-weighted images (DWI) in the hippocampi, insula, and cortex, indicating neuronal injury.[48,49] Neuron-specific enolase (NSE), which is marker of neuronal injury, is elevated in patients with status epilepticus, indicating secondary brain injury.[50,51] In the landmark study by Vespa and colleagues,[14] patients with traumatic brain injury (TBI) who had electrographic seizures were found to have ipsilateral hippocampal atrophy 6 months postdischarge. In another single-center retrospective study, patients with super-refractory status epilepticus (SRSE) were found to have global cerebral atrophy, which was related to the duration of SRSE.[52] The data are conflicting on whether the presence of seizures leads to poor patient outcomes.[27,29,53,54] However, these studies did not account for seizure burden, and there seems to be a dose-dependent relationship between seizure burden and neurocognitive outcomes. In a cohort of patients with subarachnoid hemorrhage, every 1 hour of seizure burden was associated with 10 times higher odds of disability and death and worse cognitive outcome at 6 months as measured by T-MOCA.[18] Similarly in pediatric population, seizure burden of greater than 20% per hour (12 mins per hour) was found to be associated with worse functional outcomes at discharge.[16] These findings are reflected in the newly proposed criteria for electrographic status epilepticus, which is defined as total seizure burden greater than 20% per hour,[11] indicating a threshold beyond which recurrent seizures have been shown to have detrimental outcomes.

With the recent recognition of various rhythmic and periodic patterns on cEEG, the term "ictal-interictal continuum" has been devised to remove the binary connotation of any given pattern to be either ictal or interictal.[42] Rather, these patterns are now thought to occur on a spectrum. Although the definition and spectrum of IIC continues to evolve over time, a consensus definition was recently proposed by ACNS in the 2021 nomenclature[11] to facilitate the further understanding of these patterns. Whether these patterns cause neuronal injury similar to electrographic seizures continues to be an area of active investigation. Ancillary imaging modalities such as fluorodeoxyglucose-positron emission tomography (FDG-PET), single-photon emission computed tomography (SPECT), CT perfusion, and MR perfusion are being used to assess the extent of neuronal loss caused by IIC patterns.[55] In a single-center study, patients with lateralized periodic discharges were found to have concurrent hypermetabolism on using FDG-PET scan, which resolved following treatment[13] (**Fig. 1**). Moreover, these changes of hypermetabolism directly correlated with the frequency of the LPDs, indicating dose-dependent relationship.[56] Similarly, perfusion studies using MRI and CT studies have demonstrated increased cerebral perfusion with periodic discharges similar to seizures, denoting their ictal nature.[57–59]

Advanced multimodality invasive monitoring techniques have been instrumental in understanding the physiologic underpinning of these patterns. Intracranial depth electrode monitoring has revealed that scalp IIC patterns often correlate with intracranial electrographic seizures.[7] In patients with TBI, periodic patterns greater than 2 Hz produced metabolic crisis as increased lactate/pyruvate ratio (LPR) and decreased glucose levels in cerebral microdialysate akin to electrographic seizures.[47] Similarly, in patients with subarachnoid hemorrhage with multimodality monitoring, higher frequency PDs (>2 Hz) were temporally related to reduced partial pressure of brain tissue oxygen ($PbtO_2$). There was a compensatory increase in cerebral blood flow for PDs up to 2 Hz; however, CBF did not increase for PD greater than 2 Hz, demonstrating an inadequately compensated state.[15] These findings substantiate the evidence that higher frequency PDs cause metabolic disturbances and neuronal injury similar to electrographic seizures.

Multiple prior studies have demonstrated that IIC patterns are associated with worse functional outcomes at discharge.[43,60] In patients with subarachnoid hemorrhage and acute ischemic stroke, burden of IIC patterns was found to be associated with worse functional outcomes despite adjusting for disease severity and other clinical variables.[61,62] Recent work using automated machine learning system to quantify

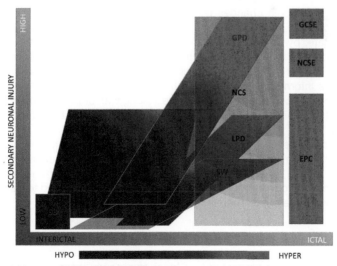

Fig. 1. Metabolic correlates of EEG patterns. (*From* Struck AF, Westover MB, Hall LT, Deck GM, Cole AJ, Rosenthal ES. Metabolic Correlates of the Ictal-Interictal Continuum: FDG-PET During Continuous EEG. Neurocrit Care. 2016;24(3):324-331. https://doi.org/10.1007/s12028-016-0245-y; with permission).

the epileptiform activity (EA) burden demonstrated that peak EA burden in the 12-hour window within the first 72 hours was associated with worse functional outcome at discharge.[63] In addition, increasing peak EA burden from 0% to 100% increases the probability of poor neurologic outcome by 35%.[63]

ANCILLARY TESTING

Decision-making surrounding the management of IIC and electrographic seizures can be complex.

Ancillary testing can help guide treatment decisions by potentially revealing evidence of neuronal injury in a patient with abnormal EEG findings. Serum NSE is the best described serum test in this regard; NSE levels will increase in any process causing neuronal injury; thus absolute levels (>20) and trends can be used to detect ongoing neuronal injury associated with an IIC pattern.[50] However, other pathologic processes of acute brain injury can affect NSE levels, independent of epileptiform activity, limiting its use in most acute neurologic disease state. NSE is also present in erythrocytes, platelets, and neuroendocrine tissues, further reducing its specificity.[51]

Neuroimaging with MRI, FDG-PET, and SPECT is perhaps the most used ancillary test in the clinical setting. DWI changes are deemed to represent increased metabolic demand and theoretically, neuronal swelling.[55] Accordingly, the presence or absence of DWI changes during IIC patterns or frequent repetitive seizures can guide decision to treat, although data on this practice are limited. MRI perfusion provides information about regional blood flow changes, which if correlates with epileptiform area on EEG, can serve as a metabolic signature of an abnormal EEG pattern. FDG-PET, another functional neuroimaging modality, measures cerebral metabolism by evaluating glucose uptake and can be particularly useful to define the nature of periodic discharges by providing good temporal and spatial resolution.[13] SPECT is conceptually similar to FDG-PET but provides lower spatial resolution.[64]

Invasive multimodal monitoring consists of various intracranial parenchymal monitors that can provide real-time information on secondary brain injury, detecting detrimental physiologic changes by tracking brain oxygen delivery-consumption, cerebral blood flow, and metabolism. Cerebral microdialysis measures extracellular glucose, lactate, pyruvate, and glutamate.[65] LPRs are useful parameters to trend, and values greater than 40 indicate metabolic distress and enhanced anaerobic metabolism.[66] Other measurements such as PbtO2 and jugular venous oxygen saturation provide information on cerebral utilization of oxygen.[66] Data obtained from these monitors are combined and interpreted along with other measurements to untangle the relationship between the abnormal EEG pattern and its metabolic and clinical impact.

It is important to keep in mind that ancillary tests provide only a metabolic and physiologic footprint, from which neuronal injury is inferred. Further, suspicion for neuronal injury related to EEG abnormality should be tempered with additional reflections as to whether the epileptiform activity is the underlying cause (as opposed to a sequalae) or the sole driving force of inferred neuronal injury.

CLINICAL CASES
Case 1

A 66-year-old man who presented to a local emergency room with acute onset of aphasia, and difficulty typing that started 1 hour prior, then had a witnessed generalized tonic-clonic seizure. Head CT was reported to be normal. Given initial suspicion for stroke at the small community hospital, he received tissue plasminogen activator, lorazepam, and levetiracetam and then transferred to the tertiary center where he presented with persistent confusion. CT angiogram showed an enhancing lesion in the left inferior parietal lobule. cEEG initially showed diffuse slowing, but within 24 hours he developed left-sided seizures progressing to focal status epilepticus (Video 1). Lacosamide was added to levetiracetam, and patient was taken to the operating room for resection of the tumor 3 days after presentation, resulting in resolution of the status epilepticus. On postoperative day (POD) #2 he developed repetitive electroclinical seizures with intermittent eye deviation with persistent confusion but was conversant, able to participate in care, and eating on his own. Phenytoin was added but he developed transaminitis. Clobazam was added subsequently and then zonisamide, finally with seizure cessation noted on POD # 5. MRI showed cytotoxic edema along resection bed. Pathology was consistent with a grade IV glioblastoma. He continued to improve in the hospital and was discharged on POD #7. At follow-up, 2 months after discharge he had remained seizure free and was doing well clinically, even tolerating his 4 antiseizure medications with a wean to fewer medications being planned.

Learning points:
- Surgery may be part of the treatment plan in focal status epilepticus related to a lesion. Sometimes, seizures may recur/persist in the immediate postoperative period.
- Not all refractory status epilepticus require escalation to anesthetic drips.
- Selecting medications based on interactions, potential side effects, and varied mechanisms of actions can be beneficial.

Case 2

A 30-year-old man with history of intravenous (IV) drug use and endocarditis presented after witnessing cardiac arrest and having received CPR for 15 minutes. Postresuscitation altered mental status, and clinical myoclonus was noted. EEG showed a burst suppression pattern initially. Bursts were associated with clinical myoclonus (Video 2), consistent with myoclonic status epilepticus. After some initial response to medications, he settled into a pattern of generalized periodic polyspike discharges ranging from 1 to 4 Hz on the ictal-interictal continuum (**Fig. 2**A, B). He was treated with multiple antiseizure medications and anesthetics including with ketamine, midazolam, propofol, and pentobarbital for a prolong period, resulting in complications such as ileus. Eventually decision was made to terminally extubate and wean antiseizure medications using medications such as amantadine/methylphenidate to promote wakefulness. Postextubation, he was noted to follow one-step commands. A witnessed seizure on 7/19 and some attempted verbalization resulted in aggressive treatment being reinitiated. He was placed back on multiple medications and reintubated. Continuous EEG again showed subclinical status epilepticus and stimulation-induced myoclonic seizures that subsided with increasing anesthetics. MRI performed on day 3 and on day 8 and head CT on day 23 were all normal. With continued treatment, EEG background steadily improved to mild slowing with continued stimulation-induced myoclonus. Patient was eventually discharged to a long-term care facility. At discharge he was awake and alert, verbalizing answers with intermittent myoclonic jerking still noted.

Learning points:
- Not all postanoxic myoclonus with burst suppression results in a bad outcome; results can be heterogeneous.[67]

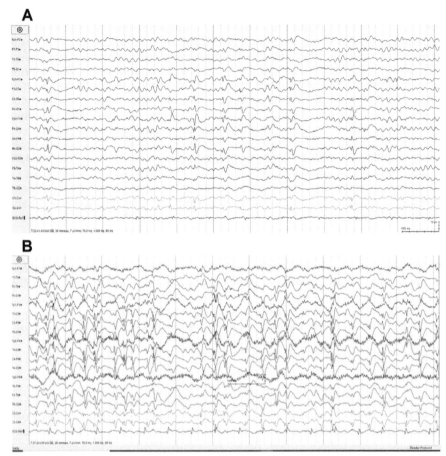

Fig. 2. (*A*) EEG background evolution on day 1 with more continuous activity noted, which then progressed to a pattern of generalized periodic polyspike discharges ranging from 1 to 4 Hz on the ictal-interictal continuum. (*B*) EEG then settled into pattern of generalized periodic polyspike discharges ranging from 1 to 4 Hz on the ictal-interictal continuum.

- Although burst suppression with identical bursts are associated with poor outcomes, background improvement to continuous EEG in the first 12 hours is strongly associated with favorable neurologic outcome.[67,68]

Case 3

A 67-year-old man with multiple cardiovascular risk factors was admitted for aortobifemoral bypass with superior mesenteric artery bypass. He had intraoperative bowel resection for ischemic bowel complicated by abdominal compartment syndrome, periapical abscesses of multiple teeth s/p dental extractions, severe acute kidney injury (on continuous variable valve timing), and then cardiac arrest, leading to intubation. A stroke code was called during admission for diffuse weakness and change in ability to follow commands with sedation wean. Patient had also been on multiple antibiotics including cefepime. Neurologic examination showed a comatose patient with eyes open, impaired leftward gaze, and no movement to pain or command. CT/CT angiography (CTA) results were reassuring against a large infarct. CEEG was started to evaluate for possible seizures and showed multifocal sharps, generalized periodic discharges, reaching 2 Hz (**Fig. 3**). Cefepime was stopped and over the next 3 days, improvement was noted on EEG with decreasing frequency and improving morphology of periodic discharges that then resolved (**Fig. 4**). Clinically also patient had improved mental status without the use of antiseizure medications. Patient was eventually discharged to a rehab center.

Learning points:
- The risk associated with IIC patterns must be interpreted within the clinical context.
- In this case, patient improved without the use of any antiseizure medications, by just withdrawing the offending medication (cefepime).

Case 4

A 67-year-old woman with stage IV melanoma and recent surgical resection of left parietal lobe metastasis presented with several days of right-sided arm and leg twitching, which progressed to a generalized tonic-clonic seizure. Two weeks before her presentation, patient had received one dose of an immune checkpoint inhibitor therapy with subsequent development of immune-mediated colitis requiring hospitalization for several days.

On presentation, patient was unresponsive with persistent right-sided arm and leg twitching. She was treated with IV benzodiazepine and was emergently intubated for airway protection. cEEG monitoring was commenced shortly after and showed continuous bilateral asymmetric LPDs lying on the IIC (**Fig. 5**). Patient was treated with sequential addition of 3 ASMs (lacosamide, phenytoin, levetiracetam) and up titration of midazolam and propofol infusions till suppression of all epileptiform abnormality. Initial workup was notable for mildly elevated protein but otherwise unremarkable cerebrospinal fluid. Brain MRI showed restricted diffusion and fluid-attenuated inversion recovery (FLAIR) hyperintensity in the left occipital and parietal lobes (**Fig. 6A–C**). Empirical IV steroid therapy was initiated in conjunction with ASMs, given suspicion for immune checkpoint–mediated encephalitis.

IV midazolam and propofol infusions were weaned and discontinued towards the end of the first week of admission. On completion of anesthetic wean, patient

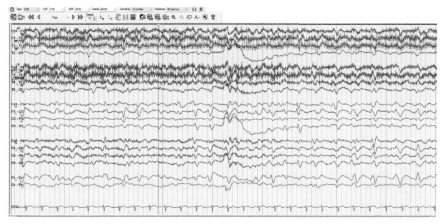

Fig. 3. EEG shows an IIC pattern with generalized periodic discharges reaching up to 2 Hz.

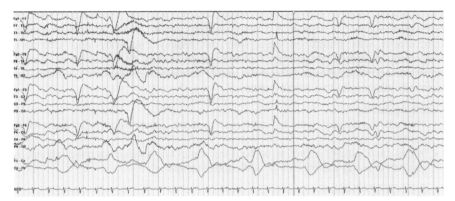

Fig. 4. Three days off Cefepime, patient's EEG background improved, with IIC pattern no longer seen.

remained stuporous, and sporadic epileptiform discharges began to reappear in left posterior quadrant, which over the course of several more days evolved into IIC pattern (LPDs with superimposed fast activity). Substitutions were made to ASMs but patient's EEG continued to worsen with emergence of BIRDs and seizures (**Fig. 7**). Ketamine infusion was commenced with quick resolution of BIRDs/seizures but persistence of IIC pattern. FDG-PET imaging along with repeat brain MRI was obtained, which demonstrated hypermetabolic foci in the left occipital lobe, bilateral thalami, and mesial temporal lobe (**Fig. 6D–F**) and persistent restricted diffusion with increased FLAIR/T2 signal in the left occipital-parietal lobe, respectively. Given imaging findings, decision was made to up titrate ketamine to achieve burst suppression.

After 24 hours of burst suppression, ketamine was discontinued, and patient was maintained on 3 ASM. Patient's mental status and EEG background began to slowly improve. However, LPDs began to reappear several days later, occasionally meeting criteria for IIC (**Fig. 8**). Given stable neurologic examination, decision was made not to escalate treatment and continue to observe patient.

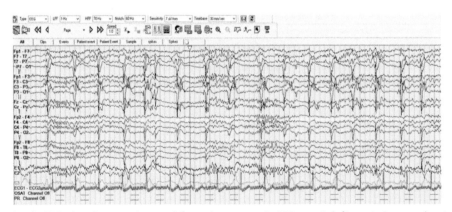

Fig. 5. EEG showing continuous bilateral asymmetric LPDs + F, left posterior quadrant maximal.

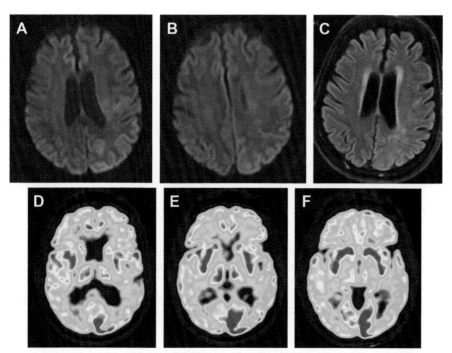

Fig. 6. Asymmetrically increased FDG uptake in the left occipital area and increased uptake in the bilateral thalami and mesial temporal lobe T2/FLAIR and DWI hyperintensity posteriorly, predominantly in the left parietal, occipital, and temporal area. (*Top row*) MRI showing DWI changes (*A, B*) in the left occipital and temporoparietal regions as well as related T2 flair hyperintensities (*C*). (*Bottom row*) (*D–F*) Asymmetrically increased FDG uptake in the left occipital region and increased uptake in the bilateral thalami and mesial temporal lobes.

Patient eventually underwent tracheostomy and was discharged to acute rehab 8 weeks following her presentation. At time of discharge, patient displayed some evidence of cognitive recovery, she was able to follow commands and was able to mouth words. EEG performed at this time showed mild to moderate slowing with sporadic sharp waves posteriorly.

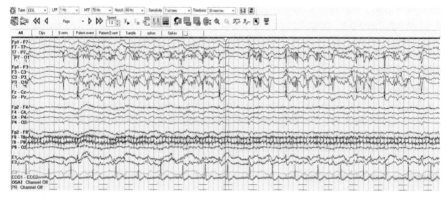

Fig. 7. Continuous periodic left posterior quadrant (P3/O1) LPD + F at 1.5 to 2 Hz with occasional focal seizures and BIRDs.

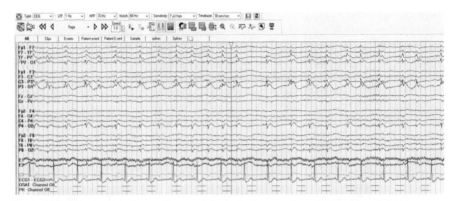

Fig. 8. EEG showing nearly continuous left posterior quadrant LPDs at 1 to 1.5 Hz.

Learning points:
- Ancillary tests such as MRI and PET-CT can reveal evidence of brain injury or metabolic impact associated with an EEG pattern and provide guidance for clinical decision-making.
- The duration of anesthetic use should be tailored to patient needs and early weaning be tried when appropriate.

Case 5

A 23-year-old, otherwise healthy woman presented with new-onset bilateral tonic-clonic convulsions. A week prior, she was noted to have worsening headache, malaise, dizziness, and flulike symptoms. Around the same time, she received multiple vaccines including for COVID. Seizure semiology was described as forced head and eye deviation to the right followed by whole body convulsions. On EEG, multiple electroclinical seizures, arising independently from right and left temporal regions were recorded (Videos 3 and 4). Extensive evaluation including MRI of brain, CTA of head and neck, and cerebrospinal fluid analysis including autoimmune and paraneoplastic panels were unrevealing. With a working diagnosis of new-onset refractory status epilepticus (NORSE) and possible seronegative autoimmune encephalitis, her treatment included empirical steroids, IV immunoglobulin, plasma exchange, multiple antiseizure medications, anesthetics, and ketogenic diet. She was eventually successfully weaned off anesthetics and status epilepticus resolved following a combination of aforementioned mention treatments, but sporadic seizures continued in the setting of illnesses, fevers in long-term care/rehab on 6 different antiseizure medications at therapeutic doses (LEV, LCM, TOP, PHB, PMP, PHT). Postdischarge, she continues to have significant cognitive and motor deficits but continues to make progress in rehabilitation.

Learning point:
- Aggressive management including an extensive workup, antiseizure medications, dietary therapy, immunotherapy, and a prolonged hospital course with supportive measures are often part of the management in these difficult cases of NORSE and FIRES (febrile infection–related epilepsy syndrome).

APPROACH TO TREATMENT

Approach to management of the critically ill patient with epileptiform abnormality is 2-fold. First, a decision must be made as to whether treatment of the abnormal EEG pattern is warranted. Second, a treatment strategy is necessary, taking into consideration various medication options and assessment of treatment response. The clinician must also decide on treatment intensity and duration, balancing potential side effects from treatment against the risk of cumulative neuronal damage, understanding that both can lead to worsened patient outcomes.

In general, clinical seizures and EEG patterns meeting criteria for electrographic seizures or NCSE warrant treatment. Patterns on the IIC require special consideration; the continuum encompass a wide range of patterns with some more on the "ictal" end than others. Although it is reasonable to approach treatment of patterns on the "ictal" end identical to seizures, data from existing literature are divided on whether IIC patterns carry the same significance and impact as seizures and status epilepticus. In addition, IIC patterns lying in the intermediate zone can also have significant clinical impact, depending on the clinical scenario and underlying disease state. Ancillary testing (described in the previous section) can provide some guidance when faced with IIC pattern of unclear significance, but these tests are not always feasible to perform and can yield indeterminate or confounding results. In the absence of reliable ancillary testing, the treating clinician can opt to initiate empirical treatment trials or continue observation of patient with cEEG monitoring, only starting treatment on evidence of clear seizures or clinical worsening.

Empirical treatment trial with low-dose benzodiazepines have historically been considered positive when both an electrographic and clinical improvement was observed.[42] However, benzodiazepine trials are frequently equivocal, with apparent electrographic improvement and no corresponding clinical improvement. This phenomenon is largely due to the sedative effect of benzodiazepines, worsening the typically encephalopathic critically ill patient. An alternate approach is to start a treatment trial with a nonsedating ASM that is rapidly titratable and has few drug interactions.[69] ASMs can then be added or substituted sequentially depending on clinical or electrographic response. Some experts advocate for starting with this method over a benzodiazepine trial to have better clarity on clinical improvement.[70,71] In some cases where there is high suspicion for a malignant IIC pattern, it may be reasonable to choose a more aggressive method, with early initiation of intravenous anesthetics in addition to ASMs. This approach carries more risk but can provide a greater chance of rapid and effective treatment to prevent secondary neuronal injury.

On initiation of treatment, empirical or otherwise, it is essential to establish treatment endpoints. The highly desired outcome is electrographic resolution of abnormal patterns with corresponding clinical improvement, achieved with the least amount of medications. However, in some critically ill patients, it can be challenging to achieve this ideal scenario, as attempts to completely suppress all abnormal EEG patterns can lead to oversedation or induced coma and paradoxically impair patient recovery.[72] Furthermore, some EEG patterns in the critically ill patient may resolve spontaneously after addressing the underlying medical disorder or exacerbating agents (eg, medications, fever, uremia).

In a similar vein, it is unclear if patients with frequent electrographic seizures should be treated as aggressively as NCSE. Although some clinical studies have shown that the total amount of time spent in ictal activity during an intensive care unit course can amount to a "seizure burden" associated with worse functional outcomes,[16,73] a recent study among acutely encephalopathic critically ill children found that electrographic status epilepticus, but not electrographic seizures, was associated with unfavorable neurobehavioral outcomes.[74] To date, there are no evidence-based studies on treatment of IIC patterns and treatment-related outcomes. Ultimately, treatment

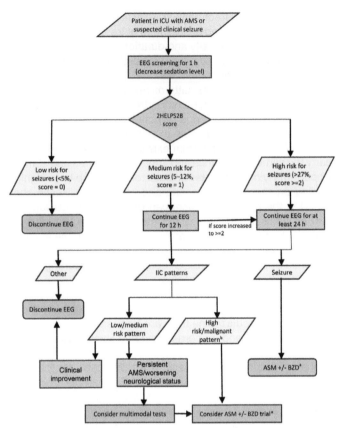

Fig. 9. Suggested management algorithm. [a]ASM (antiseizure medication) ± BZD (benzodiazepine) or escalating doses/drugs and sedatives as appropriate. [b]High-risk patterns such as BIRDS, high-frequency (>2.5 Hz) periodic discharges. See section on Ictal Interictal Continuum.

decisions should be individualized, incorporating all factors discussed in this section (**Fig. 9**).

SUMMARY

A clinician's goal in treating a critically ill patient is to orchestrate a meaningful and fast recovery with minimal long-term sequelae, thereby improving their quality of life at best or preventing deterioration at worst. The path to achieving this goal becomes increasingly complex and foggy when seizures and IIC patterns are present. The first step is identifying patients at risk for seizures and determining the timing and duration of EEG monitoring. 2HELPS2B or other risk stratification schemes may help, but the ultimate goal should be overcoming the logistical and technical barriers that prevent near-uniform EEG monitoring during critical illness, much in the same way that electrocardiogram monitoring is currently used.

Status epilepticus can cause secondary neurologic injury but the effects of discrete seizure burden and IIC patterns is still under investigation. The ambiguous nature of these EEG patterns necessitates ancillary testing where possible, such as NSE, neuroimaging with MRI, FDG-PET, or SPECT to better understand their malignant features. Treating status epilepticus, seizures, and IIC patterns is a delicate balance where the benefits and drawbacks of escalating IV anesthetic agents and ASM must be continually weighed. In addition to treating the EEG pattern, the clinician should focus on reversible causes such as metabolic disarray, offending drugs, infection, or inflammation and surgically remediable causes such as subdural hemorrhage. The optimal order and combination of ASMs and IV anesthetics is still lacking, given the complex dynamic interplay of the forces in neurocritical care. Still, one can advocate for rational polypharmacy—that is, using antiseizure medications with different mechanisms of action and compatible pharmacokinetics. Weaning of ASMs in the acute and recovery stage of critical illness is also in need of further clarification.

Answering these management questions will require an expanded use of multimodal ancillary testing, multicenter collaboration with data harmonization and innovate trial designs for a data-driven approach to neurocritical care EEG with the goal of arresting neurologic deterioration and improving neurologic recovery.

CLINICS CARE POINTS

- The incidence of seizures in critically ill patients is approximately 12%, with a majority being nonconvulsive seizures.
- Compared with clinical factors, EEG factors are more accurate predictors of patients at risk.
- Initial EEG along with seizure prognostication tools such as 2HELPS2B can guide duration of recording as well as treatment choices.

DISCLOSURE

The authors have nothing to disclose.

SUPPLEMENTARY DATA

Supplementary data related to this article can be found online at https://doi.org/10.1016/j.ncl.2022.03.015.

REFERENCES

1. Stone JL, Hughes JR. Early history of electroencephalography and establishment of the American Clinical Neurophysiology Society. J Clin Neurophysiol 2013;30:28–44.
2. Hill CE, Blank LJ, Thibault D, et al. Continuous EEG is associated with favorable hospitalization outcomes for critically ill patients. Neurology 2019;92:e9–18.
3. Claassen J, Mayer SA, Kowalski RG, et al. Detection of electrographic seizures with continuous EEG monitoring in critically ill patients. Neurology 2004;62:1743–8.
4. Varelas PN, Spanaki MV, Mirski MA. Seizures and the neurosurgical intensive care unit. Neurosurg Clin N Am 2013;24:393–406.
5. Ruiz AR, Vlachy J, Lee JW, et al. Association of periodic and rhythmic electroencephalographic patterns with seizures in critically ill patients. JAMA Neurol 2017;74:181–8.

6. Young GB, Jordan KG, Doig GS. An assessment of nonconvulsive seizures in the intensive care unit using continuous EEG monitoring: an investigation of variables associated with mortality. Neurology 1996;47:83–9.

7. Claassen J, Perotte A, Albers D, et al. Nonconvulsive seizures after subarachnoid hemorrhage: multimodal detection and outcomes. Ann Neurol 2013;74:53–64.

8. Wat R, Mammi M, Paredes J, et al. The effectiveness of antiepileptic medications as prophylaxis of early seizure in patients with traumatic brain injury compared with placebo or no treatment: a systematic review and meta-analysis. World Neurosurg 2019;122:433–40.

9. Naidech AM, Beaumont J, Muldoon K, et al. Prophylactic seizure medication and health-related quality of life after intracerebral hemorrhage. Crit Care Med 2018; 46:1480–5.

10. Jones FJS, Sanches PR, Smith JR, et al. Seizure Prophylaxis After Spontaneous Intracerebral Hemorrhage. JAMA Neurol 2021;78:1128–36.

11. Hirsch L, Fong MW, Leitinger M, et al. American Clinical Neurophysiology Society's Standardized Critical Care EEG Terminology: 2021 Version.

12. Struck AF, Tabaeizadeh M, Schmitt SE, et al. Assessment of the validity of the 2HELPS2B score for inpatient seizure risk prediction. JAMA neurology. American Medical Association; 2020. p. 77 500–507.

13. Struck AF, Westover MB, Hall LT, et al. Metabolic correlates of the Ictal-Interictal Continuum: FDG-PET During Continuous EEG. Neurocrit Care 2016;24:324–31.

14. Vespa PM, McArthur DL, Xu Y, et al. Nonconvulsive seizures after traumatic brain injury are associated with hippocampal atrophy. Neurology 2010;75:792–8.

15. Witsch J, Frey HP, Schmidt JM, et al. Electroencephalographic Periodic Discharges and Frequency-Dependent Brain Tissue Hypoxia in Acute Brain Injury. JAMA Neurol 2017;74:301–9.

16. Payne ET, Zhao XY, Frndova H, et al. Seizure burden is independently associated with short term outcome in critically ill children. Brain 2014;137:1429–38.

17. Westover MB, Shafi MM, Bianchi MT, et al. The probability of seizures during EEG monitoring in critically ill adults. Clin Neurophysiol 2015;126:463–71.

18. De Marchis GM, Pugin D, Meyers E, et al. Seizure burden in subarachnoid hemorrhage associated with functional and cognitive outcome. Neurology 2016;86: 253–60.

19. Swisher CB, Shah D, Sinha SR, et al. Baseline EEG pattern on continuous ICU EEG monitoring and incidence of seizures. J Clin Neurophysiol 2015;32:147–51.

20. O'Connor KL, Westover MB, Philips MT, et al. High risk for seizures following subarachnoid hemorrhage regardless of referral bias. Neurocrit Care 2014;21: 476–82.

21. Carrera E, Claassen J, Oddo M, et al. Continuous electroencephalographic monitoring in critically ill patients with central nervous system infections. Arch Neurol 2008;65:1612–8.

22. Viarasilpa T, Panyavachiraporn N, Osman G, et al. Electrographic Seizures in Patients with Acute Encephalitis. Neurocrit Care 2019;30:207–15.

23. Newey CR, Kinzy TG, Punia V, et al. Continuous Electroencephalography in the Critically Ill: Clinical and Continuous Electroencephalography Markers for Targeted Monitoring. J Clin Neurophysiol 2018;35:325–31.

24. Gilmore EJ, Gaspard N, Choi HA, et al. Acute brain failure in severe sepsis: a prospective study in the medical intensive care unit utilizing continuous EEG monitoring. Intensive Care Med 2015;41:686–94.

25. Crepeau AZ, Fugate JE, Mandrekar J, et al. Value analysis of continuous EEG in patients during therapeutic hypothermia after cardiac arrest. Resuscitation 2014; 85:785–9.

26. Mani R, Schmitt SE, Mazer M, et al. The frequency and timing of epileptiform activity on continuous electroencephalogram in comatose post-cardiac arrest syndrome patients treated with therapeutic hypothermia. Resuscitation 2012;83: 840–7.

27. Lee H, Mizrahi MA, Hartings JA, et al. Continuous electroencephalography after moderate to severe traumatic brain injury. Crit Care Med 2019;47:574–82.

28. Vespa PM, O'Phelan K, Mirabelli J, et al. Acute seizures after intracerebral hemorrhage: a factor in progressive midline shift and outcome. Neurology 2003;60: 1441–6.

29. Claassen J, Jetté N, Chum F, et al. Electrographic seizures and periodic discharges after intracerebral hemorrhage. Neurology 2007;69:1356–65.

30. DeLorenzo RJ, Waterhouse EJ, Towne AR, et al. Persistent nonconvulsive status epilepticus after the control of convulsive status epilepticus. Epilepsia 1998;39: 833–40.

31. Alvarez V, Drislane FW, Westover MB, et al. Characteristics and role in outcome prediction of continuous EEG after status epilepticus: A prospective observational cohort. Epilepsia 2015;56:933–41.

32. San-Juan OD, Chiappa KH, Costello DJ, et al. Periodic epileptiform discharges in hypoxic encephalopathy: BiPLEDs and GPEDs as a poor prognosis for survival. Seizure 2009;18:365–8.

33. Struck AF, Osman G, Rampal N, et al. Time-dependent risk of seizures in critically ill patients on continuous electroencephalogram. Ann Neurol 2017;82:177–85.

34. Moffet EW, Subramaniam T, Hirsch LJ, et al. Validation of the 2HELPS2B seizure risk score in acute brain injury patients. Neurocrit Care 2020;33:701–7.

35. Singla S, Garcia GE, Rovenolt GE, et al. Detecting seizures and epileptiform abnormalities in acute brain injury. Curr Neurol Neurosci Rep 2020;20:42.

36. Orta DSJ, Chiappa KH, Quiroz AZ, et al. Prognostic implications of periodic epileptiform discharges. Arch Neurol 2009;66:985–91.

37. Gaspard N, Manganas L, Rampal N, et al. Similarity of lateralized rhythmic delta activity to periodic lateralized epileptiform discharges in critically ill patients. JAMA Neurol 2013;70:1288–95.

38. Osman G, Rahangdale R, Britton JW, et al. Bilateral independent periodic discharges are associated with electrographic seizures and poor outcome: A case-control study. Clin Neurophysiol 2018;129:2284–9.

39. García-Morales I, García MT, Galán-Dávila L, et al. Periodic lateralized epileptiform discharges: etiology, clinical aspects, seizures, and evolution in 130 patients. J Clin Neurophysiol 2002;19:172–7.

40. Newey CR, Sahota P, Hantus S. Electrographic Features of Lateralized Periodic Discharges Stratify Risk in the Interictal-Ictal Continuum. J Clin Neurophysiol 2017;34:365–9.

41. Reiher J, Rivest J, Grand'Maison F, et al. Periodic lateralized epileptiform discharges with transitional rhythmic discharges: association with seizures. Electroencephalogr Clin Neurophysiol 1991;78:12–7.

42. Chong DJ, Hirsch LJ. Which EEG patterns warrant treatment in the critically ill? Reviewing the evidence for treatment of periodic epileptiform discharges and related patterns. J Clin Neurophysiol 2005;22:79–91.

43. Foreman B, Classen J, Abou Khaled K, et al. Generalized periodic discharges in the critically ill: a case-control study of 200 patients. Neurology 2012;79:1951–60.

44. Yoo JY, Marcuse LV, Fields MC, et al. Brief Potentially Ictal Rhythmic Discharges [B(I)RDs] in Noncritically Ill Adults. J Clin Neurophysiol 2017;34:222–9.

45. Struck AF, Ustun B, Ruiz AR, et al. Association of an electroencephalography-based risk score with seizure probability in hospitalized patients. JAMA Neurol 2017;74:1419–24.

46. Vespa PM, Miller C, McArthur D, et al. Nonconvulsive electrographic seizures after traumatic brain injury result in a delayed, prolonged increase in intracranial pressure and metabolic crisis. Crit Care Med 2007;35:2830–6.

47. Vespa P, Tubi M, Classen J, et al. Metabolic crisis occurs with seizures and periodic discharges after brain trauma. Ann Neurol 2016;79:579–90.

48. Szabo K, Poepel A, Pohlmann-Eden B, et al. Diffusion-weighted and perfusion MRI demonstrates parenchymal changes in complex partial status epilepticus. Brain 2005;128:1369–76.

49. Chatzikonstantinou A, Gass A, Förster A, et al. Features of acute DWI abnormalities related to status epilepticus. Epilepsy Res 2011;97:45–51.

50. DeGiorgio CM, Correale JD, Gott PS, et al. Serum neuron-specific enolase in human status epilepticus. Neurology 1995;45:1134–7.

51. DeGiorgio CM, Heck CN, Rabinowicz AL, et al. Serum neuron-specific enolase in the major subtypes of status epilepticus. Neurology 1999;52:746–9.

52. Hocker S, Nagarajan E, Rabinstein AA, et al. Progressive Brain Atrophy in Super-refractory Status Epilepticus. JAMA Neurol 2016;73:1201–7.

53. De Herdt V, Dumont F, Hénon H, et al. Early seizures in intracerebral hemorrhage: incidence, associated factors, and outcome. Neurology 2011;77:1794–800.

54. Rabinstein AA, Chung SY, Rudzinski LA, et al. Seizures after evacuation of subdural hematomas: incidence, risk factors, and functional impact. J Neurosurg 2010;112:455–60.

55. Herlopian A, Struck AF, Rosenthal E, et al. Neuroimaging correlates of periodic discharges. J Clin Neurophysiol 2018;35:279–94.

56. Subramaniam T, Jain A, Hall LT, et al. Lateralized periodic discharges frequency correlates with glucose metabolism. Neurology 2019;92:e670–4.

57. Venkatraman A, Khawaja A, Bag AK, et al. Perfusion MRI can impact treatment decision in ictal-interictal continuum. J Clin Neurophysiol 2017;34:e15–8.

58. Royter V, Paletz L, Waters MF. Stroke vs. status epilepticus. A case report utilizing CT perfusion. J Neurol Sci 2008;266:174–6.

59. Strambo D, Rey V, Rossetti AO, et al. Perfusion-CT imaging in epileptic seizures. J Neurol 2018;265:2972–9.

60. Claassen J, Hirsch LJ, Frontera JA, et al. Prognostic significance of continuous EEG monitoring in patients with poor-grade subarachnoid hemorrhage. Neurocrit Care 2006;4:103–12.

61. Tabaeizadeh M, Aboul Nour H, Shoukat M, et al. Burden of epileptiform activity predicts discharge neurologic outcomes in severe acute ischemic stroke. Neurocrit Care 2020;32:697–706.

62. Zafar SF, Postma EN, Biswal S, et al. Effect of epileptiform abnormality burden on neurologic outcome and antiepileptic drug management after subarachnoid hemorrhage. Clin Neurophysiol 2018;129:2219–27.

63. Zafar SF, Rosenthal ES, Jing J, et al. Automated annotation of epileptiform burden and its association with outcomes. Ann Neurol 2021;90:300–11.

64. la Fougère C, Rominger A, Förster S, et al. PET and SPECT in epilepsy: a critical review. Epilepsy Behav 2009;15:50–5.

65. Citerio G, Oddo M, Taccone FS. Recommendations for the use of multimodal monitoring in the neurointensive care unit. Curr Opin Crit Care 2015;21:113–9.

66. Bouzat P, Sala N, Payen J-F, et al. Beyond intracranial pressure: optimization of cerebral blood flow, oxygen, and substrate delivery after traumatic brain injury. Ann Intensive Care 2013;3:23.
67. Cloostermans MC, van Meulen FB, Eertman CJ, et al. Continuous electroencephalography monitoring for early prediction of neurological outcome in postanoxic patients after cardiac arrest: a prospective cohort study. Crit Care Med 2012; 40:2867–75.
68. Hofmeijer J, van Putten MJ. a. M. EEG in postanoxic coma: Prognostic and diagnostic value. Clin Neurophysiol 2016;127:2047–55.
69. Lee JW. EEG in the ICU: what should one treat, what not. Epileptologie 2012;29: 210–7.
70. Jirsch J, Hirsch LJ. Nonconvulsive seizures: developing a rational approach to the diagnosis and management in the critically ill population. Clin Neurophysiol 2007;118:1660–70.
71. Rossetti AO, Bromfield EB. Levetiracetam in the treatment of status epilepticus in adults: a study of 13 episodes. Eur Neurol 2005;54:34–8.
72. Kapinos G, Trinka E, Kaplan PW. Multimodal Approach to Decision to Treat Critically Ill Patients With Periodic or Rhythmic Patterns Using an Ictal-Interictal Continuum Spectral Severity Score. J Clin Neurophysiol 2018;35:314–24.
73. Topjian AA, Gutierrez-Colina AM, Sanchez SM, et al. Electrographic status epilepticus is associated with mortality and worse short-term outcome in critically ill children. Crit Care Med 2013;41:215–23.
74. Fung FW, Wang Z, Parikh DS, et al. Electrographic Seizures and Outcome in Critically Ill Children. Neurology. 2021 Apr 23;10.1212/WNL.0000000000012032.

Rescue Treatments for Seizure Clusters

Robert J. Kotloski, MD, PhD[a,b,]*, Barry E. Gidal, PharmD[c]

KEYWORDS

- Seizure cluster • Acute repetitive seizure • Epilepsy • Benzodiazepines
- Antiseizure medication

KEY POINTS

- For individuals with epilepsy who continue to have seizures, nearly half experience seizure clusters. Seizure clusters cause harm, worsen quality of life, and increase usage of the health care system.
- FDA-approved treatments are available for seizure clusters, including rectal (Diastat) and intranasal (Nayzilam, Valtoco) formulations of benzodiazepines.
- A seizure action plan (SAP) is a written document that provides individuals with epilepsy, caregivers, and health care providers with a predetermined response after a seizure.
- SAPs may involve recording/reporting the seizure, use of rescue medications, and/or seek immediate medical attention.

INTRODUCTION

Epilepsy is a prevalent condition with more than half of those affected continuing to have seizures.[1] For individuals with persistent seizures, nearly half experience seizure clusters (defined as ≥3 seizures within 24 h).[2] Seizure clusters cause additional worsening of the quality of life for those with epilepsy and their caregivers,[3] and lead to increased health care utilization, emergencydepartment visits, and hospitalizations.[2] As compared with those with epilepsy without clusters (who themselves have a significantly increased risk over the general population), seizure clusters are associated with a 3.5-fold increase in risk of premature death, and a 2.5-fold increase in the risk of sudden unexplained death in epilepsy (SUDEP).[4] Given the clinical need, seizure rescue treatments have been developed to ameliorate the risks of repeated and/or prolonged seizures and the potential to progress to status epilepticus, as well as to use additional

---

[a] Department of Neurology, University of Wisconsin School of Medicine and Public Health, 1685 Highland Avenue, Madison, WI 53705-2281, USA; [b] Department of Neurology, William S Middleton Memorial Veterans Hospital, 2500 Overlook Ter, Madison, WI, 53705, USA; [c] University of Wisconsin School of Pharmacy, 777 Highland Avenue, Madison, WI 53705, USA
* Corresponding author. Department of Neurology, University of Wisconsin School of Medicine and Public Health, 1685 Highland Avenue, Madison, WI 53705.
E-mail address: kotloski@neurology.wisc.edu

Neurol Clin 40 (2022) 927–937
https://doi.org/10.1016/j.ncl.2022.03.016
0733-8619/22/© 2022 Elsevier Inc. All rights reserved.

antiseizure treatment when future seizures can be anticipated.[2,5,6] Recently approved seizure rescue treatments are significant improvements toward the goal of a therapy which is easy and safe to administer, effective at small doses with a large therapeutic index, and exhibits rapid onset of action that can be sustained for several hours.[7]

Seizure clusters exist within the duration spectrum for ictal activity, which ranges from isolated seizures lasting seconds to refractory status epilepticus lasting days or longer. Within this spectrum, there is no clear consensus for a definition of seizure clusters, though more than 2 to 3 seizures in a day or with an inter-seizure interval of less than 6 to 8 hours are often used. The mechanisms underlying the clustering of seizures are generally unknown, though hormonal changes during the menstrual cycle can result in seizure clustering in catamenial epilepsy.[8] Seizure clusters are more likely to occur with frontal and temporal epilepsy, posttraumatic epilepsy, and intractable epilepsy of long duration.[9,10] Finally, with the advent of responsive neurostimulation treatments for epilepsy, chronic recordings of brain activity are now available and may provide new insights into seizure clustering.[11]

Seizure rescue treatments face several challenges. As seizure rescue treatments are intended to be used during a seizure or early in the postictal period, alterations in mental status often preclude swallowing oral medications. Before FDA approval of diazepam rectal gel, caregivers were offered parenteral diazepam to be used for outpatient rectal administration. However, this approach involved risks of dosing errors and safety concerns as the formulation was not intended for use by nonmedical caregivers in an outpatient setting.[12,13] The efficacy and safety of diazepam rectal gel for the treatment of seizure clusters was established by pivotal randomized, double-blind, placebo-controlled clinical trials which demonstrated significant reduction in seizure frequency along with acceptable safety and tolerability.[12,13] Somnolence was the most common adverse event (AE), seen in 13% to 16% of patients, and importantly respiratory depression was not seen following treatment.[12,13] However, despite the ability to improve outcomes, including decreasing risk of progression to prolonged seizures and potential avoidance of emergency room admissions, rescue therapies designed for use by nonmedical caregivers have been underused, particularly in the adult population.[2,14] After approval of diazepam rectal gel but before the approval of nasal formulations, only 43.5% of those with seizure clusters had received a benzodiazepine rescue medication.[15] Social and institutional constraints, and at least perceptions regarding willingness to receive rectal administration, were likely significant barriers to the use of diazepam rectal gel[14,16]

While diazepam rectal gel provides a safe and effective option for the treatment of seizure clusters, it also has significant limitations which hampered use. Therefore, intranasal formulations were developed as an alternative, despite the significant challenges related to pharmacology, solubility, and bioavailability.[17] Notwithstanding these difficulties, intranasal delivery has several advantages including the microvilli and elaborate vascular network of the nasal cavity which are ideal for drug absorption.[17] Furthermore intranasal delivery avoids first-pass metabolism and can reduce pharmacokinetic variability associated with food consumption seen with oral or rectal diazepam.[18,19] Finally, a nasal spray device allows for self-administration, a significant advancement over rectal diazepam.[20]

In addition to these FDA-approved options, agents using other routes of administration (eg, oral or buccal benzodiazepines) are used off-label for nonmedical caregiver use. In a 2017 study, while FDA-approved diazepam rectal gel was used by 7.8% of those with seizure clusters, off-label benzodiazepine use was common, with oral lorazepam used most frequently (28.9%), followed by oral diazepam (7.0%), midazolam formulated for injection given intranasally via an atomizer (6.9%), and oral clonazepam

(5.4%).[21] Lorazepam, tablets or liquid Intensol, and clonazepam orally disintegrating tablets may have been prescribed to adolescents and adults to minimize social concerns when the only approved treatment was rectal diazepam.[2] However, these approaches have not been formally established to be effective for the treatment of seizure clusters in large, well-designed clinical trials. Moreover, oral benzodiazepines possess other challenges, such as difficulty swallowing and the potential for aspiration.[5]

Benzodiazepine Pharmacology: Mechanisms of Action & Relevance to Seizures

γ-Aminobutyric acid subtype A ($GABA_A$) receptors are heteropentameric chloride channels with 8 identified subunits (α, β, γ, δ, ε, π, θ, and ρ). $GABA_A$ receptor activation leads to increased chloride conductivity, with chloride influx leading to the hyperpolarization of the neuronal cell membrane and reduction in excitability. The specific physiologic functioning of the $GABA_A$ receptor is dependent on subunit subtypes forming the channel.[22] For instance, the type of $\gamma 2$ isoform expressed (long [$\gamma 2L$] vs short [$\gamma 2S$] forms) and its modifications (eg, phosphorylation status) can modulate $GABA_A$ receptor currents, synaptic clustering and dispersion, internalization, trafficking, and degradation.[23] Furthermore, repetitive seizures can modify the physiologic function of $GABA_A$ receptors through altered subunit localization and trafficking, as well as through disruptions to intracellular chloride homeostasis.[24–26]

Benzodiazepines are positive allosteric modulators of $GABA_A$ receptors and are used therapeutically to attenuate the excessive neuronal excitation that occurs during a seizure. Benzodiazepine-induced modulation of $GABA_A$ can occur with receptors containing $\alpha 1$, $\alpha 2$, $\alpha 3$, or $\alpha 5$ subunits, along with β and $\gamma 2$ subunits,[27] with specific effects mediated through particular subunits. For example, anxiolytic-like effects are mediated through $GABA_A$ receptors that contain $\alpha 2$, $\alpha 3$, and/or $\alpha 5$ subunits but not $\alpha 1$ subunits.[28] In contrast, locomotor function is attenuated and sedation induced through $GABA_A$ receptor activation when the $\alpha 1$ subunit is present in the receptor complex, while the activation of $\alpha 2$, $\alpha 3$, and/or $\alpha 5$ does not affect locomotor function or sedation.

The antiseizure mechanism of action for benzodiazepines, although not fully elucidated, involves binding at the benzodiazepine site of the $GABA_A$ receptor and resultant potentiation of GABAergic neurotransmission.[29] Several factors are known to influence the central nervous system effects of benzodiazepines, including dosing, route of administration, and the presence or absence of other therapies.[30–33] Evidence from animal and human studies demonstrate that epilepsy and seizures provoke changes in $GABA_A$ receptor composition and function, which may contribute to tolerance or adverse effects to treatment.[29] Benzodiazepine administration over time has also been associated with reductions in $GABA_A$ receptor subunit expression in animal models,[34,35] which could contribute to tolerance. Further, evidence suggests that tolerance to intermittent benzodiazepine exposure in patients with seizure clusters is infrequent.[36–38]

Benzodiazepine Formulations

Pharmacokinetic and pharmacodynamic considerations

The different routes of administration for rescue therapy have potential advantages and disadvantages.[17] The recently approved intranasal formulations offer the opportunity for rapid administration relative to intravenous (IV) and rectal formulations, as well as improved patient/caregiver satisfaction and resultant usage relative to rectal formulations, without compromising efficacy or safety.[39] The approved intranasal midazolam formulation uses several organic solvents to increase the solubility of midazolam while maintaining the pH in the range of 5 to 9^{32}. However, organic solvents may cause nasal irritation.[18,40] The approved diazepam nasal spray formulation contains DDM (Intravail A3; 0.25% weight/volume concentration) to enhance nasal absorption and vitamin E as a solvent.[17]

The timing for the onset of action of rescue therapies for seizure clusters may be determined by drug plasma level associated with a reduction in spike counts,[41] rather than time to maximum plasma concentration (t_{max}) or other pharmacokinetic parameters. Early efforts to develop a rectal formulation of diazepam had detected a reduction in spike-wave activity after 10 to 20 minutes (per electroencephalogram [EEG]) despite peak serum levels being achieved after 15 to 90 minutes, suggesting that EEG response occurs much earlier than t_{max}.[42] A subsequent study of oral diazepam conducted in healthy volunteers noted a similar response, with EEG effects (fraction of total EEG amplitude within 13–31 Hz) detected 15 minutes following administration, whereas t_{max} occurred approximately 1 hour after administration.[43] Although brain electrical activity can exhibit responsiveness to relatively low plasma concentrations of benzodiazepines before achieving maximal concentrations, the clinical efficacy of low concentrations to terminate or prevent seizures is difficult to characterize owing to patient heterogeneity. Plasma concentrations of diazepam in excess of 200 ng/mL have been associated with successful termination of seizure clusters (serial seizures) in adult patients,[44] as well as seizures and malaria-induced convulsions in pediatric patients.[45,46]

In a phase 1 open-label crossover study of an intranasal midazolam formulation dosed at 2.5, 5.0, or 7.5 mg compared with midazolam IV solution (given intranasally or intravenously) in 25 healthy adults, t_{max} was rapid with midazolam nasal spray at 10 to 12 minutes across the 3 doses, with maximum plasma concentration (C_{max}) values of 59, 73, and 93 ng/mL for the 2.5-, 5.0-, and 7.5-mg doses, respectively.[47] The pharmacokinetics of the approved diazepam nasal spray have been assessed across several studies. In a randomized phase 1 crossover study comparing diazepam nasal spray and an intranasal suspension versus IV diazepam in 24 healthy adults,[48] pharmacokinetic parameters for the solution included C_{max} of 272 ng/mL and t_{max} of 1.5 hours. Similarly, in a dose-ranging crossover pharmacokinetic study of single nasal spray doses (5, 10, and 20 mg) and a 2-dose regimen (2 × 10 mg, 4 hours apart) of diazepam nasal spray in 33 healthy adults,[49] single-dose median t_{max} was 1.4 to 1.5 hours and mean C_{max} values were 85.6, 133.6, and 235.3 ng/mL, respectively, for the 5-, 10-, and 20-mg doses. When the bioavailability and safety of diazepam nasal spray (15 or 20 mg) were compared with those for diazepam rectal gel and oral diazepam (reference formulation) in 48 healthy adults,[33] median t_{max} was 1.25 hours for both doses of diazepam nasal spray. Geometric mean C_{max} values were 226 and 186 ng/mL, respectively, for diazepam nasal spray at 15- and 20-mg doses.

Currently Approved Benzodiazepine Rescue Formulations

Clinical effectiveness

Currently, three rescue therapies are approved by the US Food and Drug Administration (FDA) for the acute treatment of intermittent, stereotypic episodes of frequent seizure activity (ie, seizure clusters, acute repetitive seizures) that are distinct from the usual seizure pattern for individuals with epilepsy (**Table 1**).[30–32] In 1997 diazepam rectal gel (Diastat) was approved for individuals ≥2 years of age,[30] in May 2019 midazolam nasal spray (Nayzilam) was approved for individuals aged ≥12 years,[32] and in January 2020 diazepam nasal spray (Valtoco) was approved for individuals aged ≥6 years.[31]

Diazepam rectal gel. Diazepam rectal gel (Diastat, Bausch Health US, LLC) was the first rescue therapy approved by the FDA for acute treatment of seizure clusters in patients

Table 1
Rescue therapies for the acute treatment of intermittent, stereotypic episodes of frequent seizure activity

Drug	Delievery Method	FDA-Approved Products	Dosing	Pharmacokinetics
Diazepam	rectal	• Diastat (Bausch Health US) • generic formulations	• Age 2–5 y (0.5 mg/kg) • Age 6–11 y (0.3 mg/kg) • Age 12+ years (0.2 mg/kg) • Round to nearest 2.5 mg increment. • Maximum dose 20 mg.	• 1.5 h to peak • Half-life 45–46 h, 71–99 h for desmethyldiazepam • Half-life may be prolonged in the elderly • No adjustment for renal or hepatic impairment
Midazolam	nasal	• Nayzilam (UCB)	• Age 12+ years all weights, 5 mg	• 10–12 min to peak serum concentration • Half-life 2.1–6.2 h • No adjustment for renal or hepatic impairment
Diazepam	nasal	• Valtoco (Neurelis)	• Age 6–11 y (0.3 mg/kg) • Age 12+ years (0.2 mg/kg) • Round to nearest 5 mg increment. • Maximum dose 20 mg. • Administered using 2 sprayers from a single blister pack (ie, 2 sprays of 7.5 mg for 15 mg total dose or 2 sprays of 10 mg for 20 mg total dose; one in each nostril).	• 1.5 h to peak • Half-life ~49 h, 71–99 h for desmethyldiazepam • No adjustment for renal or hepatic impairment

with epilepsy ≥2 years of age.[30] This formulation is packaged as a prefilled, unit-dose delivery system. Doses range from 5 to 20 mg based on age and weight, with target doses of 0.5 mg/kg (patients aged 2–5 years), 0.3 mg/kg (6–11 years), and 0.2 mg/kg (≥12 years). If needed, a second dose can be administered after 4 hours.

Two randomized, double-blind, placebo-controlled studies, including a total of 239 treated patients, showed reduced seizure frequency per hour ($P < 0.001$) with diazepam rectal gel. One study discontinued treatment owing to an AE for 2 patients each in the diazepam (lethargy, rash) and placebo (sedation, seizure) groups,[13] whereas the other study reported that no patients discontinued treatment owing to an AE.[12] No cases of respiratory depression were reported in either study.

In a long-term safety study (N = 149 treated; 48.3% were ≤11 years of age), 1578 seizure clusters were treated and approximately 48% of patients participated for ≥2 years.[50] In 23% of treated seizure clusters, further seizures occurred within 12 hours of dosing. There was limited provision for the second dose in this study. Somnolence was the most common AE (occurred in 17% of patients and was considered treatment related in 9% of patients), but the investigators noted that it was difficult to distinguish from postictal somnolence. No respiratory compromise or serious

AEs were attributed to diazepam rectal gel, and 3 patients (2%) withdrew owing to AEs possibly related to treatment.[50,51] When compared with treatment before enrollment in the study, caregivers and investigators were satisfied with diazepam rectal gel treatment at 12- and 24-month follow-up visits.[50] However, despite the efficacy and safety of this rectal formulation, this route of administration is associated with social considerations, and alternative routes of administration were an unmet need, particularly for adolescents and adults.[7]

Midazolam nasal spray. Midazolam nasal spray (Nayzilam, UCB, Inc.) is approved by the FDA for the treatment of seizure clusters in patients aged $\geq$12 years.[32] The drug is packaged in a single-use sprayer with a premeasured 5-mg dose (used for patients of all ages and weights). If needed to control an ongoing cluster, the second dose of midazolam nasal spray can be administered 10 minutes after the initial dose. For patients at risk of respiratory depression, a test dose, given under the supervision of a health care professional, is recommended.

In a double-blind study, 292 patients received an open-label test dose (total of 10 mg of midazolam nasal spray) to assess safety, and 262 patients were subsequently randomized to receive midazolam or placebo, with 201 proceeding with the study drug.[52] During the randomized comparative phase, the primary, composite endpoint of seizure termination within 10 minutes of dosing and no further seizures between 10 minutes and 6 hours after treatment was significantly higher in the active drug group compared with placebo (53.7% vs 34.4%; P = 0.0109). Thirteen patients discontinued the test dose phase owing to a drug-related treatment-emergent AE (8 owing to sedation-type AEs), including 3 patients with serious AEs. Two of these 3 patients had clinically meaningful respiratory depression. During the comparative phase, no patients discontinued owing to an AE, and none had respiratory depression.

In the long-term safety study (N = 161 treated, 5.0% were <18 years of age), 1998 seizure clusters were treated across a median of 16.8 months.[38] Second doses were used in 38.5% of clusters within 6 hours of the first dose. Fifty-seven patients (35.4%) experienced $\geq$1 treatment-related AE over the course of the trial ($\geq$12 months). The most common AEs were nasal discomfort (12.4%) and somnolence (9.3%), and there were no reports of respiratory depression. Four patients (2.5%) experienced $\geq$1 serious AE that was categorized as potentially treatment related (all classified as "unlikely related"), and 2 patients (1.2%) discontinued owing to treatment-related AEs (1 case each of nasal discomfort and somnolence, both nonserious).[38] Patient satisfaction and anxiety as assessed with questionnaires improved over time in patients who received midazolam nasal spray.[53]

Diazepam nasal spray. Diazepam nasal spray (Valtoco, Neurala, Inc.) is approved by the FDA for the treatment of seizure clusters in patients aged $\geq$6 years.[31] Diazepam nasal spray is provided in premeasured, single-use sprayers. Doses range from 5 to 20 mg based on patient age and weight, with target doses of 0.3 mg/kg for patients 6 to 11 years of age and 0.2 mg/kg for patients $\geq$12 years of age.[31] The 15- and 20-mg doses both require the use of 2 sprayers in a single blister pack to provide the full dose (ie, 2 sprays of 7.5 or 10 mg; 1 in each nostril). A second dose may be administered if needed at least 4 hours after the first dose, which would require a new blister pack. The formulation includes benzyl alcohol, dehydrated alcohol, n-dodecyl beta-D-maltoside (DDM), and vitamin E. The excipient DDM increases absorption across mucosa.[54] Vitamin E is used to promote the nonaqueous solubility of diazepam.[55]

In a pharmacokinetic study, intra-patient variability was found to be lower for patients receiving diazepam nasal spray compared with diazepam rectal gel (%

geometric coefficient of variation of area under the curve, 42% to 66% compared with 87% to 172%).[33] Respiratory depression was not reported in a pharmacokinetic study of patients with epilepsy who were treated with diazepam nasal spray, nor was it observed in previous studies of healthy subjects.[55]

The long-term safety study for diazepam nasal spray was recently published.[56] A total of 163 patients (27.6% $\leq$ 12 years) were treated for 3853 seizure clusters, and a second dose was used for 12.6% of clusters within 24 hours of the first dose. Thirty patients (18.4%) experienced $\geq$1 treatment-related AE; among these, treatment-related nasal discomfort occurred in 6.1% of patients, whereas treatment-related somnolence occurred in 1.8% of patients. No patients withdrew owing to a treatment-related AE, there were no treatment-related serious AEs, and no cases of respiratory depression were observed.[56] Analyses in subpopulations of this study based on the frequency of use,[57] use of concomitant benzodiazepines,[58] and history or concomitant treatment of seasonal allergies or rhinitis[59] reported results similar to those reported in the overall study. A survey conducted as part of the study found that patients and caregivers were satisfied with diazepam nasal spray and were more comfortable using it in public situations compared with diazepam rectal gel, and some patients (as young as 11 years) reported self-administration of diazepam nasal spray.[20]

Future rescue therapies

In addition to rectal and most recently intranasal rescue therapies, the development of benzodiazepine formulations delivered via alternative routes continues. A rapidly dissolving, buccal diazepam film that can be applied to the inner cheek is in late-stage development (Libervant, Aquestive Therapeutics).[60] This buccal formulation appears well-tolerated and displays a favorable pharmacokinetic profile.

Inhaled alprazolam (Staccato, UCB) has also demonstrated promise in early clinical trials. In a model using photosensitive epilepsy, inhaled alprazolam reduced epileptiform activity recorded as soon as 2 minutes following inhalation,[61] which is similar to IV administration of benzodiazepines. This suggests that this formulation could have utility in aborting an ongoing seizure.[62] Of note, alprazolam is approved for use in anxiety disorders but has no current epilepsy indication.

SUMMARY

For individuals with epilepsy who continue to have seizures, nearly half experience seizure clusters.[2] Seizure clusters worsen the quality of life for individuals with epilepsy and their caregivers, increase health care utilization, emergencydepartment visits, and hospitalizations.[2,3] FDA-approved treatments, in the form of benzodiazepines delivered rectally or nasally, are available to treat seizure clusters. While all current rescue therapies demonstrate clinical efficacy, overall effectiveness will be dependent not only on the pharmacology of the active drug, but the ease (and ultimately, acceptability) of drug delivery. No doubt, the recent development of alternatives to rectal administration has advanced our armamentarium.

CLINICS CARE POINTS

- Treatments for seizure clusters are available, with newly approved nasal delivery options.
- Treatment of seizure clusters is important to avoid the harm of prolonged and/or repeated seizures.

- Every individual with epilepsy and caregivers for individuals with epilepsy should know how to respond to a seizure. A seizure action plan (SAP) is an excellent option for formalizing this response.

DISCLOSURE

R.J. Kotloski- Nothing to Disclose; B.E. Gidal – Speaking/Consulting: Eisai, Greenwich, SK Life Sciences, Aquestive, UCB, Neurelis; Dr B.E. Gidal is a consultant for Aquestive, Eisai Inc., Greenwich, Neurelis, Inc. Dr Kotloski has no conflicts of interest to disclose.

ETHICAL PUBLICATION STATEMENT

The authors confirm that they have read the Journal's position on issues involved in ethical publication and affirm that this report is consistent with those guidelines.

REFERENCES

1. Zack MM, Kobau R. Morbidity and mortality weekly report national and state estimates of the numbers of adults and children with active epilepsy-United States. Morb Mortal Wkly Rep 2015;66(31):821–5.
2. Jafarpour S, Hirsch LJ, Gaínza-Lein M, et al. Seizure cluster: definition, prevalence, consequences, and management. Seizure 2019;68:9–15.
3. Penovich PE, Buelow J, Steinberg K, et al. Burden of seizure clusters on patients with epilepsy and caregivers: survey of patient, caregiver, and clinician perspectives. Neurologist 2017;22(6):207–14.
4. Sillanpää M, Schmidt D. Seizure clustering during drug treatment affects seizure outcome and mortality of childhood-onset epilepsy. Brain 2008;131(Pt 4):938–44.
5. Gidal B, Klein P, Hirsch LJ. Seizure clusters, rescue treatments, seizure action plans: unmet needs and emerging formulations. Epilepsy Behav 2020;112: 107391.
6. Haut SR, Shinnar S, Moshe SL, et al. The association between seizure clustering and convulsive status epilepticus in patients with intractable complex partial seizures. Epilepsia 1999;40(12):1832–4.
7. Agarwal SK, Cloyd JC. Development of benzodiazepines for out-of-hospital management of seizure emergencies. Neurol Clin Pract 2015;5(1):80–5.
8. Herzog AG. Catamenial epilepsy: update on prevalence, pathophysiology and treatment from the findings of the NIH progesterone treatment trial. Seizure 2015;28:18–25.
9. Haut SR. Seizure clusters: characteristics and treatment. Curr Opin Neurol 2015; 28(2):143–50.
10. Ferastraoaru V, Schulze-Bonhage A, Lipton RB, et al. Termination of seizure clusters is related to the duration of focal seizures. Epilepsia 2016;57(6):889–95.
11. Karoly PJ, Nurse ES, Freestone DR, et al. Bursts of seizures in long-term recordings of human focal epilepsy. Epilepsia 2017;58(3):363–72.
12. Cereghino JJ, Mitchell WG, Murphy J, et al. Treating repetitive seizures with a rectal diazepam formulation: a randomized study. Neurology 1998;51(5): 1274–82.
13. Dreifuss FE, Rosman NP, Cloyd JC, et al. A comparison of rectal diazepam gel and placebo for acute repetitive seizures. N Engl J Med 1998;338(26):1869–75.

14. Tatum WO. Adult patient perceptions of emergency rectal medications for refractory seizures. Epilepsy Behav 2002;3(6):535–8.
15. Chen B, Choi H, Hirsch LJ, et al. Prevalence and risk factors of seizure clusters in adult patients with epilepsy. Epilepsy Res 2017;133:98–102.
16. Terry D, Paolicchi J, Karn M. Acceptance of the use of diazepam rectal gel in school and day care settings. J Child Neurol 2007;22(9):1135–8.
17. Cloyd J, Haut S, Carrazana E, et al. Overcoming the challenges of developing an intranasal diazepam rescue therapy for the treatment of seizure clusters. Epilepsia 2021;62(4):846–56.
18. Ivaturi VD, Riss JR, Kriel RL, et al. Bioavailability and tolerability of intranasal diazepam in healthy adult volunteers. Epilepsy Res 2009;84(2–3):120–6.
19. Yamazaki A, Kumagai Y, Fujita T, et al. Different effects of light food on pharmacokinetics and pharmacodynamics of three benzodiazepines, quazepam, nitrazepam and diazepam. J Clin Pharm Ther 2007;32(1):31–9.
20. Penovich P, Wheless JW, Hogan RE, et al. Examining the patient and caregiver experience with diazepam nasal spray for seizure clusters: results from an exit survey of a phase 3, open-label, repeat-dose safety study. Epilepsy Behav 2021;121(Pt A):108013.
21. Chen C, Lee DS, Hie SL. The impact of pharmacist's counseling on pediatric patients' caregiver's knowledge on epilepsy and its treatment in a tertiary hospital. Int J Clin Pharm 2013;35(5):829–34.
22. Ghit A, Assal D, Al-Shami AS, et al. GABAA receptors: structure, function, pharmacology, and related disorders. J Genet Eng Biotechnol 2021;19(1):123.
23. Lorenz-Guertin JM, Bambino MJ, Jacob TC. gamma2 GABAAR trafficking and the consequences of human genetic variation. Front Cell Neurosci 2018;12:265.
24. Goodkin HP, Joshi S, Mtchedlishvili Z, et al. Subunit-specific trafficking of GABAA receptors during status epilepticus. J Neurosci 2008;28(10):2527–38.
25. Kapur J, Coulter DA. Experimental status epilepticus alters gamma-aminobutyric acid type A receptor function in CA1 pyramidal neurons. Ann Neurol 1995;38(6):893–900.
26. Naylor DE, Liu H, Wasterlain CG. Trafficking of GABAA receptors, loss of inhibition, and a mechanism for pharmacoresistance in status epilepticus. J Neurosci 2005;25(34):7724–33.
27. Mohler H. GABAA receptor diversity and pharmacology. Cell Tissue Res 2006;326(2):505–16.
28. Rowlett JK, Platt DM, Lelas S, et al. Different GABAA receptor subtypes mediate the anxiolytic, abuse-related, and motor effects of benzodiazepine-like drugs in primates. Proc Natl Acad Sci U S A 2005;102(3):915–20.
29. Greenfield LJ Jr. Molecular mechanisms of antiseizure drug activity at GABAA receptors. Seizure 2013;22(8):589–600.
30. Bausch Health US L, Diastat® C-IV. diazepam rectal gel [Internet]. 2021. 2021. Available at. https://www.bauschhealth.com/Portals/25/Pdf/PI/Diastat-PI.pdf.
31. Neurelis Inc. Valtoco. diazepam nasal spray [Internet]. 2021. 2021. Available at. https://www.valtoco.com/sites/default/files/Prescribing_Information.pdf.
32. UCB Inc, NAYZILAM®. midazolam nasal spray [Internet]. 2021. 2021. Available at. https://www.ucb-usa.com/_up/ucb_usa_com_kopie/documents/Nayzilam_PI.pdf.
33. Hogan RE, Gidal BE, Koplowitz B, et al. Bioavailability and safety of diazepam intranasal solution compared to oral and rectal diazepam in healthy volunteers. Epilepsia 2020;61(3):455–64.

34. Chen S, Huang X, Zeng XJ, et al. Benzodiazepine-mediated regulation of alpha1, alpha2, beta1-3 and gamma2 GABAA receptor subunit proteins in the rat brain hippocampus and cortex. Neuroscience 1999;93(1):33–44.

35. Kang I, Miller LG. Decreased GABAA receptor subunit mRNA concentrations following chronic lorazepam administration. Br J Pharmacol 1991;103(2):1285–7.

36. Cascino GD, Tarquinio D, Wheless JW, et al. Lack of observed tolerance to diazepam nasal spray (Valtoco®) after long-term rescue therapy in patients with epilepsy: interim results from a phase 3, open-label, repeat-dose safety study. Epilepsy Behav 2021;120:107983.

37. Mitchell WG. Status epilepticus and acute repetitive seizures in children, adolescents, and young adults: etiology, outcome, and treatment. Epilepsia 1996; 37(suppl 1):S74–80.

38. Wheless JW, Meng TC, Van Ess PJ, et al. Safety and efficacy of midazolam nasal spray in the outpatient treatment of patients with seizure clusters: an open-label extension trial. Epilepsia 2019;60(9):1809–19.

39. Haut SR, Seinfeld S, Pellock J. Benzodiazepine use in seizure emergencies: a systematic review. Epilepsy Behav 2016;63:109–17.

40. Ivaturi VD, Riss JR, Kriel RL, et al. Pharmacokinetics and tolerability of intranasal diazepam and midazolam in healthy adult volunteers. Acta Neurol Scand 2009; 120(5):353–7.

41. Dhir A, Rogawski MA. Determination of minimal steady-state plasma level of diazepam causing seizure threshold elevation in rats. Epilepsia 2018;59(5):935–44.

42. Milligan N, Dhillon S, Oxley J, et al. Absorption of diazepam from the rectum and its effect on interictal spikes in the EEG. Epilepsia 1982;23(3):323–31.

43. Friedman H, Greenblatt DJ, Peters GR, et al. Pharmacokinetics and pharmacodynamics of oral diazepam: effect of dose, plasma concentration, and time. Clin Pharmacol Ther 1992;52(2):139–50.

44. Remy C, Jourdil N, Villemain D, et al. Intrarectal diazepam in epileptic adults. Epilepsia 1992;33(2):353–8.

45. Agurell S, Berlin A, Ferngren H, et al. Plasma levels of diazepam after parenteral and rectal administration in children. Epilepsia 1975;16(2):277–83.

46. Ogutu BR, Newton CR, Crawley J, et al. Pharmacokinetics and anticonvulsant effects of diazepam in children with severe falciparum malaria and convulsions. Br J Clin Pharmacol 2002;53(1):49–57.

47. Bancke LL, Dworak HA, Rodvold KA, et al. Pharmacokinetics, pharmacodynamics, and safety of USL261, a midazolam formulation optimized for intranasal delivery, in a randomized study with healthy volunteers. Epilepsia 2015;56(11): 1723–31.

48. Agarwal SK, Kriel RL, Brundage RC, et al. A pilot study assessing the bioavailability and pharmacokinetics of diazepam after intranasal and intravenous administration in healthy volunteers. Epilepsy Res 2013;105(3):362–7.

49. Tanimoto S, Pesco Koplowitz L, Lowenthal RE, et al. Evaluation of pharmacokinetics and dose proportionality of diazepam after intranasal administration of NRL-1 to healthy volunteers. Clin Pharmacol Drug Dev 2020;9(6):719–27.

50. Mitchell WG, Conry JA, Crumrine PK, et al. An open-label study of repeated use of diazepam rectal gel (Diastat) for episodes of acute breakthrough seizures and clusters: safety, efficacy, and tolerance. North Am Diastat Group. Epilepsia. 1999; 40(11):1610–7.

51. Pellock JM. Safety of Diastat, a rectal gel formulation of diazepam for acute seizure treatment. Drug Saf 2004;27(6):383–92.

52. Detyniecki K, Van Ess PJ, Sequeira DJ, et al. Safety and efficacy of midazolam nasal spray in the outpatient treatment of patients with seizure clusters-a randomized, double-blind, placebo-controlled trial. Epilepsia 2019;60(9):1797–808.

53. Fakhoury T, Chen L, Bass A, et al. Treatment satisfaction, anxiety level, and confidence about traveling with midazolam nasal spray in patients with seizure clusters: phase III, open-label extension trial (1704). Neurology 2021;96(15 suppl): 1704.

54. Rabinowicz AL, Carrazana E, Maggio ET. Improvement of intranasal drug delivery with Intravail® alkylsaccharide excipient as a mucosal absorption enhancer aiding in the treatment of conditions of the central nervous system. Drugs in R&D 2021;21(4):361–9.

55. Hogan RE, Tarquinio D, Sperling MR, et al. Pharmacokinetics and safety of VALTOCO (NRL-1; diazepam nasal spray) in patients with epilepsy during seizure (ictal/peri-ictal) and nonseizure (interictal) conditions: a phase 1, open-label study. Epilepsia 2020;61(5):935–43.

56. Wheless JW, Miller I, Hogan RE, et al. Final results from a phase 3, long-term, open-label, repeat-dose safety study of diazepam nasal spray for seizure clusters in patients with epilepsy. Epilepsia 2021;62(10):2485–95.

57. Miller I, Wheless JW, Hogan RE, et al. Consistent safety and tolerability of Valtoco® (diazepam nasal spray) in relationship to usage frequency in patients with seizure clusters: interim results from a phase 3, long-term, open-label, repeat-dose safety study. Epilepsia Open 2021;6(3):504–12.

58. Segal EB, Tarquinio D, Miller I, et al. Evaluation of diazepam nasal spray in patients with epilepsy concomitantly using maintenance benzodiazepines: an interim subgroup analysis from a phase 3, long-term, open-label safety study. Epilepsia 2021;62(6):1442–50.

59. Vazquez B, Wheless J, Desai J, et al. Lack of observed impact of history or concomitant treatment of seasonal allergies or rhinitis on repeated doses of diazepam nasal spray administered per seizure episode in a day, safety, and tolerability: Interim results from a phase 3, open-label, 12-month repeat-dose safety study. Epilepsy Behav 2021;118:107898.

60. Seinfeld S, Gelfand MA, Heller AH, et al. Safety and tolerability associated with chronic intermittent use of diazepam buccal film in adult, adolescent, and pediatric patients with epilepsy. Epilepsia 2020;61(11):2426–34.

61. French JA, Wechsler R, Gelfand MA, et al. Inhaled alprazolam rapidly suppresses epileptic activity in photosensitive participants. Epilepsia 2019;60(8): 1602–9.

62. Lahat E, Goldman M, Barr J, et al. Comparison of intranasal midazolam with intravenous diazepam for treating febrile seizures in children: prospective randomised study. BMJ 2000;321(7253):83–6.

UNITED STATES POSTAL SERVICE®

Statement of Ownership, Management, and Circulation
(All Periodicals Publications Except Requester Publications)

1. Publication Title	2. Publication Number	3. Filing Date
NEUROLOGIC CLINICS	000 – 712	9/18/2022

4. Issue Frequency	5. Number of Issues Published Annually	6. Annual Subscription Price
FEB, MAY, AUG, NOV	4	$343.00

7. Complete Mailing Address of Known Office of Publication *(Not printer)* *(Street, city, county, state, and ZIP+4®)*

ELSEVIER INC.
230 Park Avenue, Suite 800
New York, NY 10169

Contact Person
Malathi Samayan

Telephone *(Include area code)*
91-44-4299-4507

8. Complete Mailing Address of Headquarters or General Business Office of Publisher *(Not printer)*

ELSEVIER INC.
230 Park Avenue, Suite 800
New York, NY 10169

9. Full Names and Complete Mailing Addresses of Publisher, Editor, and Managing Editor *(Do not leave blank)*

Publisher *(Name and complete mailing address)*

DOLORES MELONI, ELSEVIER INC.
1600 JOHN F KENNEDY BLVD. SUITE 1800
PHILADELPHIA, PA 19103-2899

Editor *(Name and complete mailing address)*

STACY EASTMAN, ELSEVIER INC.
1600 JOHN F KENNEDY BLVD. SUITE 1800
PHILADELPHIA, PA 19103-2899

Managing Editor *(Name and complete mailing address)*

PATRICK MANLEY, ELSEVIER INC.
1600 JOHN F KENNEDY BLVD. SUITE 1800
PHILADELPHIA, PA 19103-2899

10. Owner *(Do not leave blank. If the publication is owned by a corporation, give the name and address of the corporation immediately followed by the names and addresses of all stockholders owning or holding 1 percent or more of the total amount of stock. If not owned by a corporation, give the names and addresses of the individual owners. If owned by a partnership or other unincorporated firm, give its name and address as well as those of each individual owner. If the publication is published by a nonprofit organization, give its name and address.)*

Full Name	Complete Mailing Address
WHOLLY OWNED SUBSIDIARY OF REED/ELSEVIER, US HOLDINGS	1600 JOHN F KENNEDY BLVD. SUITE 1800 PHILADELPHIA, PA 19103-2899

11. Known Bondholders, Mortgagees, and Other Security Holders Owning or Holding 1 Percent or More of Total Amount of Bonds, Mortgages, or Other Securities. If none, check box ▶ ☐ None

Full Name	Complete Mailing Address
N/A	

12. Tax Status *(For completion by nonprofit organizations authorized to mail at nonprofit rates)* *(Check one)*
The purpose, function, and nonprofit status of this organization and the exempt status for federal income tax purposes:
☒ Has Not Changed During Preceding 12 Months
☐ Has Changed During Preceding 12 Months *(Publisher must submit explanation of change with this statement)*

PS Form 3526, July 2014 *(Page 1 of 4 (see instructions page 4))* PSN: 7530-01-000-9931 PRIVACY NOTICE: See our privacy policy on www.usps.com.

13. Publication Title	14. Issue Date for Circulation Data Below
NEUROLOGIC CLINICS	MAY 2022

15. Extent and Nature of Circulation			Average No. Copies Each Issue During Preceding 12 Months	No. Copies of Single Issue Published Nearest to Filing Date
a. Total Number of Copies *(Net press run)*			237	218
b. Paid Circulation (By Mail and Outside the Mail)	(1)	Mailed Outside-County Paid Subscriptions Stated on PS Form 3541 (Include paid distribution above nominal rate, advertiser's proof copies, and exchange copies)	119	111
	(2)	Mailed In-County Paid Subscriptions Stated on PS Form 3541 (Include paid distribution above nominal rate, advertiser's proof copies, and exchange copies)	0	0
	(3)	Paid Distribution Outside the Mails Including Sales Through Dealers and Carriers, Street Vendors, Counter Sales, and Other Paid Distribution Outside USPS®	74	65
	(4)	Paid Distribution by Other Classes of Mail Through the USPS (e.g., First-Class Mail®)	0	0
c. Total Paid Distribution *(Sum of 15b (1), (2), (3), and (4))* ▶			193	176
d. Free or Nominal Rate Distribution (By Mail and Outside the Mail)	(1)	Free or Nominal Rate Outside-County Copies included on PS Form 3541	26	24
	(2)	Free or Nominal Rate In-County Copies included on PS Form 3541	0	0
	(3)	Free or Nominal Rate Copies Mailed at Other Classes Through the USPS (e.g., First-Class Mail)	0	0
	(4)	Free or Nominal Rate Distribution Outside the Mail (Carriers or other means)	0	0
e. Total Free or Nominal Rate Distribution *(Sum of 15d (1), (2), (3) and (4))* ▶			26	24
f. Total Distribution *(Sum of 15c and 15e)* ▶			219	200
g. Copies not Distributed *(See Instructions to Publishers #4 (page 83))* ▶			18	18
h. Total *(Sum of 15f and g)* ▶			237	218
i. Percent Paid *(15c divided by 15f times 100)* ▶			88.12%	88%

* If you are claiming electronic copies, go to line 16 on page 3. If you are not claiming electronic copies, skip to line 17 on page 3.

16. Electronic Copy Circulation	Average No. Copies Each Issue During Preceding 12 Months	No. Copies of Single Issue Published Nearest to Filing Date
a. Paid Electronic Copies ▶		
b. Total Paid Print Copies (Line 15c) + Paid Electronic Copies (Line 16a) ▶		
c. Total Print Distribution (Line 15f) + Paid Electronic Copies (Line 16a) ▶		
d. Percent Paid (Both Print & Electronic Copies) (16b divided by 16c × 100) ▶		

☒ I certify that 50% of all my distributed copies (electronic and print) are paid above a nominal price.

17. Publication of Statement of Ownership

☒ If the publication is a general publication, publication of this statement is required. Will be printed ☐ Publication not required.
in the NOVEMBER 2022 issue of this publication.

18. Signature and Title of Editor, Publisher, Business Manager, or Owner		Date
Malathi Samayan - Distribution Controller	*Malathi Samayan*	9/18/2022

I certify that all information furnished on this form is true and complete. I understand that anyone who furnishes false or misleading information on this form or who omits material or information requested on the form may be subject to criminal sanctions (including fines and imprisonment) and/or civil sanctions (including civil penalties).

PS Form 3526, July 2014 *(Page 3 of 4)* PRIVACY NOTICE: See our privacy policy on www.usps.com

Printed and bound by CPI Group (UK) Ltd, Croydon, CR0 4YY

03/10/2024

01040404-0009